Island Boy

AN AUTOBIOGRAPHY

Tom Davis,
Pa Tuterangi Ariki

with illustrations by the author

ISBN No. 982-02-0071-7

Publication was supported by a contribution from the Government of Japan to the USP Endowment Fund.

Maps by Tony Shatford.

Published jointly by:

The Institute of Pacific Studies
University of the South Pacific;

The Macmillan Brown Centre for Pacific Studies
University of Canterbury;

The Centre for Pacific Studies
University of Auckland.

Typeset in 10/11 Times Roman
by the University of Canterbury, Christchurch.

Printed in New Zealand.

Contents

168°W

156°W

⚬ PENRHYN

• RAKAHANGA   — 10°S
″ MANIHIKI

PUKAPUKA ⚬

• NASSAU

⚬ SUWARROW

COOK   ISLANDS

PALMERSTON ⚬

• AITUTAKI
MANUAE •
TAKUTEA ⚬ ⸱ MITIARO
ATIU ⸱ MAUKE

RAROTONGA •

• MANGAIA   — 22°S

Airstrip
Arutanga
AIRPORT   AVARUA

ARUTANGA ●   MATAVERA ●

NGATANGIIA ●
AKAIAMI   ● ARORANGI
RAROTONGA

AITUTAKI

MURI ●

TITIVAEKA

The Cook Islands

Illustrations

PART ONE

Home Ground

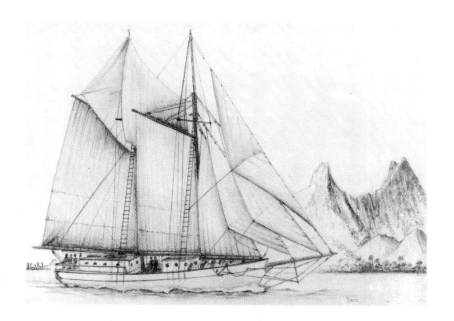

CHAPTER ONE

Growing Up

"The children are no longer yours. They must be shared with those on shore and each child must have many mothers."   JAMES A. MITCHENER

Rarotonga, where I was born, is a small island at Longitude 157 degrees 55 minutes east and Latitude 21 degrees 21 minutes south. It is the largest of the fifteen Cook Islands. The small nation stretches about 1300 kilometres north/south and 650 kilometres east/west with only 256 square kilometres of land area. Over half of the 17,000 people live on Rarotonga. Cook Islanders are Polynesians, most of whom also have some European heritage, and there are some Europeans.

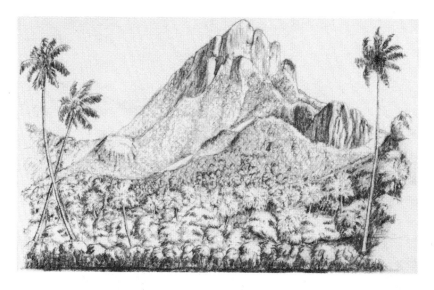

The islands separate into a Southern Group of eight high volcanic islands and a Northern Group of seven coral atolls. The Exclusive Economic Zone (EEZ) is over 2 million square kilometres. The nearest neighbours are French Polynesia with its capital Tahiti 1,200 kilometres to the north-east, the Samoas about 1,600 kilometres to the north-west and New Zealand about 2,400 kilometres to the south-east.

Rarotonga is a beautiful high island with lush vegetation and fertile flat lands ideal for the production of fruits and vegetables. Michener considered it one of the most, if not the most, beautiful island of the Pacific. Despite its small area of about ten by six and a half kilometres and a substantial mountainous region, Rarotonga has been called the Market Garden of the Pacific.

From before I was born in 1917, until the depression of the 1930s, Rarotonga
·was in its economic heyday as a result of several ships a month enabling a
healthy export of agricultural products to New Zealand and imports from both
New Zealand and the United States. The shipping bonanza had been created
some years before by the Sydney /Auckland/Rarotonga/Tahiti/San Francisco
shipping service operated by the Union Steam Ship Company (USSCo) using
two liners crossing each other in opposite directions between Rarotonga and
Tahiti. The Tahiti/San Francisco bound ship arrived in Rarotonga on a Friday
and the Auckland/Sydney bound boat arrived the following Monday once every
four weeks. They maintained their schedules like clockwork. During the winter
months, from March to August, an extra USSCo cargo vessel carried oranges,
bananas and tomatoes from Rarotonga and the other islands of the Southern
Group to the winter market in New Zealand. Some went to Tahiti also. Efficient
production and efficient shipping was the basis for an effective economy.

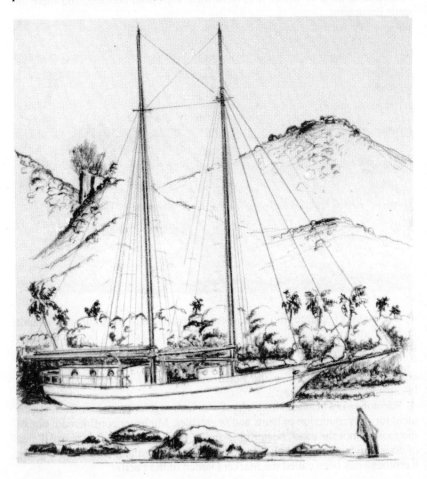

My grandfather, Captain Thomas Harries, operated his schooners around the islands working out of Rarotonga and Tahiti, from the 1880s until 1918. Other schooners operated until the 1940s. Copra, pearl shell and gem pearls were the prime outward cargoes, with trade goods being the bread and butter of the inward trade. As a result of extensive trading in pearls and pearl shell both in the Northern Cook Islands and the Tuamotu Islands, my grand father was known as the Pearl King of the Pacific. His operations and our own planting for the export trade kept my family in fairly good economic circumstances after his death in Tahiti in 1918.

My family consisted of my mother, my sister Mary and myself. My mother and father divorced soon after I was born. My mother later married Raitia Tepuretu and I grew up in Rarotonga with three sisters. Mary, Reureu and Tepaeru.

Our mother being half Polynesian and our stepfather full Polynesian, we grew up in the Polynesian way. Once brought up this way, you are unlikely to be anything but Polynesian in your fundamental ways. I have never regretted it.

Mary, being the eldest, went off to school in New Zealand first, followed by me in 1930 and then Reureu and Tepaeru. My sisters all went to St. Cuthbert's while I went to King's College, both in Auckland. Mary married Ian Harvey of Alex Harvey Ltd which later became AHI.

Mary was Papa's pet as well as everybody's pet. I do not believe anybody thought ill of her for this as she thoroughly deserved this special position. Tepaeru, or Paeru for short, was a real tomboy when she was little and was often my companion in things we could do together. She now lives in Rarotonga with her retired husband, Jack Whitta. Reureu was a gentle and female soft girl. She had been a good friend of the present King of Tonga as my mother had been a friend of his mother, Queen Salote, before him. The King, his younger brother and I, through these earlier family associations and our many personal contacts since 1950, also became good friends. Misfortune befell Reureu in her twenties and she died of a bowel form of the "scourge of the Pacific", tuberculosis. It was then a Polynesia wide problem.

Until the early 1900s, the Polynesians were a dying race and not just in odd spots, but throughout Polynesia. Early in the 1900s the population levelled out and in the following decades reversed and began to grow. Again the reversal occurred throughout Polynesia. There were several probable reasons: one was the growing immunity to infectious diseases. Mumps and measles during the early years of contact had been fatal to enormous numbers. Tuberculosis must have been another factor as it was, at the height of its effects, the major cause of all deaths.

In the 1950s, for not very clear reasons, tuberculosis started to disappear from the Polynesian Islands. Doctors can claim that it was due to vaccination with BCG and better medical care, but this was not the case for all Polynesian Islands which exhibited this same decline. Neither can this be satisfactorily explained by any significant improvement in standards of living. At about this time leprosy also started to reduce but the reasons for this were clearer because streptomycin was proving to be an effective agent against it.

It was only later that I realised that growing up in the Polynesian way had been a growing up in a special way. Under the classificatory kinship system, cousins are treated as brothers and sisters, uncles and aunts are like fathers and mothers and so on. Therefore, one always had aunts, uncles, grandmothers, grandfathers, big brothers, big sisters, little brothers, little sisters at hand to take care of you or for you to take care of. And there were always chores to do wherever you were. The first chore a child must share once he or she is able to walk is picking up rubbish or koi tita in the vernacular. From this simple beginning all other chores were added as one grew older.

Because aunts, uncles, grandmothers, grandfathers, sisters and brothers were always in profusion, a child was seldom afraid of adults because they were most likely relations. That is why Polynesian children are not usually afraid of strangers. Anthropologists call these extra family members facilitatory relatives. There is no equivalent in western society and we have to get by the best way we can with strangers by using the terms nieces and nephews, uncles and aunts as equivalents. This is not satisfactory, but it is the best we can do because not to recognise a facilitatory son as a son would be much worse.

Because there was usually a big sister, a big brother or adults keeping an eye on you, you were given more opportunity than is usual in other societies to get into trouble and be bailed out when you had a taste of what could happen to you. There was a disciplinary requirement that you be home by night fall, but no one needed to worry if you were not because there was always somebody to take care of you. This did not necessarily prevent the hiding you got for not being home when you were supposed to be. Everybody in sight of a child was considered responsible for it. There was collective responsibility for the welfare of all children as well as careless adults who are most likely to be visitors from elsewhere.

Our toys were usually home-made, either by our own efforts or with the help of a big brother or sister. Each month had its particular toy, which was indulged in by all and sundry until the craze for it wore off. At that time, the playthings were in most cases traditional in nature and ranged from topi (tops), titiraina (model yachts), patapata (marbles), teka (cane javelin throwing), rore (stilts), ana (archery), tupakere (a game of throwing pebbles in the air and catching the falling pebbles on the back of the throwing hand), pere toka (a game like drafts, played on lines and not squares), tukutuku manu (kite flying), ipana (a game of casting a stick laid across a hole in the ground for distance), tupe (a deck quoits type of game), pinipini ta'ae (the ubiquitous game of hide and seek), tupaoro'oro (tobogganing and surfing) and many others now almost extinct. Swimming, surfing and other water sports were always popular in the summer which is the hurricane season when the big rollers come in from the north. These are called the "children's waves" and belong to the children only.

Tradition says that no adult can participate, nor interfere with children playing in these waves, and that if these rules are broken, a child will drown. For the uninitiated adult to witness children surfing in these wild conditions, especially in the middle of a full cyclone, can be unsettling. It is difficult to restrain strangers from interfering, but no child ever got into trouble which is probably the reason we have no deaths from hurricanes. What is a hurricane to one who has surfed the waves of a cyclone as a youngster? The only death recorded in our many hurricanes was that of a European trying to save agricultural records in the 1935 hurricane. During hurricane Sally in 1987, on the afternoon before the night of its greatest destructive force, I watched children aged from 6 to 15 surf the waves coming around the end of the western breakwater of the Avatiu Harbour. In this respect not much had changed over the years. As we grew older, we played the usual games of which rugby and cricket were at the top of the list with tennis not far behind.

* * *

One of the more important ways affecting one's later outlook on life was the special place of children in society. They were never excluded from involvement in social and community affairs which are considered the domain of adults in many societies. It was up to the child whether he or she participated. Children did things as everywhere in the world according to their age, but they were never excluded if they chose to participate before the age they were expected to.

I remember attending dances and a ball or two along with other children and participating in other social get togethers. There has, as far as I know, never been any serious generation gap between adults and young people. However, changes in life-style as a result of employment, other than on the family land, have brought independence and commitments which demand new outlooks, new skills and new ways of spending one's time. These have strained parent-child relationships.

New songs, styles, hair-dos, fashions and new ways of doing things dreamt up by a mentally and physically healthy youth have never been a matter of unfavourable concern to the older generation as it seems to have done in other societies. In fact, members of the older generation are more likely than not to be interested in the new things and what makes them so interesting to the new generation. Having satisfied their curiosity, the older generation may take them up or regard them as not their cup of tea and ignore them.

* * *

There were numerous opportunities for play and learning all sorts of things the fun way. Various ways of fishing could be indulged in with little effort. My mother's half brother was a master of all the Polynesian fishing techniques. My cousin Willie and I learnt as much as we could from him. He was the last of those who fished the whales using the methods brought us by the Nantucket and New Bedford whalers. I have regretted very much that Willie and I were too young to have been part of the crew that went out when the whales were passing Rarotonga on their way to their feeding grounds in the Bering Sea. The boat they used is preserved in our National Museum and the whales still come by in July and August. Thankfully they are no longer molested in our waters and the human whale watchers are beginning to appear amongst us.

Except for the very modern fishing methods used by purse seiners, there are few methods used anywhere that were not used here in Polynesia. Fishing, using all the many methods available to us, occupied a great deal of our time, so we had little of it to spare in our busy young lives. It was a great growing up time.

The mountains of Rarotonga are high, steep and majestic. The highest peak is only 670 metres, but because of the small base upon which they stand and the steepness of their slopes, they seem much grander than their height would

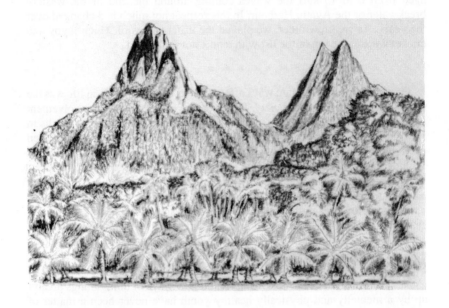

indicate. I climbed most of the peaks in those early days, but found some beyond my youthful abilities. Nevertheless, we managed to range over the accessible parts, setting snares for the beautifully coloured wild cocks brought here by the early Polynesian settlers. They are like the Malayan breed from which they originated thousands of years ago.

The traditional snares catch birds alive. We used to set twenty to fifty at a time. We let the hens go and kept the cocks for cock fighting. We little kids indulged in this sport. Occasionally little kids here still do. It is not a generally popular sport but it was and is practised throughout Polynesia to some degree. It was harmless because the fights, as normal in nature, end up by one cock running away before any damage was done. We did not use artificial spurs or confinement of a pit or selective breeding which does the damage of the sophisticated cock fights practised elsewhere.

Many things we did were frowned upon by our elders. These gave us that feeling of excitement that makes forbidden things worthwhile. We made home-brew like adults did and drank our concoctions like adults did, usually before the brew matured into one with significant alcohol content. The brew was usually made from orange juice, squeezed and left to ferment. We probably got more vitamin C than alcohol out of it! Like all kids the taste of the fully matured brews did not appeal. We often wondered why adults drank the stuff. At that age, we did not understand the funny things that happen to adults that seemed to make them need it.

Like kids everywhere, we raided orchards. Melon patches were our favourite targets. Nobody really cared whether we took oranges or mangoes or most fruits, but a patch of watermelons was a good economic crop on the local market and raiding them was quite a challenge. In this respect we were not different from kids elsewhere in the world, but I think we were unique in the water and in catching fish. We were unique also in the numbers of intimate relatives and our ability to dance anyone off their feet. It was a good way to grow up.

* * *

At about nine years of age, I repaired and started to use our one man family outrigger canoe to venture out on the open ocean. I had wanted to do this for a long time. My first literary purchase had been a Whitcombe & Tombs World Atlas. It was a glorious book with all the magic places in the world. It also had a two page spread of the map of the world showing every island, country and port of the world. It helped satisfy my day-dreams of sailing the world in my own imaginary boat. On its pages, I could draw courses of the many voyages I was going to take. That atlas got a real beating with courses marked every which way on its pages.

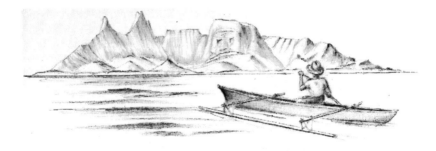

These persistent day-dreams were intensified when Bill Robinson sailed the little Svaap into Avatiu Harbour in Rarotonga on his way around the world and stayed for several weeks. At about the same time, George Beltran, about three years my senior, started going beyond the reef in his little outrigger canoe. What was good for Bill Robinson and George was good enough for me and for several years George and I tried to emulate the great cruising yachtsman. In our own little way, we cruised the world in the confines of the waters around Rarotonga, he in his dainty dug-out and I in my planked canoe, both with outriggers. I don't know whether George had the same dreams and imaginings as I had, but it was comforting to think so.

At first we went on these ventures together, but my consuming ambition was to paddle out as far as I could in the hope of reaching that magic place on the ocean where Rarotonga could no longer be seen over the horizon. George never going over the horizon was an all consuming obsession. But no matter how far out to sea I went, the high mountains would not go below the horizon. No matter how early in the morning I started, time always ran out for that having-to-get-home-before-dark requirement. Little wonder, Rarotonga can be seen from eighty kilometres out to sea. The best I could manage was to have the houses along the beach disappear.

For the several years I went on these ocean cruises they were kept a secret from my mother. She rightly would have imagined the worst of perils awaiting me and firmly brought them to a shuddering, screeching halt. These frequent ventures on to the ocean blue did result in some horrendous moments of dire peril from sudden changes of weather, hissing squalls and threatening reefs to the lee. Somehow I survived, developed good paddling muscles and heightened my self assurance from the successful escapes.

* * *

The thing that gave us all, young and old alike, the greatest joy were the "Pictures". The "Movies" to Americans. Pictures were shown three times a week and all who could, went and enjoyed themselves regardless of how bad the pictures were. They were silent pictures. The fun and games on picture nights started about four o'clock in the afternoon, when (facilitatory) Uncle Willie Browne, the proprietor of the theatre, would climb on to one of his trucks (the one that was in working order) with a sheaf of mimeographed notices about that night's showing and, with numerous members of his drum band, start around the Island. While the drums beat out a hot Cook Islands' drum tune, Uncle Willie, sitting like a king in an armchair, would cast the mimeographed notices to those that the beat of the drums had brought to the roadside. More often than not, those waiting on the roadside would not be able to resist the drums and spontaneous dancing would break out with great abandon.

There being no street lights, everybody went to the pictures carrying flashlights which in even older days had, by law, to be carried between members of the opposite sex walking side by side. From the further out villages, trucks brought loads of people, all of whom wore eis and ei katu(s) (leis and head wreaths), singing and dancing all the way to the picture theatre.

One could always tell when the show was about to start for Uncle Willie would stride in and enter his specially constructed platform to the left front of the upstairs seating area, sit in his armchair and signal Fred Story in the projection room to dowse the house lights, fire up his carbon arcs and get the show rolling.

At this point there would be cheers and whistles and at least a hundred flashlights would cast their beams on the screen. As soon as the show started, Uncle Willie would begin narrating what was happening on the silent screen.

* * *

At twelve years of age I was shipped off to King's College in Auckland, New Zealand, for an English type of Public School education. There was no high school in the Cook Islands in those days. I believe that the Public School system was designed to insure that those who make it through the system will never ever again find anything in life that cannot be taken in one's stride with aplomb, equanimity and forbearance. That probably makes it worth a great deal. Life is not always a bed of roses. In truth public school was not that bad. I can look back on it with some pleasure, many chuckles and a great deal of pride.

In the beginning I was homesick. The new environment and my having come from an entirely different world, now very far away, made what might have been a simple homesickness into a desperate longing, overlaying a feeling of utter loneliness. At that time there were few Cook Islanders in New Zealand and none I could turn to for a little bit of home.

To an island boy New Zealand had some surprises. Although I, like other Cook Islanders, knew a great deal about New Zealand second-hand from school books and the teaching of New Zealand ways in schools, it was nevertheless a surprise to see no coconut trees, in fact not many trees that I could recognise and name.

The houses were different. In the Cook Islands at that time there were still indigenous style huts thatched with plaited coconut leaves but, even our 'European style' houses were different. They had wide verandahs all around where most of the living and entertainment and feasting was done. Despite being European style, they tried to follow the Polynesian traditional practice of having three distinct areas or actual structures based on the custom that one did not live where one slept and one did not cook or eat where one lived or slept.

The paved roads of New Zealand were a delight. They made me remember the dusty coral roads of home that were always full of pot-holes. The electricity as a means of lighting the streets and houses was fascinating, particularly the fact that one could get light simply by flipping a switch.

I became an addict of all things electrical and electronic. Electricity was not new to me, because I had often sneaked into the projection room of Uncle Willie's theatre to help Fred Story tend the arc lights of the projector and in the bargain see a picture-show free. At home, the smelly kerosene lamps needed seemingly endless attention, cleaning their lamp glasses and topping up the kerosene fuel while the hissing pressure benzine lamps needed constant tending and pumping.

I received many jolts in examining the properties of electricity and finding out what it could and could not do. Many things in New Zealand were familiar in a second hand way, but were exciting on first hand acquaintance; not the least were street cars and the puffing monster steam engines of the trains.

What was most surprising of all was saying "hello" to people you passed in the street and receiving nothing more than a surprised or sometimes belligerent glare. Occasionally, I received a smile and a hello back which only reinforced my continuance of this Cook Islands custom of greeting to all you met in the street. Finally, I was firmly told that one did not do this in New Zealand or elsewhere in the world.

Although the English language is used in the schools in Rarotonga, at home and generally we spoke Rarotongan. The Polynesian languages are very expressive and, for that and other reasons, probably will not be readily displaced. Ours is becoming a more dynamic language as time passes and responds to the changing context. However, some families in Rarotonga have not taught it to their children in the mistaken belief that more Maori means less English, when in fact one language enhances the other.

By Cook Islands' standards, I spoke English pretty well. But it was a source of huge amusement to everybody in my new environment. For example, in Polynesian, the plural is not used unless it needs to be emphasised and, when this happens, several words are available to convey the reason you are emphasising the plural. These words indicate a variety of plural connotations including rank, clique, family relationship, organisational groupings, and more. Therefore, it is difficult for us to get into the habit of using a plural which conveys nothing more than plurality as is the case with English and other languages. As a result we tend to unconsciously confuse our use of plurals in English, either using the singular for both cases or adding esses where they are not supposed to be. When we use the simple English plural, we unconsciously feel that something is missing and create problems when we add or compensate for what we feel is missing. Our intonation also gets all confused. These and more were a source of a great deal of banter which was not always in good humour.

* * *

My first year at King's was difficult all round. It was no less difficult for other Cook Islanders in similar circumstances. Some even left their schools in New Zealand and came home for this reason. My athletic career was better than my academic career. The rigidity of a boarding school was hard to take and at first harder to understand. The freedom I was used to was gone, but at no time did I consider quitting because I had already chosen what I was going to do with my life. I was going to be a Doctor of Medicine and to achieve this, I must subject myself to the requirements. This resolution did not make things easier. Feelings of "to heck with it all", kept surfacing both then and many times later.

King's used the cane, as did all schools at that time. A whacking was not new to me, but during that first year, I seemed to get caned every day. I had a great deal to learn and I seemed to infringe rules wherever I turned: in school, on the playing field, in the dining room and in the dormitory. There seemed to be rules for everything and for every minute of the day. I bore all this without malice because I did not then, nor do I now, believe that the one whack I got a day was given for anything else than to draw my attention to the fact that there were innumerable rules. That first year goes down in my memory as the "year of the cane". I personally approve of the judicious use of the cane. It is quick, the point is made with no arguments. There are no after emotional effects and both parties are quickly back into business as usual. It is a pity that some have abused the use of this otherwise fairly good mode of communication. It is probably far less traumatic than other modes of disciplinary communication which have replaced it.

I worked hard to adjust to my new environment. My English improved and I slowly but surely climbed the fortnightly academic lists from the bottom of the first list of the year to the top of the last list of the year. I was proud at Prize Giving to receive my first academic prize for the most improved pupil of the school. It was not so great because there was really no way for me to go but up. There were to be four more academic prizes, but my athletic accomplishments were better with three championships under my belt. More importantly I made some close friends who remain good and loyal friends until today.

* * *

That first New Zealand winter had a lasting effect on me. Not only did I feel it, I did something about it which later formed the foundation of a large part of my basic scientific research work. Daytime was bad enough with me all bundled up and miserable with cold. Prior to this I had never experienced a temperature for any length of time below 60 degrees F (15.5 degrees C) and that very rarely. In Rarotonga we lived most of the time at temperatures averaging 72 degrees F (22. degrees C) in the winter and much warmer in the summer (84 degrees F, 27 degrees C). The first New Zealand winter came down on me like a frozen bolt. At night it was a nightmare of shivering. I just could not control it. I used all the blankets available to me with my rug on top and wearing my dressing gown under it all.

It was painfully obvious that the other boys in the dormitory were unaffected. Asking them about it confirmed that they were not going through what I was. They just laughed it off with a "Don't worry, you'll get used to it." That remark sparked off a train of thought that led me to the strangest of activities in the strangest of places in the world for a significant part of my professional life.

My misery with the cold created sympathy from the kindly Matron of my House, St. John's House. Her efforts with extra blankets for the night and extra singlets under my flannel shirt, tweed jacket and long pants for the daytime helped a great deal, but not enough to extinguish that spark set off by the remark "You'll get used to it." I thought I would give "Getting used to it" an extra push. So, against the pleadings of Matron, I discarded the extra clothing and faced the winter elements with open-necked shirt, shorts, socks and boots.

Within a couple of weeks or so, I was sleeping soundly with nary a shiver and took the cold shower winter record from 10 minutes to 42 minutes. I swore that, if the opportunity came my way and if nobody had done anything about it, I would put some effort into defining the bodily processes and, if possible, the bodily mechanisms involved in "Getting used to it". At that time it became clear to me that I had experienced an adaptive process first hand. This was later to lead me into the sometimes bizarre world of science, research and strange, interesting places.

* * *

I came home in January 1933 with Mary who had just completed her schooling at St. Cuthbert's. We were both coming back for a month's holiday.

On that last night at sea, I looked forward with unexpected anticipation to seeing Rarotonga again. I could not sleep.

Although I had no means of first hand comparison, I had always been impressed by the steep and craggy mountains of Rarotonga. From the back verandah of our Ruatonga home in Avarua, one could see, from left to right, soaring Ikurangi (Tail of the sky), Te Manga (The Branching), part of the ridged, straight back of Te Kou (The Misty One), and almost straight ahead the broad, sphinx-like face of Maunga Tea (White Mountain). I was even more impressed at the sight of the profile of Rarotonga in those days when I looked back at her from far out at sea during my canoe voyages in search of that magic place over the horizon where I could not see these craggy peaks and spiny ridge-backs.

As we neared Rarotonga on that slick calm ocean before day-break, I remembered. I placed myself in the bow of R.M.S. "Tahiti" and waited for a sight of Rarotonga, also known to Polynesians by the expressive names of: Tumu Te Varovaro (Source of Echoes and Thunderclaps), Nuku Tere (The Busy Crossroads), Avaiki Raro (The Centre of Culture to the South) and Avaiki Tautau (Fairyland Avaiki).

I watched and waited. At first there was only the hiss and swishing cadence of the bow wave as the steel stem of the liner rose and fell, responding to the force and counterforce of buoyancy and inertia. The ocean moved from the colour of nothing much to gun metal blue through slate and, after the sun had exploded through the glory of its dawn colours, there lay Rarotonga, capped by its companion cloud, standing clear on the horizon, dead ahead, surrounded by a sea of incredible blue. A lump climbed from the depths of my emotions and lodged in my throat.

Both Mary and I had a wonderful holiday. Our reception at the dock was a royal one. The elderly ladies, as was the custom, went down on their knees wailing real tears on to our feet and wiping them off with their long gray hair. For me it was a most unnerving and humbling experience.

From there we went to Makea's Palace to be formally welcomed back and to have morning tea with the Paramount Chief and his immediate family. The crowd was large and the food was, as was the custom, abundant. But the seating was just for the immediate family, my mother, Mary and I, again as was the custom. From there we went to our home in Tupapa and took our rest, but fully conscious of the activity of many relations preparing for the great feast for the guests that evening, of whom there must have been two hundred or more. There was a band and after everybody had eaten and after the formal speeches, there was great jollity and dancing. It was a grand welcome home.

The month was filled with activity every day with feasts, picnics, swimming in the lagoon and in the freshwater pools of Papua. There were parties at a different home each night with feasting and dancing. At the end of the month I was exhausted, but managed to last the pace until it came time to go back to school and go through that always wrenching occasion, a Polynesian farewell with the sad farewell songs, the wailing and the tears. I felt I could not have lasted another day and that my having to leave was the saving of my life. Mary seemed as fresh at the end of it all as at the beginning.

During the visit, my mother did not miss the opportunity to spend a significant period of our time together to take me through my paces as to what was expected of a son of her family. This had been impressed on me for years and it was unrelenting in its persistence. Many of us had already gone through this before being sent off to school, while at school, and after we had returned home to face responsibilities with only a high school education behind us.

Our respective families considered that a high school education was all that was needed to meet their expectations of us. I could at that time count a number of those of us who had gone before me and had come back and turned into wrecks for seemingly no other reason than that too much was expected of them with too little grounding to achieve it. Most took to drink, one or two took to drugs. Our colonial masters were not much help. They did not want educated Pacific Islanders in positions of responsibility in their own home islands.

The girls who were educated were never pressed in this manner. They were not expected to be more than a secretary for a short time and then a dutiful wife. As a result their confidence in themselves was never shaken to the core and they were, for the most part, not forced to, or even wanted to, take responsibility for more than this. However, our women are no less capable than women of other countries.

* * *

When I informed my parents that I was going to become a medical doctor, they were happy as long as I went to the Central Medical School in Fiji. That would have meant coming out as an Assistant Medical Practitioner with a life sentence to the limited medical scene of the Pacific Islands, always at the beck and call of a fully qualified doctor from elsewhere. That was not my idea and never would be. But I kept quiet about what would have been interpreted as an act of defiance and rebellion. And when it came out what I was really after, my motives were under suspicion. I had disrupted the order of things set by the colonial masters. Their displeasure had already been made apparent. It is still on record. We had no say as the Cook Islands was what was then known as a Dependency of New Zealand. We had no elected or even appointed representatives and all decisions were made by officials in Wellington or by New Zealand officers in Rarotonga.

After King's I went to medical school in Dunedin, New Zealand. Medicine had been my choice for a long time. It also seemed to me to be the best way for me to be of service to my people as was expected of me in one form or another. I was about nine years old when I decided that medicine was what I wanted to do in life. The path to achieve this goal was not to be an easy one.

The relatively affluent life that we had had before 1930 came to an end due to the economic crash of 1929, though the full impact did not strike our part of the world until 1932. The Sydney/Frisco shipping schedule came to an end as did the in-between fruit boat. Things were harder than I had realised, especially when Reureu and Paeru had to have their turn at boarding school.

For the holidays we usually had friends who took us to their homes. In my case the home that became for me a home away from home was Mercury Island.

Through Pat Mizen, his family became as much a family to me as it was for Pat and his two sisters, Joan and Anne. On Mercury Island I learnt a great deal about sheep and cattle farming, enough to appreciate it as a way for somebody else to make a living.

To communicate with the mainland, Skip, Pat's father, and Joan took a course in radio communication and operation and kept schedules with Auckland. The family also had a 35 foot launch and later a 50 foot working vessel with accommodation and cargo capacity below decks and a capability to transport stock on deck. Both of these vessels, each in their time, allowed Skip and me to indulge to our hearts content our mutual love of the sea, practice coastal navigation and pry into the mysteries of celestial navigation. All of this stood me in good stead in the future small sailboat sea voyages and ocean races I took part in.

Medical school looked a mighty long way away. The depression was still on and prospects did not look very good for anything except staying on the farm for God knows how long. I spent a while thinking about it all and at last I decided that the move towards a medical career had to be made. I asked Skip for a loan of fifty pounds which should, I thought, be enough for a train ticket to Dunedin where the medical school was, enough for the first year's fees with a little over for a little place to sleep and a little to eat. As it turned out it was all too little for too long a time. It was soon after this that I leaned heavily on the saying, "The Lord will provide." Strange as it may seem, He always did then and has always done so since.

CHAPTER TWO

Medical School

It takes only a minute to write an error of fact into a textbook but it takes twenty years to remove it. PERCY GOWLAND

These were the hard years. The depression was in full swing. Life was not easy for anybody, especially a penniless medical student. Some money came from home, but it was not enough to keep body and soul together. I shared a room with a school friend, Tom Fraser. He was an exemplary room mate and we managed quite well together. But my relationship with our elderly retired bank clerk landlord and his good lady was strained.

There are people who come into my life with whom I am unable to reach an even reasonable relationship no matter how much I try. There is a gulf between us that is uncrossable. This was the case with my landlord couple. When this phenomenon occurs I am usually unable to explain it in a logical manner. The problem was solved while I was away staying with a friend for the May term holidays. I received a curt note summarily instructing me to pick up my things and leave. With such short notice, I had no place to go, but as usual things worked out and the good Lord provided.

* * *

The quaint city of Dunedin is well down towards the south of the South Island of New Zealand near 45 degrees Latitude. Its residents were of Scottish descent and most spoke with a brogue. The buildings were, in the tradition of Scottish towns, substantial but smaller copies of buildings from its namesake, Edinburgh, in Scotland.

The university buildings were attractive in their old world architecture of stone with the expected stone tower, four faced clock and a weathercock perched on top. This architecture was repeated in several places around the town, notably the Cathedral and several other churches, The Exchange, The Grand Hotel, Knox College, the Railway Station and way out of town, Larnach's Castle. In between, there were all sorts of buildings, mostly square in their utilitarian purposes. These included the Public Hospital with its obvious additions over the years, its close neighbour, the Medical School and near neighbour, the museum, and other structures scattered elsewhere, falling gently into the architectural category of nondescript.

Surrounding the city was the Town Belt where most of the virgins of the town were initiated into a new life and many a bairn was conceived. Beyond this haven bequeathed by past farseeing city fathers were the low hills that supported, with a degree of misty, picturesque grace, the more important nearby suburbs. Dunedin's deep inletted harbour, guarded by Port Chalmers at its entrance, provided some exciting small boat sailing from winds driven down in sudden gusts from the surrounding hills. Little wonder that Dunedin has given

New Zealand some notable yachtsmen on both the national and international scene.

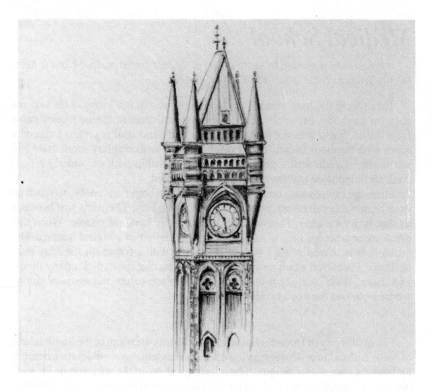

It was a university town. Its forbearance of students was legendary. We, the students, can bear witness to that. Short of arson, armed revolution and murder, our goings on were tolerated. Even a fantastic murder hoax was treated with dignified court justice which made its perpetrators humbly repentant and made any further such depredations on the hospitality of our hosts unthinkable.

* * *

My next digs had a much friendlier atmosphere and our kindly landlady made room for a seemingly large number of us. There were several training college students, two dental students and a labourer. We all got along very well. Usually with this number of people living close together, there is one who is always out of tune with the rest, but in our case there was no one in this category.

The labourer, Percy, out of his working duds, was an elegant and well mannered person and he and I became good friends for many years until our paths were geographically separated by our respective callings. I was always short of money and it was fortunate for me that Percy and I were good friends. He was able to get me jobs which helped pay for my board and lodgings and generally keep the wolf from the door with a little over with which to indulge myself.

These were not easy jobs. The depression saw to that. As a student, I was allowed only casual status. Off and on I worked on the roads, in ditches, in the manure works of Kempthorne and Prosser, on the presses of the wool stores and the wool dumps and for one short time, I was foreman of the gang that tarsealed the Caledonia Grounds Bicycle Race Track. I became foreman only because most of my other jobs required the use of a shovel and I was the best spreader of gravel over hot tar on that first day.

To give an idea of how physically demanding some of these jobs were, I was often prevailed upon by other students for work and few could last more than a day or so. At the beginning I found the work as equally demanding as they, but they probably had less need of a job than I, who had to grin and bear it.

* * *

I acquired a taxi driver's license, but taxi driving was no easier than the other jobs had been - its price was lack of sleep. I would drive from 5 pm to 3 am and then get up to attend lectures at 9 am and twice a week at 8 am. During the day, I learnt to sleep on the floor, on benches and anything I could find that would allow me to stretch out for a few minutes, better still, for as long as possible. I later learnt to doze off in any position, including standing up. I did posters and any art work that came my way. One summer I went back farming as a teamster on a sheep station in Taras, Central Otago. It was a 4,000 acre "station" and the acres I was responsible for putting under cultivation were extensive enough to keep me busy all summer.

Apart from working with the horses, which I have always liked, the job had little to recommend it. The rabbiter was supposed to milk the cows, but more often than not it fell to my lot to do this as well. Rabbiters are a pretty independent lot, depending more on the proceeds from rabbiting than other jobs demanded of them. The pittance our rabbiter was paid to milk the cows was small by comparison.

He was a good friend to me and helped me out whenever he could and his nice homely wife was always good to me. Her pies, fresh from the oven, were delicious. They had three children of varying ages, too young to be of any great help in their hand to mouth type of existence. My friend's problem was the bottle and when he made the effort to collect enough rabbits and sell their skins, most of the proceeds went for booze. At these times, which were only too frequent, besides being the teamster, I also became the milkman.

Since there were only six house cows, I did not mind doing this for my friend, but sometimes I was so tired that I was careless with Daisy, the only Jersey cow in the bunch of Holsteins. She would take every opportunity to kick out at me or worse still plant a carefully gauged kick at a full bucket of milk. Daisy was a beautiful looking Jersey cow. Her innocent brown doe-like eyes belied her calculating nature.

At milking time she would put her head in the right place for the restraining mechanism, but until she was leg roped, which had to be done with skill and speed, she would watch her opportunity for a well timed and positioned sideways cow kick. The same would happen when she was released. But her most favourite time was after the milking when she, along with the other cows, were walked out from the byre. Invariably at such times I would be carrying the last cow's bucketful of milk and Daisy would seem friendly and hang back. If I was tired and not as alert as I should be, her timing and judgement of distance would be perfect and the bucket of milk would go flying.

I tried everything I knew to make a good woman of her, but to no avail. Kindness did no good. A swift kick would be met with a swift kick back. A thump on her rump with a handy stick was a pure waste of time. In the end her innocent eyes won out and the game she wanted to play went on without any real malice. It made me jealous that her attentions were not exclusively for me. Anyone who did the milking got the same thing.

Except for Dinah and Sheilah, the horses were great. Big Mack, the Clydesdale, was everything a Clydesdale should be - big, strong, willing, considerate and good natured. He was the only pure bred, the rest were half draughts from obscure origins. Sheilah was a quarter draught and branded an outlaw. Dinah was lazy, underhand, jealous and fractious. Boss would do anything you asked of her. The rest were just nice decent horses. The rig I used was a four-horse chain pulley affair with an outrigger that turned it into a five horse rig when needed. With it you could hitch on to a five furrow plough, a triple set of discs, a wide-spanning harrow and anything else that needed beef to move it. The chains ran through pulleys in such a manner that any horse which did not pull its weight found its heels banging against the swingle tree.

Because of Dinah's evil nature, I put her in the outrigger where it was more difficult for her to nip and annoy the others. Here, when she failed to pull her weight, the outrigger would get out of shape and force her to get moving, assisted by some choice words from me. With this rig and the big strides of Big Mack, we covered a lot of ground each day. At night when we were all unharnessed and deserved a good feed, Dinah would get into her daily feed time act which consisted of chasing the others from the feed boxes and grabbing everything she could for herself. It lengthened my day because I felt I had to stick around and force her to behave and allow others to get their share. This I did by grabbing the root of her tail and making her drag me like a water skier round and round the corral. After this she would behave and let the others eat in peace. In time it was not necessary for me to do my water-skiing act. A word was enough.

Sheilah was a different kettle of fish. She had earned her reputation as an outlaw by not being able to be harness broken and I was warned not to use her. Like most outlaws, she was friendly until you asked her to do something. Her quarter draught ancestry showed and she was big and rangy. Since I had only the bare minimum of horses to do the job, she was needed to give the other horses a rest, one at a time. So I started to handle her and get her used to me and she responded quite well, but her 'mad as a hatter' nature would show through now and then and she would become nervous and edgy for no apparent reason. Otherwise she was quite amenable.

I thought that if I put her alongside good old steady Big Mack, she might be usable. Accordingly, when nobody was around, I harnessed her next to him, but she was not going to have any of it. She reared in the chain traces and tried every way to free herself but only succeeded in getting herself tangled in the traces and the swingle tree. However, the time I had spent handling her paid off because I could hold her head and talk her into quietening down. When she pulled, she did so with great jerking, uncoordinated gusto and managed to break two trace chains. I repaired these with many windings of fencing wire and continued to work her. Finally she and Big Mack, side by side, proved to be good working mates and dragged the rest of the team behind them, forcing them to put in an honest day's work. If there had been a team pulling competition, I would have entered them with confidence.

* * *

As a medical student I was not always welcomed as a labourer or even a farm hand. There were those who felt that I was taking up space that belonged to one of the brethren. Fortunately I gained staunch friends who saw to it that these prejudicial attitudes did not get too far out of hand. But in the early stages I often had to face situations which fortunately I was able to handle without the need for resorting to physical violence. Mostly my physical dimensions and sometimes my reputation as a boxer were a sufficient deterrence. However, after turning up for the line-up for casual and seasonal work time after time, I was finally accepted as one of the brethren.

* * *

As a taxi driver I never had a problem handling awkward situations with belligerent or drunken passengers, although things got sticky on occasions. However, I was not so lucky in avoiding the attentions of the law. We were particularly susceptible to speeding and other traffic violations on a rainy Friday or Saturday night, when brisk business gave us an opportunity to make a record take. God knows why because we got paid the same for a big take as for a small one. I guess it was the competitive spirit.

I was never to make the top position. On occasion I made fourth or third or even second place. We accused the few who had the knack of beating the rest of us of cheating, though the only way to cheat that I could see was to make up the take by putting in money from their own pockets. This did not make sense, because there was no cash prize for being top dog.

The only other way was to abandon courtesy on the road by scaring every driver who had the right of way at intersections, out of crossing before you. Such situations gave us the jump over kindly civil drivers. We had fun racing back from an outlying depot at the end of a night shift in the early morning. In this I was the champ. I had a 1938 Plymouth with gearing just right for acceleration in the straights and speed in the corners for me to stay in low gear, with occasional shifts into second, all the way back to the main depot. There were no prizes for this either.

My falling foul of the law was much more subtle and innocent. The first time was on a Saturday with a Ranfurly Shield rugby game, just two weeks after I started driving. Anyone familiar with New Zealand knows that this is a rugby day of days. Teams from all districts of the country compete for this Shield over the year. On this day, the final was to be played in Dunedin. The city was clogged with visitors. At ten thirty, I was alone in one of the town depots across from Ma Blaney's Hotel. Despite the many visitors in town, things were quiet. Most of the visitors were nursing their morning-after sore heads before the game, due to start at 2.00 pm that afternoon with a curtain raiser.

I was sitting in my taxi waiting for action, when an elderly dapper little man weaved his way towards me. Without a beg your pardon, he climbed into the front passenger seat and ordered me to take him to the bright lights and a woman. With only two weeks on the job, I was not at all sure what my duties to customers were, especially in this respect, but somewhere along the line I had been told that the customer was always right. I called the dispatcher who had always been kind and helpful, and he said, "Oh! That. Take him to No 1 .... St. "My passenger showed me his wad of notes saying, "Sonny, there's 77 quid (pounds) here, one for each year of my life and I intend to have a good time."

In all innocence I did what I was told. It was a very nice neighbourhood. The house was an attractive bungalow with neatly cut lawns, decorative bushes and a display of roses. My passenger ordered me to go find out the "score". I was reluctant to do this because, in my innocence, I could not believe that I had been sent to the right place, but he insisted. I decided to use an oblique approach that would mean a lot to the right party and nothing at all to the wrong party. I was pleased with my subtle ploy and went to the front door and knocked. A luscious lady of about thirty or so years opened the door and asked me what I wanted. I slipped my oblique ploy and blurted out, "There's a man out there."

She peered past me trying to make out what he was like and said, "He looks pretty old. Has he got any money?"

I pleaded ignorance. She sighed and said, "Bring him in and come in yourself."

I walked back to the taxi and informed the old man that this was the right place. I helped him out of the taxi and assisted him up the path, lined on both sides with roses, and led him into the house. Noticing my hesitation to leave, he reached for his roll and peeled off a pound note. Our luscious lady intervened and told him to give me three pounds and that I was to go and fetch them a dozen large bottles of beer and some deep fried oysters. She accompanied me to the door and told me "I was a bit of all right" and she would like me to be her partner. I gathered that what she meant was that I was to bring her customers and we would split the earnings.

By now it was lunch time and I was getting peckish myself. So off I went to get the order. When I returned the lady informed me that she had done her stuff and the old codger had paid her six pounds. She further informed me that he had a lot more where that came from. The old boy looked as though he had been dragged through a hedge backwards and it seemed that all he wanted to do was sleep. I had more change from the oysters and beer than I needed for the fare.

So I went to give our friend his change but our lady made it plain that he would be a stinkpot if he took it.

"We're all going on a pub crawl," she announced. Arm in arm they weaved their way to the street and climbed into the back and we drove off to the nearest pub. The old boy was most disinterested and lay back with his eyes closed.

At the first pub, she got out, shook the old boy awake saying, "Give us a quid, Pop." Sleepily he pulled out his roll, which looked a good bit thinner than when I first saw it, and peeled off a note. She grabbed it and went into the pub and returned with a half bottle of Johnny Walker Red Label and placed it on the empty front seat. And so we went from pub to pub with the same routine starting with, "Give us a quid, Pop". But now she, with a pretence of giving me instructions, would get out, open the front door, pick up the half bottle of Johnny Walker, go into the pub for a drink, return with what seemed to be the same half bottle, put it back on the front seat, climb in the back and off we would go to the next pub to repeat the procedure.

We must have done this at seven or eight pubs. When I informed her that I was due off at five, she told me to return to her home where she repeated her offer of a partnership. On the way home, I thought about how this lady had worked her customer over and realised that he would be lucky if he got back to his hotel with any of that roll still intact. For me it was fascinating and it did cross my mind that, as an upstanding citizen, perhaps I should have saved the old boy from himself. I salved my conscience by the thought that perhaps he was getting his money's worth.

Next morning, the landlady woke me for the phone. Still half asleep, I picked up the phone and heard a voice say, "This is Detective Sergeant Berry, did you pick up a fare from etc, etc, etc." I weakly answered, "Yes," to which he said, "shall we pick you up, or will you come in to the Dunedin Police Station yourself." To this I replied tremulously, "I'll come in myself." That was the end of what was to have been a beautiful, restful Sunday.

The old boy had ordered a taxi at 11 pm that night from our lady's home and the driver had brought him to the police station because he had no money for the fare. She had been brought in and both she and the old boy, according to Detective Sergeant Berry, had accused me of having taken the old boy's money. I was facing a likely charge of theft as well as aiding and abetting prostitution. My story of my innocent involvement seemed to have held up, but it was several months before I was told that I was off the hook and they had not been able to charge her. I sweated through those months and since that time I have kept the ladies of the trade at a respectful arm's length.

All my close calls with the police while taxi driving were innocent, but they were sufficiently frequent for the police each time to say, "Oh! It's you again!" The last time was a beautiful warm, sunny Sunday. My customers had been to church and were now back home. It was the quiet time that repeated itself every Sunday. My customers had just about finished their Sunday dinner with their families and, were contemplating an afternoon outing to the beach or an afternoon nap with the kids out of the way at the park nearby.

It was my custom on such quiet Sundays to have my text books on hand and do some desultory reading and learning, usually with no enthusiasm at all. I was half asleep in the back seat with a neglected tome just about to fall out of my sleepy fingers when there was a gentle tap, tap beside my sleepy right ear. I came fully alert and struggled out of the taxi to confront a dapper elderly gentleman. Gentlemen to whom I fall victim are always dapper and falling victim to them has happened often enough for me to have learnt to recognise them, but I never have.

He indicated that he would be most obliged if he could hire me to assist him in his great need. His circumlocution should have warned me, but instead, I indicated that the pleasure was all mine. We drove to the south end of King Street which was full of unused buildings which might have been little stores at one time.

We stopped at one of these. He hopped out, opened the door of one of these places, went inside and returned with a heavy bundle of used newspapers all neatly tied up. He repeated this manoeuvre with another bundle of newspapers. The third he was sweating and breathing hard, so I asked him how many bundles were there. He told me, "As many as we can get into the taxi." So I took off my jacket and helped him pile these bundles of paper in the trunk, in the back seat and between us in the front seat until we could get no more in. The taxi was well down on its springs.

We drove to the Chinese fish shop near the junction of Pitt Street and George Street and with the help of the Chinaman, we laboriously unloaded the bundles of paper. The Chinaman paid my new found friend who in turn paid me the fare and we went our separate ways.

Next morning, dum di dum dum, "Did you yesterday etc., etc., etc.," "Yes I did." .... "No, you don't have to pick me up." .... "Bye, see you."

It turned out that I and my dapper friend had broached the Salvation Army's paper collection depot, an important part of their war effort for recycling used paper. We were both facing a charge of breaking and entering and theft. Before hiring me he had broken the lock so that he could walk in as though he had every right to do so. Fortunately a number of my taxi driver mates had been conned into doing the same thing and they testified to that effect. I was saved from another of my dapper gentlemen.

* * *

I hated learning, I considered it an assault on my creativity that I had to passively sop up knowledge by the bucketful and give nothing creative of myself to it and, whenever I did, the reaction from my mentors was horrendously unappreciative. The utter boredom of sopping up knowledge like pig swill found its cure in an array of extracurricular activities. By careful assignment of my time (it was not really that careful), I was able to attend parties, be a labourer and drive a taxi in turn.

I had early in life discovered that I had a fairly good visual and auditory memory and, if I attended the lectures, demonstrations and practicals, I did not need to pore over notes and books to get by. Unfortunately, some of my high school teachers in the first instance and, later, university professors, knew about this trait and my extracurricular activities were a source of annoyance to them. On occasion I would have to give them up to appease someone's wrath and go to the top of the class for a little while. On the whole, however, I enjoyed the loose way things managed themselves to be.

Often, contemplation of the eons of time and the bucketfuls of boredom it was taking to obtain a medical degree made me consider giving it all away. But the thought of what was expected of me back home and the alternatives of having to work for someone else, like I was having to then, would bring me to my senses. Only very much later, after I found that I could creatively add to the sum total of knowledge, did I find learning stimulating and enjoyable. It was only then that I would regret my past intolerance to passively sopping up knowledge.

While at Medical School I acquired some good friends, a dog named Tiger, a 1926 500cc flat tank Norton motor-bike named the Iron Duke, a wife named Lydia, a 1929 Austin Roadster automobile, a son named John, a great deal of extra curricular knowledge which included what was needed to support life in outer space and an experiment with conclusions on the possible mechanism of acclimatisation to cold. These were not necessarily acquired in that order. Our lives, acquisitions, aspirations and accomplishments at this time and for many years later are covered in an autobiography Lydia and I co-authored and published in 1954.[9] It is out of print. So I may be forgiven for reviewing some of the more important things that happened at this time. Of special note are those things, not previously thought relevant to mention, but which eventually led to things which occupied my time and effort after *Doctor to the Islands* was published.

* * *

Lydia and I were married in 1940. In 1942, John was born to us followed by two more sons, Tim in 1947 and Teremoana in 1954. After 26 years of marriage and for probably paltry reasons we separated and finally divorced in 1972. While in the United States, Lydia had made it explicit that she did not like to live in the Cook Islands where my own life had always been tied for reasons that were very much my own.

I thought I had conveyed these reasons to Lydia over the years. Lydia believed that we, and particularly I, had no future in the Cook Islands. To me it was not a matter of a future. It was a matter of obligation which, if not fulfilled, would become a serious matter of conscience. This I was unable to convey to her or, for that matter, to many others. Lydia now lives in Wellington, New Zealand. Tim has an insurance company of his own in Indiana. John works for Xerox in Rochester, New York. Teremoana does his own things in the Cook Islands. Owning a bar is one of them. Each of our sons has blessed Lydia and me with a grandchild each.

* * *

I acquired Tiger, after he had bitten his owner who was going to shoot him. Tiger and I became inseparable friends for many happy years. In his prime, he weighed just over 90 pounds, but reached 110 pounds when Mary, my sister, looked after him for three weeks. She was unable to get over her mistrust of his fierce mien and fed him constantly in the belief that, if she did, he would not add her to his diet.

Tiger was a fearsome looking animal. He was supposed to be a mixture of a dark coloured German Shepherd and a black Labrador, but he bore little resemblance to either. The hair along his back started faintly black just behind his head and got darker towards his tail so that his rump and tail was almost black. From his back down his flanks, towards his belly, the dark colour gradually lightened to light fawn on his under belly. His eyes were a bright yellow. He could not have had any other name than Tiger.

Tiger was extremely intelligent. I hesitate to talk about his intelligence for it threatens my credibility. We understood each other perfectly. He would go to the butcher to purchase his own meat with a threepenny bit carried in his mouth. What he obtained for this paltry amount was always enough for both of us for a couple of days.

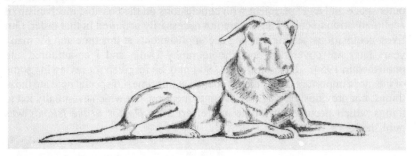

He loved children and would leave me for days while he visited them in the various neighbourhoods in which we had digs (low cost accommodation) in the past. The children's parents did not understand this relationship and the seemingly fearsome mock battles that the children had with him caused them enough alarm to call the police and write unfavourable letters to the editor about him in the local papers. That is how I found out where he disappeared to. To get where he wanted to go, he rode the street cars and, according to the conductors, he made the right changes from one street car to another to get where he was going.

You might ask how Tiger was able to go freely with me from one digs to another. In a few minutes, while negotiations were going on, he was able to charm any landlady or landlord into wanting him to be the lodger. I just went along for the ride and to pay the rent. I guess there were those who did not like him for, after six years of good companionship, someone poisoned him with strychnine.

* * *

In 1942, soon after John was born, we lived in an upstairs flat above a barber's shop. Nobody should have been allowed to live in such a place. Its clapboard walls in places were open to the outside environment and that winter we shovelled snow out of the living room. The toilet was outside in an outhouse which was also used to store wood and coal for the open fire place.

In these quarters I spent a number of happy hours pursuing the extracurricular activity of demonstrating to myself and my friends that we had the means for man to live in a closed environment in outer space. My friends thought this was a useless activity, especially since there were no space vehicles to drive it into space, but they were used to my aberrations into Fantasy Land. The idea to delve into this problem came about after several visits to the Children's Ward at the Dunedin Public Hospital in the course of my obligations as a medical student.

This ward always had a good supply of comics, with Flash Gordon and other space heroes among them. I was already an addict of science fiction and my visits to the children's ward were not always for professional reasons. These interests led me to ask myself whether we had the technology to support life in outer space. The conclusion of my efforts clearly showed that we did. I was to put this information to good use in the early years of space research in the United States between 1956 and 1961.

* * *

This flat, being next to the hospital and the medical school, was most convenient for me, but in other respects, it left much to be desired. Lydia, who was working for the Crown Solicitor, found highly desirable quarters with the most delightful landlord and landlady in Onslow Street in the elite neighbourhood of St. Clair. This proved to be fortuitous for following up my interest in pursuing the subject of acclimatisation and exposure to cold, sparked by my first experience of cold while boarding at King's.

In Onslow St. we were only two streets from the fine surfing beach of St. Clair. A number of medical student friends were addicts, as I was, of "body shooting" the formidable waves of St. Clair Beach. Since the waves rolling on to St. Clair Beach were huge during the winter, we were contemplating extending the season of our sport into the cold months. What better opportunity than this, my friends thought, for using Tom's and Lyd's place as a base from which to enjoy their sport in both summer and winter. What better opportunity than this, I thought, for using my friends for my experiments.

The price I extracted for this service was that they were to be human subjects for an experiment to measure the effects of their exposure to the cold water of these latitudes. St. Clair Beach is about 45 degrees Latitude south. Unhappy as they were at this turn of events, they agreed and my first research into my favourite subject then and in future years was on.

I bought a number of rectal thermometers. When I could obtain their co-operation, my friends were required to insert these thermometers rectally for five minutes before entering the water. While in the water they were, at a signal from me on shore, to read their thermometers every five minutes and call their readings to me for recording in my note book. It was quite a sacrifice, but enough data were obtained to arouse all of our interests and co-operation with the demands of the experiment.

We had thought that the body temperature would gradually fall and that, after leaving the water, it would rise as each subject warmed up. Almost the opposite was observed. At the first five minute reading, after getting into the water, the temperatures shot up from an average of about 37 degrees to an average of about 39.5 degrees centigrade. At the ten minute immersion it dropped to around 38.5C degrees and remained there until the subjects returned to the dressing shed. After immersion, the temperature fell slowly and the ten or twenty minute post-immersion temperature readings would read as low as 35.5 degrees, returning to normal between one to two hours after a slight overshoot. The water temperature remained around 3 degrees during the experiments. The period of immersion was 20 to 25 minutes. During and after each immersion, there was little or no shivering exhibited by the subjects and the warm up period was luxuriously relaxing. Sitting close to the fire, or the consumption of hot drinks or food, comforts which none of my subjects would forego, made little difference to the pattern of temperature changes during the post-immersion period.

None of the subjects were exposed to the limit. They had been very co-operative and I did not have the heart to ask anyone to find out the limit of exposure. I reserved this dubious privilege for myself. Instead of getting out of the water when I thought I had had enough, I persevered. At between the 35 and 40 minute readings, I felt uncomfortable and the next reading confirmed my feeling that I was now losing body heat. After this I had the uncontrollable urge to get out of the water, but I hung on for another two more readings, taking the total immersion to 50 minutes. During the post-immersion period the temperature continued to fall to 34.6 degrees and did not return to normal for about 8 hours.

Walking the two blocks back home was like walking on air. My feet felt nothing. I was sure my cerebration was impaired, but no one seemed to notice this. My colour vision seemed to be impaired and did not return to normal until the next day. However, there was no objective testing of this. The luxurious relaxed feeling of the post immersion period experienced after lesser periods of exposure was absent. I did not feel well or normal until the next day. Sleep that night was restless, but I have little memory of it. These reactions were not much different to those I had experienced on the completion of my winter record cold shower exposure of 42 minutes at King's.

St. Clair during the blustery and miserable winter months, unlike the gay, busy months of summer, closed its busy shops and boarded itself against the cold winds and spume of the southern winter. We should have been safe from the prying eyes of passers-by, but word got around and, after a humorous piece in the press, spectators joined in the spirit of things and cheered when thermometer reading times came around. Some shops opened and a proprietor or two thanked me for attracting an off-season trade.

The results were not earth shaking, but it gave me an insight into what was needed in the future, if the chance to work on the subject ever came my way. Literature I was able to peruse in the Medical School Library indicated that no one had done scientific research into the subject, though there was mention that Claude Bernard, the famous French physiologist, had 160 years previously proposed a chemical component in addition to the muscular activity component of shivering in heat production, induced by exposure to cold. This fitted very well with my school boy and St. Clair Beach observations of the disappearance of shivering on acclimatisation to cold.

Since there was no shivering in my inured subjects and since the body temperature increased significantly on exposure to cold water, heat was being generated by the body. This had to be what Claude Bernard had referred to as "Chemical Heat Production". Over the years, researchers on the subject had not been able to demonstrate Claude Bernard's proposal and three eminent scientists, Alan Burton of Canada, Otto Edholm of the Medical Research Council of Great Britain and James Hardy of Harvard in a joint publication subsequently refuted the possibility of chemical thermogenesis. In 1955, using new techniques, Professor Jean Mayer, then of Harvard, and I revived the possibility of its existence in a storm of controversy which led me into a great deal of research effort to support this possibility.

* * *

My requirements for the degree in medicine finally came to an end. At the end of 1943, Lydia and John went to my second home in New Zealand, the Homestead of the Mizens on Mercury Island, while I went to Seacliff Mental Hospital to learn a little about psychiatry.

In March 1944, I started work at the Auckland Public Hospital. It was work from early morning to dark at night with many nights up to deal with emergencies. During a period of particularly heavy night and day work, I came down with virus pneumonia which at least gave me a little respite. Respite also came about with secondments to the Rotorua Hospital and Greenlane Hospital. At Greenlane Hospital I had the privilege of working with Douglas Robb, later Sir Douglas, and we became good friends.

At last, what I had been waiting for appeared in the press: an advertisement for the post of Medical Officer to the Cook Islands. I applied. I was turned down. The notice appeared again. I applied again and was turned down again. It appeared a third time. I was turned down a third time. On the fourth round, they could not ignore me. Who else would want to go to be Medical Officer to the Cook Islands? Much later I found out that I was not turned down because of my professional abilities, but because it was a colonial policy of New Zealand not to employ educated Cook Islanders in the Cook Islands. They were likely to be troublemakers. I also found out that I had particular traits which had been identified as prone to becoming the worst kind of trouble maker.

When Douglas Robb and others heard that I was off to Nevernever Land, never to be heard of again, all arguments were put forward why this was the worst professional decision I could possibly make. My arguments to the contrary made no impression. It was an obligation which, if not fulfilled, would become a problem of conscience. In December 1945, Lydia, John and I with our chattels sailed in the tiny "Maui Pomare" via Tonga, Samoa and Niue to Rarotonga. The islands were all then, and had been for sometime, "The Forsaken Isles", as aptly expressed around that time by the man who became my predecessor as Prime Minister, Albert Henry.

CHAPTER THREE

Doctor To The Islands

The impact of its beauty of mountains and lush green vegetation, framed in a pure white setting of surf bursting on an encircling reef, was almost too much to admire at that early hour. RONALD SYME

"Who is able to treat diseases now?" It is uncertain. For actual treatment is now mixed with superstition and spiritualism and mere lies. JOHN PAPA I'I

The medical treatment of the sick was a matter that belonged to the gods. DAVID MALO

The excitement of seeing Rarotonga again was no different from that first home-coming twelve years before, but added were the mixed emotions brought about by coming back as a fully qualified medical doctor. I was no longer the simple island boy. I was taking on something no Island boy had attempted. Deep down I knew that it had an unsettling effect on our people. I was up at day-break and as we approached Rarotonga, with its familiar rugged peaks where I had snared wild fowl and hunted flying fox, the nostalgia of one who had been long away surged through me. As we approached the anchorage, the offshore breeze brought us the scent of frangipani and tiare maori, the native gardenia, beloved of every South Sea Islander. Mother was the first to greet us. She came towards me with outstretched arms. She had not changed, a little thinner perhaps, but her hair was just as dark and her face as unlined as when I had seen her last twelve years before. She had the same proud bearing and her face had lost none of its characteristic determination. Although her welcoming kiss was warm, I knew by her eyes that her opinion of me was guarded. The question in them was, "Will he come up to our expectations?" Others no doubt were asking the same question. I formally introduced mother to Lydia and John. Her welcome of John was a grandmother's welcome. John was rather awed by her, but he took it like a man.

While we four were caught up in the intimacy of this reunion, I was aware of the genuine emotion of those in the background, for, to a Polynesian, a welcome is as serious and as much a matter for tears as a farewell. There were relatives with eis of frangipani and gardenia on their arms waiting their turn to bedeck us and welcome us home. The welcoming feast later at our Tupapa home was no less sumptuous than that which welcomed Mary and me home twelve years before.

My eagerness to come home was not solely motivated by my wish to serve my people. Though given the choice, they were the ones I would choose above others. The other motive was a selfish one, based on the fact that in growing up, I had had the best of all worlds. I had been the favourite son of my aunts and uncles and seemingly everybody else also. My mother was hard on me in the matter of discipline, but everybody else made up for it and when I did things which they knew would get me in trouble with mother, they would go to no end of effort to protect me from her wrath. The care and love that everybody gave me, bound me to them as nothing else could. I could never do enough to show them my love and loyalty in return.

I had access to anywhere and anything my little heart desired. I could visit and stay with many aunts and uncles, real and facilitatory. And I could partake of what they had to my fill, either in the home or in the fields.

I also had access to the world of sea captains, sailors, sailing ships, steamers and the small boats that served them. The big ones were too big to enter our two little harbours, Avarua and Avatiu, between which I was born. They anchored in the open sea. In those days Avarua was the harbour where most of the action took place. On shipping days, I was first on the 35 foot launch, Takuvaine, skippered by Papa Manuela, towing four or five lighters at a time between the Avarua wharf and the steamers anchored beyond the reef. I rode the launch to and fro between ship and shore. When I tired of this, I climbed one of the mooring ropes to which the lighters clung for loading and unloading, clambering aboard the steamer to find new things to explore and shipboard food to eat. But at noon I would make it to shore and line up for my piece of salt pork and hard tack (ship's biscuits). For me it was always a meal fit for a king, for its connotations of the sea if not for the taste.

When the schooners moored to the great anchors stuck and held tight by the growing coral on each side of the harbours, I would try to help the divers who made the mooring lines fast to them. Some of them had been laid by my grandfather years before. Or I made a nuisance of myself in other ways, but nobody ever seemed to complain. I was accepted as part of the scene until I went to school in New Zealand.

Once, a four masted barquentine, came into Avatiu harbour to unload. I think it carried cement and timber from the United States or Canada. I bust with joy when I was allowed to have a go at working one of the steam donkey engines controlling the hoists of the two cargo booms needed to handle the cargo laden nets or slings. The right hand control wound open to lift the load out of the hold straight up. The left hand control was to sweep the load across the deck, clearing all structures that might be in the way. Then, the controls were reversed and both were wound in sensitive unison to lower the cargo gently into the waiting lighter. When the coast was clear, my friend who normally worked the controls would move over for me to take over. I was proud I was the only kid allowed to do this, but then, it seemed I was the only one interested in doing it. This schooner was particularly large, at least to the eyes of us kids. It was, therefore particularly suitable to tie a rope to the outer end of its main cross yard on the foremast, swing out from the ratlines in a great arc and, high in the air just at the end of the swing, let go and dive into the sea. Some of us could do somersaults and body twists on our way into the sea. One after another we would take our turn until we found some other interesting thing to do.

Our house in Ruatonga was where the sea captains came with their peaked caps with removable white covers for tropical climes and their white double-breasted jackets buttoned with bright brass buttons. I ate every word they spoke when they talked of their adventures or when they just gossiped.

When there were no ships around we took to the hills mainly with Johnny Webb whose Tahitian mother was friends with my family. Sometimes we were joined by Don O'Brien who was born here and spoke Rarotongan like a native. My two dogs and Johnny's two dogs would join us on these inland sorties. Our dogs and especially my smelly goat, Billy, were banned from the school environs, but the dogs could always find us later, no matter where we went. When I lived in Tupapa, my friends were the Kamana boys who were nephews of my stepfather. Tau the eldest would take me on our horse, Beauty, and we ranged all over the land.

The special position my mother held in this society exposed me to all the facets of community life, both Maori and European, and I seemed to live fully in both worlds and in many smaller worlds of the various clans and cliques, religious denominations and occupations, that confined many others to restricted experiences. In part it was all of these, I believe, that made Rarotonga a place to come back to. It was coming back to where one had been loved and cared for by so many. In a way, I suppose this world was for me an escape back to the comfort and security of the womb.

* * *

As demanded by protocol, next morning I presented myself to the Resident Commissioner. I remembered him from old. Though born in New Zealand, he had worked his way up in the Cook Islands from an office boy, as only a perfect bureaucrat can, to the exalted official position of Resident Commissioner, the highest in the land. His exposure to the world, even to the limited world of Rarotonga, was as limited as that of anyone in similar circumstances.

At last, when I stood before him in his large office, he stared at me with that twisted grimace I remembered so well and said in as stern a voice as he could summon, "You are not here. I have not been informed of your coming." After a moment of stunned silence, I realised that he meant every word of what he said. "But I am here," I said. No you're not," he bellowed. This was getting us nowhere. So with as much dignity as I could muster, I said, "Sir, I will come back when I arrive." and left, but not without first seeing the rage I was leaving behind. Next day I was summoned back and the conversation we had was on a much better plane.

I cannot say that I got on well with the Resident Commissioner during the many years we were together. He had the entrenched views of a dyed in the wool colonialist and that alone would have put us on a continuous collision course which took some adept manoeuvring, mostly on my part, to avoid. Not all collisions could be averted. His views on how I should conduct myself as the only qualified medical doctor in the Cook Islands were extraordinary to say the least.

In his view, I was to take less heed of the medical problems the people faced and pay more attention to the social amenities that went with my high official status. He inferred that since they were only natives, there was not much that could be done for them anyway. I had no answer to this. He was either joking or he had failed to read me as a person and as a doctor. I could not be sure.

I was left in little doubt when three weeks later he called me back to his office and severely berated me for not taking his advice. I quietly advised him that the ethics of my profession could not allow me to take his advice, no matter how well intentioned it was. At this he displayed irritation at my attitude and neither of us ever brought the subject up again.

* * *

The same boat that brought us was also to take away the retiring doctor. After that first visit with the Resident Commissioner, I kept my appointment with the retiring doctor to get first hand information that I felt would stand me in good stead for the responsibilities I was about to take over from him. He was to show me the hospital and the Sanatorium. This he did with a flourish. He presented me to the Matron and the three of us first toured the hospital which had been designed for thirty two beds. From the outside, one could not see the hospital properly because it was surrounded by a veritable jungle. A beautiful jungle, but scarcely hygienic when one remembers that such a jungle harbours the mosquito vector for filariasis and dengue fever. It was not a good example for the populace. Creepers, trees, tangled masses of flowering shrubs and flower beds springing up unexpectedly before one, all forming a design which made no horticultural or artistic sense.

When the doctor noticed my interest in the jungle, he remarked, "Yes, isn't it beautiful. It's Matron's pride and joy." Our round of the handful of patients reduced me to silence. There were fifteen of them, almost all, according to the good doctor, suffering from Filariasis. As he led me from bed to bed, it became clear that, if they were suffering from filariasis, they also had things wrong with them of a more urgent nature.

Nearly all the patients were elderly. In my experience, of the many things which scream of poor delivery of medical care, one is a low daily bed rate and the other a high proportion of chronic elderly patients. If both occur at the same time, things are not what they should be. If the third indicator, an undue presence of self styled medicine men or outright medical charlatans are in evidence, the bottom of the barrel of poor delivery of medical care has been struck. If, in addition, the medical profession uses their presence as an excuse for not delivering professional medical care, the bottom of the barrel of poor delivery of medical care is being scraped. We have seen it all here in the Cook Islands.

While we were making the rounds, the doctor said, "Tom, we are very lucky here. We have no cancer, no rheumatic fever, no poliomyelitis, not even mumps!" I had to suppose that it was easier to call everything filariasis. It saves a lot of trouble. There being no specific cure for it, you're off the hook if the patient dies.

I had a fairly good impression of Matron, but years in the outback of Australia and some years in the Pacific Islands had taken their toll of her knowledge of modern medical nursing. She believed that natives had a special biological make-up which made them non-responsive to modern drugs represented by

Sulpha and Penicillin. She had no problems with this kind of thinking because it was the popular thinking of officialdom in general. She also did not believe in asepsis. To overcome this last was a major problem, but overcome it we did. The nurses came off the street as they used to in England before the days of Florence Nightingale. There was no attempt to give them any training.

She informed me that no Islander would let anyone stick a needle into them. I thought this strange because I did not remember them being particularly afraid of anything. Later in conversation with some old friends and people in general, I gleaned their opinion of the medical service. In regard to injections it was simple. When patients were moribund, it was the custom of the doctor to give them an injection of morphine, "To ease their going," Matron explained when I talked to her about it later. Naturally, some Islanders assumed either that the patients were dying as a result of the injections or that it was a last resort. It was in effect a pronouncement of death.

· From the inside, the jungle looked even worse than from the outside. In the bushes were empty tins, half coconut shells and other small containers which are the breeding places for the Aedes Polyensiensis, the vector for filariasis in our area, and Aedes Aegypti, the vector for dengue or breakbone fever. There could not be a better example of the filarial vector/host relationship than right here at the main hospital of the Cook Islands.

There were no receptacles for rubbish and no ash trays. The result was a profusion of empty meat tins, half coconut shells, orange and banana peel, discarded paper, cigarette butts, discarded cigarette and tobacco containers. I mentioned this to Matron and she assured me that the natives were naturally dirty and the last thing they would use would be a rubbish container or an ash tray. The hospital floors were strewn with rubbish. The inside walls of the hospital were painted blue because, said the Matron, "That colour keeps the mosquitoes away." This further darkened the already jungle-darkened hospital rooms. I had no illusions that I had a fight on my hands to hygienize and sanitize the hospital.

This was all upsetting to me. The Doctor and the Matron had forgotten that I was just an Island boy and had given me their thoughts on my people without restraint. The picture they gave was founded on prejudice, not fact. I was again learning the low opinion with which European officialdom regarded our people. I knew otherwise and was to confirm over and over again that our people had a great deal more going for them than they were given credit for. I would not have returned then and again later if I did not believe this.

I said I would like to see the operating theatre. "Oh! You don't want to see that, Doctor. We never do surgery here. The tropics you know. Every thing goes septic no matter what you do and, with all the filariasis about, all sorts of complications are likely to occur."

While she was chattering, I found the theatre myself. Flaking calcimine painted walls and ceilings and general neglect told their story. Again a rationalisation had been found to deny my people even a modicum of surgical services. Although there was a reasonable array of surgical instruments, there were no retractors and no light to operate under. I wondered what further rationalisations were dreamt up when a surgical emergency operation was not done and the patient died.

The Xray unit was a dental unit and was run by an expatriate school teacher. It was not working because it was giving everybody who touched it a severe shock. I gingerly tested it and received a good enough shock to throw me some way across the room. Being electronically minded, I washed the machine with methylated spirits and there were no more shocks. The hospital being on the sea shore, the machine had become caked with salt and leaked high voltage everywhere. The equipment had been neglected even for a wipe down. Later I was surprised at the reasonable Xray pictures of anatomical structures other than teeth this unit was able to produce and the chest Xrays were acceptable. Much later I obtained a fine unit left by the American armed forces on Aitutaki some 250 kilometres to the north. When I returned twenty years later this unit was still in operation. In a place where so many deaths were due to tuberculosis, an Xray unit which could do a good job was a necessity.

"May I see the laboratory please, Matron." I asked.

"Sorry, Doctor, there is no Laboratory." Matron replied.

Our next stop for the three of us was the Sanatorium, seven kilometres from the Hospital, where the main hospital is now situated. Although tuberculosis is a thing of the past, this hospital is still called the Sanatorium. As he drove, the doctor spoke with irritation about the native medicine men and women.

"Tom," he said, "You have no idea how many of these people, including Europeans, take their illnesses to the medicine men. They know there is a law against it, but they go right on doing it. We do our best to stop it by reporting them and fining them in the courts, but it does not seem to do any good." I could not help thinking that, if the Medical Department did its job, it would win hands down over the medicine men.

After a climb of about a kilometre, there was the Sanatorium, high inland above "Te Reinga", the place whence the spirits of the dead traditionally took off for the next world. It was a great site for a sanatorium with a cool breeze and a great view. It was also a place Cook Islanders associated with the spirits of the dead and avoided. Nevertheless, in true Polynesian style, everybody used the pool at Black Rock, as Te Reinga is now commonly known, as a salt water swimming hole.

The doctor now, for the first time, informed me that the Sanatorium had no patients, even though it had been open for over a year. He added that it was likely not to have any for a long time. He said the people believed the place to be haunted and no amount of cajoling would get anybody to be a patient there. The Sanatorium had been fully staffed ever since it opened, but no patients. The jinx became apparent to him only after the Sanatorium was built.

I was now fed up to the teeth with all the silly problems entailed in bringing even the poorest of medical services to our people. I made up my mind that I was going to tackle each of the jobs staring me in the face one by one and God help anybody who got in my way. It was not going to be popular, at least in the beginning, because nobody thought that anything was wrong with the medical service. Nobody knew better. I did not come back and give up a good future in medicine to be stalled by ignorance, superstition and professional incompetence.

On our way back, I asked the Doctor about the Assistant Medical Practitioners trained in Fiji.

"They're not worth a damn," he said.

"That's right" Matron chimed in, "The poor Doctor has to do everything himself, but they are useful for the Outer Islands."

I could not quite see how they would be useful in one place and not in another. I was dropped off at the Otera (Hotel) Rarotonga, now the site of the "Banana Court".

Physically and emotionally drained, I took time to sit down and review the day's happenings. The sanitary conditions at the main hospital were appalling. The jungle had to go. The number of relatives attending patients would have to be reduced to one at a time. In the absence of an adequate number of staff and proper medication, they were some help, but in the end they would have to be replaced by adequately trained staff. Much else had to be done first. I would have to make full use of the Assistant Medical Practitioners. Rubbish containers and ash trays were a must. The operating theatre had to be upgraded. Aseptic techniques would have to be learned and adhered to.

The general hospital would have to cease being no more than a place for chronic cases and the elderly. It was against all medical experience that, in the population of Rarotonga alone, there were no cases requiring the professional skills of modern medicine. The local Medicine Men were lording it over the Medical Department only because they were doing a better job in dealing with people's real and imagined medical ills. They did not have to do well to do that. The trick was not to fine or denigrate them, but to try to fit them into the scheme of things. The actions being taken against them were turning them into saints in the eyes of the populace.

The new chemotherapeutic agents and antibiotics, proper medical, surgical and every other kind of care were going to be the weapons to deal with most of the problems that had exploded before me that day. The Tuberculosis Sanatorium was like a new pin. It had a full complement of nursing staff, kitchen staff, groundsman, laundry staff, vehicles, but no patients. And, strangest of all, no Xray equipment. The immediate need was to break the jinx that the place was haunted. Polynesians are not all that superstitious unless they want to be.

My own people had no yardstick to measure anything by. They did not know that anything was wrong and that there was a better way of doing things. For a long despairing moment, I harked back to what Sir Douglas Robb had said and thought of the joy of going back to the saner world of medicine. The "Maui Pomare" was still lying at anchor off the reef and there was time for me to say, "To Hell with it all", climb back aboard and leave. But good sense or sheer stupidity and, I must admit, the challenge of it all, made me remind myself that it was for this that I had so painfully prepared myself, no matter what the odds. I excused myself from Lydia and John, looked up some old friends and acquired a hangover.

On my first day in charge, I went to the hospital at 8 am, the hour I was accustomed to start my medical day. By this time any hospital should be clean and ready for the day's work. The cigarette butts and the other debris I had noticed the day before were all there. There were unmade beds, dirty dishes, unwashed enamel and general havoc. It seemed no one expected me or was this the usual way things were?

I had a quick look at the patients and had definite ideas of what could be done for some of them. When I indicated this to the Matron, she assured me that I need not worry because nothing could be done for them. This repeated strain I was beginning to find irritating and I began to show it. The lack of order, routine and cleanliness was beginning to irk me, but I decided to bide my time.

Matron indicated that I ought to be getting to the out-patients as there was a crowd gathering there. I meekly followed her and was astounded at the size of the crowd around what I guess was out-patients and my office. I could not help sticking my chest out a little more than usual, believing that my fame as a doctor had preceded me.

On noticing my astonishment, Matron said, "Oh! Doctor, this is nothing. Wait till Friday, we really get the crowds before the weekends. "I felt let down. This was the usual thing. My fame had nothing to do with it. However, this was cheering, perhaps the stories I had heard of people refusing medical treatment were an exaggeration. The crowd was pressing in at the doors and windows. How was privacy to examine patients to be achieved? When I seated myself at my desk, Matron installed herself firmly by my side with a pink covered booklet in hand which I took to be an out-patients' record book. Here at last was efficiency.

"Ready to begin, Doctor?" said Matron rustling starchily.

"Let 'em come," I replied.

"Come in, whoever got here first. Doctor's a busy man. No dawdling there."

"Good morning, What can I do for you?" I said in the vernacular which goes something like this, "Kia orana, akape'ea au e tauturu ia koe?"

In reply I got the one word, "Pamati."

I did not understand the word and glanced towards Matron. She was writing busily in her little pink covered book. She tore out a page and placed it before me.

"Sign here, Doctor," she said pushing a pen into my hand.

To cover my ignorance of this mysterious symptom or disease. I picked up the piece of paper and read:

I hereby certify that...Uti......requires..1 bottle....of whiskey... for G.H.P.

Signed...................

Medical Officer

Turning to matron I asked, "What's this?"

Her reply was lengthy and full of detail, the upshot being that my duties during out-patient clinic time was to include the dishing out of liquor permits. Now I understood the meaning of pamati, it was the Rarotongan for permit. Early in the period of the London Missionary Society influence, the Cook Islands had been declared "dry". Nobody could get an honest drink without a medical prescription from the Medical Officer. "G.H.P." was short for "General Health Purposes". I, as the only qualified medical officer in the Cook Islands, was the sole and autocratic controller of the consumption of liquor for the whole of the Cook Islands. This duty also extended by mail to the Outer Islands. Since few wanted the medical services of the hospital anyway, this, for a while, was my main function during "Out-patients".

When the French, next door in French Polynesia, heard about this, they roared with laughter and could not be convinced that I was not the richest man in the Cook Islands. "Even at 10 francs a time....Oo La La," they knowingly chimed.

In time, I made other arrangements to circumvent the law and ease the load of this function as my medical duties started to increase. Circumventing a law of this nature was not difficult. There were many precedents. The law which required that you carry a light between you and a female companion walking on the road was, like many other of the "Blue Laws", still on the books, though not enforced.

* * *

While I was busily attending to this onerous "medical" duty, the Assistant Medical Practitioners were sitting on the verandah rail laughing and talking with the crowd of "non-patients", joking back and forth and roaring with laughter at some remark, as only Polynesians can. I smiled to myself at the thought that they had better laugh while they can, for I was planning to put them to full use. They were going to fetch up hard against cases they never thought existed and, if they did, they never believed that they would become professionally responsible for in the strongest sense of the word.

Out there among the population were medical cases requiring our skills, even cases of cancer, chest diseases, rheumatic fever, poliomyelitis, acute appendicitis and the rest. They were hidden from the medical department and were in the perhaps more compassionate, but medically limited hands of the medicine men. In the mean time, I patiently signed one pamati after another and stocked up with the medical armamentarium that makes doctors what they are. Professional compassion is not the least of these.

No laboratory, no surgery or Xrays of any consequence had been done for some time, little parenteral therapy (various forms of injections), no blood transfusion had ever been done and no blood typing reagents stocked, no therapeutic injections or intravenous therapy were administered. And the list went on. The miracle sulpha drugs and the recently discovered antibiotic, penicillin, were absent. Neither had been considered of any use in the Cook Islands. I could see twenty years of work ahead to educate, cajole and convince both the people and officialdom to bring about the changes required. And this is not to mention all the public health programmes that needed to be planned and implemented.

Some of the problems were easy to solve, some took longer than others, some were never solved even when solutions were at hand, some were solved more by accident than by good management. One that I thought might never be solved was in this last category and was solved almost immediately.

One of the fifteen patients whose condition had been diagnosed as filariasis looked very anaemic to me and, if she had filariasis, she also had anaemia. She had been sent from the island of Aitutaki by the Americans with a diagnosis of perforated gastric ulcer.A perforated peptic ulcer is an emergency condition, but fortunately for the lady, the diagnosis had been wrong or she would have been dead. However, she was moribund and needed urgent attention.

There was no problem of getting blood via a prick of the finger, and the blood showed that the patient had the typical blood picture of Megaloblastic Anaemia. Further inquiry confirmed that there was none of the magic medication for this condition on the Island. The only alternative to hold off progression of the condition was to give her a blood transfusion to stabilise things until medication could arrive by the once a fortnight flight of a DC3 New Zealand Government plane that took three days via Fiji, Tonga, Samoa and Aitutaki to reach Rarotonga. "Matron," I said, "I would like you to set up a blood transfusion and a donor for Mrs Teariki." "Blood? Blood, you say? Really, Doctor Davis, what next? You can't give blood transfusions to natives. Where will you get the blood? There's no blood bank in the islands. Natives believe that they will drop dead if you take blood from them. Even if you can find a donor, how do you think you are going to get a needle into Mrs Teariki.? Please remember that you are in the islands now."

At my look of pained exasperation, she continued breathlessly, "It's a pity, but Mrs Teariki will just have to die. Her illness is so complicated with filariasis that blood will not do her any good."

"Matron, let me have a word," I finally managed. "If the natives believe they are going to drop dead from loss of a pint of blood, we've got to teach them that they won't. Islands or no islands, we're not going to let Mrs Teariki die because of her and everybody's ignorance of medicine.You go ahead and set up. I will find the blood."

Matron was flustered. "Doctor," she said forlornly, "There is no blood transfusion apparatus."

As forlornly, I said, "We'll make one."

Matron suddenly got a glint in her eye and immediately became noisily and spectacularly enthusiastic. Even though she did not seem to hold out much hope of finding a donor, her enthusiasm for making do was unquestionable.

"You just tell me what you need and I'll dig it up from somewhere."

In a few minutes she proudly laid out everything we needed; a rubber suction bulb from the back of a dispensary drawer, perished somewhat, but still serviceable, a clean bottle and cork from her own bathroom, a length of glass tubing, some questionable rubber tubing and an assortment of hypodermic needles in various stages of sharpness. We'd also found some sodium citrate to keep the blood from clotting. We were all set to go.

"Now, Matron, you've got blood and I've got blood."

Matron sighed, "That means that I will have to be the donor. You'll have to do the transfusion."

"No, we won't do it that way. This is too good an opportunity to teach the people that it won't harm them to give their blood. I don't mind you sticking a needle into me and I am sure that you won't mind me sticking a needle into you, but this time we're going to let somebody else be the donor." Our preparations had taken time and now it was night. Matron and I had become so engrossed in what we were doing that time had flown.

*   *   *

People hang around the hospital at all hours of the day and night. They may be visiting a patient or just dropping in for a chat with anybody who might be around. As luck would have it, I recognised a friend of the family. One of the nurses had told everybody hanging around what she understood was the problem with Mrs Teariki and what I wanted to do.

. Like all peoples of the world, we are intensely curious and always want to know what is going on. Our situation was worse than most because there were no newspapers and one could get the news only by getting around and talking. If you don't believe this just try to imagine yourself without a newspaper or radio, you'd be hanging around any place you thought you could get news or even gossip. What goes in one end and what comes out the other may not be the same. It may be better. Usually the gist of the facts is there. We call it "Coconut Wireless" and until we printed a newspaper, that is all we had. It was not bad.

My friend was only too anxious to learn more and do what he could. I asked him where I could get volunteers to give blood, explaining that out of these, I would have to find one that matched the blood of the patient. He told me that he would get me all the donors I needed within a half hour. I thought he was exaggerating the simplicity of the task, but he was a Mataiapo, clan chief, and the mana (authority) that went with it could just do the trick.

He was as good as his word. He accomplished this miracle by going to the local picture theatre, stopping the performance, giving the picture goers his version of what I had told him and demanding volunteers in a dramatic plea from centre stage. In a matter of minutes almost the entire audience shifted from Uncle Willie's picture theatre to the hospital verandah and grounds with the overflow milling over Matron's flower beds and jostling for a place in the front of the queue. For once, Matron forgot to scream at the vandals in her garden. There must have been two hundred volunteers and spectators at the hospital that night.

As for Uncle Willie, he rued the day that the talkies came into being. He could have woven this event into his narration not once, but several times and on several occasions. The loss of his clientele did not bother him either for, as he said, they'd already paid and he was going to have an earlier night home than usual. Also he could show the movie again and charge the same price.

I did a direct cross match on several volunteers and found a match. We hitched him up directly, venous system to venous system as it were, to Mrs Teariki and pumped what, as best as we could judge, was a pint of blood from donor to recipient. The crowds would not disperse until they were assured that the deed had been done and both were doing well. After that night, blood transfusions became common place and a pool of volunteers was always on hand. No problems were ever encountered until Jehovah's Witnesses became part of the Cook Islands scene, but this problem was confined to them only. For the rest of my six years in the Cook Islands as a medical officer and as the Chief Medical Officer, I never again encountered another case of this type of anaemia. Moreover, Mrs Teariki recovered fully. Having played her role in overcoming prejudices against parenteral therapy, she retired from the scene to continue a normal healthy life.

* * *

Mrs Teariki, coming from the outer island of Aitutaki, was luckier than most outer islanders. Aitutaki had an airport built by the Americans and there were military doctors there who freely gave of their medical skills. Furthermore, in such emergencies, an aeroplane was at hand to fly patients to Rarotonga as with Mrs Teariki. This was not, however, the case with other outer islands. There were no such facilities. It was by sea or not at all.

During the hurricane season from December 1 to March 31, all shipping left our waters. Local schooners holed up in either Papeete, Tahiti, 735 nautical miles to the north-east or Penrhyn our most distant outer island, 755 miles to the north. Shipping from overseas did not come at all. This was an overkill because a hurricane which bothered the Southern Cook Islands occurred on an average of once every 10 years. But hurricane warnings did not exist and the risk was ever present. My grandfather lost one schooner in Avatiu Harbour as a result of his practice of ignoring hurricanes and doing a roaring trade in the absence of other shipping.

When the island of Atiu was struck with an epidemic affecting the young children in the middle of the hurricane season, a request for urgent help was morse-coded to Rarotonga. There was a cargo boat passing through our waters, but my request to the Resident Commissioner to divert it to allow me to respond to Atiu's request for medical assistance was refused. By the time I and the continuing messages from Atiu convinced him of the severity of the problem, the ship was beyond recall.

We were now forced to fall back on our own resources. I called on Ron Powell, Fred Story and John Pratt who were all sailors at one time or another to see what could be done. We decided that our only recourse was to use the Union Steamship Company's 35 foot launch, the Takuvaine, to reach Atiu some 140 nautical miles to the north-east. We would need to cover the forward cockpit and rig two masts and sails borrowed from the Sailing Club's racing outrigger canoes. We decided that the crew would have to be minimal, because space was at a premium. The only shelter was over the 35 horse power diesel and there was just room for one person to squeeze into it. Any others would have to sit in the open cockpit. Therefore, we concluded that Louis Wohler, who normally ran the engine of the launch, myself as the Doctor and maybe one or at the most two others would be sufficient.

We took our thoughts to the Resident Commissioner who exploded with his usual negativism and vetoed our plan. But we did not give up. We knew his great fear of having to shoulder blame for anything, which exhibited itself by indecision and doing nothing as the best course for self preservation. In this matter he was caught betwixt and between. His refusal to divert a passing ship was a matter of record, as was the barrage of messages for medical assistance. I did not spare him on how it would look for him if he continued to refuse assistance. He looked at me with sadness mixed with anxiety, fear and anger as though the whole matter was our fault. He capitulated, but insisted that a Union Steamship Company man travel with us to insure that if anything went wrong the Company could not sue the Administration. He insisted that all four of us navigators go along and that I take a medical assistant. He also instructed that we take six drums of fuel that far exceeded our requirements.

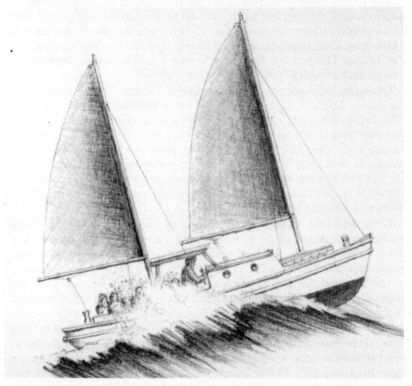

Already some of the children had died and time was at a premium. In less than twenty four hours we were ready: masts stepped, forward cockpit covered and provisions in the form of vacuum flasks of hot coffee, sandwiches and other goodies supplied by our wives. The weather was not at all to our liking. As usual at this time of the year, the south-east trades turns into north-east trades and it was on the nose for travelling to Atiu. The wind was blowing at about 25 knots with seas and white caps to match.

It took two wet and uncomfortable days for the Takuvaine to fight her way to Atiu. The cramped open quarters forced us to remain in a sitting position at all times. We sat, we ate, we slept in fits and starts in this position. We managed our physiological functions as best we could and the constant movement of pitching into the head seas took its physical toll. Frequent inundation with head-on breaking seas kept us constantly wet and chilled to the bone.

Vainerere and his Boys Brigade on Atiu kept a fire burning constantly on the highest point on the island which assisted us greatly in making a landfall. My assistant, Tere Williams, and I went ashore through some abominable surf, treated the remaining patients and made a provisional diagnosis of meningitis which was confirmed by laboratory tests on the samples of cerebro-spinal fluid I brought back with me. I left Tere in Atiu to continue treatment and he was able to arrest the progress of the disease and further deaths. However, before leaving Atiu, I was requested to attend a woman in labour. I delivered her of a baby boy which she named Papa Tom Davis. Recently I was unfortunate in not being able to attend his daughter's twenty first birthday. However, my wife attended and gave my apologies.

The return trip was a sleigh ride under full sail. Apart from a compass affected by the magnetism of the redundant drums of fuel, causing us to over-run Rarotonga and fight our way back upwind, the voyage back was by comparison a nice sail. But the total venture had taken heavy toll on our physical and mental resources and we landed in Rarotonga exhausted, but pleased with the success of our mission. As in other situations of this nature we were at a loss to explain the appearance of this disease in this isolated manner other than that the organism had been lurking in the population waiting for conditions to be right for its propagation.

* * *

As the days went by, the hospital started to fill with patients and not just chronics and old people. There was, however, a problem in that people who came to the hospital and patients within it would not allow anybody other than myself to treat them or give them intravenous or intramuscular or subcutaneous therapy. Their fear of injections was gone, but they would accept a parenteral injection only from me.

In those early days of penicillin, it had been worked out that injections had to be given every three hours to keep up the desired blood levels. That old bugbear of mine, enough sleep, again became a problem of the first order. Something had to be done. Again I tried to have patients accept injections from Matron and the nurses, but this was roundly rejected. I tried to have them accept the ministrations of the AMPs, but this was rejected even more severely. I was at my wit's end.

Eventually I was forced to give the 24 hour total of eight divided doses in four doses, over a period of 12 hours during the day time. The rationale for higher doses per single injection did not bother me, because it had been demonstrated that high concentrations of penicillin in the blood caused no side effects.

I was literally forced into this regimen when the hospital was filled to over capacity with children with pneumonia. By the time I had gotten through doing all the injections for one dose, the time for the next dose was due. I kept a close eye on the efficacy of the medication using the new regimen to make certain that I was not short changing my young patients. Penicillin is so effective that the drama of its curative effect is unmistakable.

My new six hourly regimen was just as effective as the three hourly recommended treatment. I experimented with only three and two injections a day and there was no apparent loss of efficacy. I made the three injections during twelve hours of the daytime period the routine to be followed. I felt that I could have reduced the total dose and the medication would still have been effective, but I would not experiment this far. I have always drawn a clean line between research to find the truth, and clinical treatment of patients.

In the end, I was able to induce patients and their relatives to accept treatment from others in my presence, and after a little while, when I was not present. Eventually we began, as a staff, to work as a team.

Because surgery had not been done except when a visiting surgeon happened to pass by once in a blue moon, neglected cases began to appear out of the wood work. But these, in these very early days, were not of an acute nature and it takes an emergency to penetrate entrenched prejudices.

It irked me to know that the prejudices were more those of the staff than of the patients. The fear of septic wounds as well as inadequate facilities and equipment reinforced these prejudices. The "cold" as opposed to the acute or "hot" cases were occurring mostly in women and consisted mainly of ovarian cysts, prolapses, uterine retroversions and uterine fibroids. Having received, more by chance than design, a good grounding in the surgery, management and care of these conditions, I was itching to get at them and relieve the women of the discomfort and threatening possibilities of these conditions.

* * *

Then one day the opportunity arose. Ron Powell, then in his forties and now in his eighties, came in with an "acute on chronic" appendicitis. He had had several typical attacks over the years, but these had been diagnosed and treated as gastritis. I did not relish going in surgically because, with that kind of history, the appendix would be surrounded by a mass of adhesed fibrous tissue which would have to be cut through and tied off for bleeders. The surgery could take a long time.

Just as he had recovered from previous attacks, so was it likely that he would recover from this one, but the ethical thing to do was to remove the focus of present and future trouble. There was no choice but to take this ethical position. Fortunately, it was daytime and, with the use of flash-lights, we could manage.

Appendicitis can be one of the easiest surgical procedures and it can be one of the most difficult. It is also a condition which epitomises the existence of several schools of thought. At one extreme, there are those who regard surgery as unwarranted, saying that most cases of appendicitis are medically treatable. This is true, but the rub is, which ones, and are they treatable this way by the time they come to one's notice? Misdiagnosis and no surgery caused Ron severe intermittent problems for many years. Since you do not know which case will give trouble in the future and which case will rupture and cause peritonitis and even death, and which case will subside and cause no more problems, the wise course is surgical intervention in all cases of acute or chronic appendicitis.

There was a good variety of instruments, but no retractors, so I went to see Fred Story, always a good standby for the mechanical and electrical and innovative needs of the health service, and together we constructed some retractors out of aluminium.

One of the AMPs gave the anaesthetic by the good old "Rag and Bottle" method and, as I suspected, it was a two hour job with sweat running off us in all directions and cords of adhesions to wade through to reach the fibrously encapsulated inflamed appendix and remove it from a retrocaecal position. Ron made a fine recovery and word got around. I took the opportunity to mount a beautiful theatre operating light which, I was only now told, had been sitting at Public Works for some years. We also scraped off the flaking calcimine from the ceiling and the walls and repainted them with real paint which could be washed down without destruction. For this operation, I personally supervised the sterilisation and preparation of the theatre and the wound sepsis bogeyman did not appear, much to everybody's surprise. Our elation was temporary. We had not put this bogeyman to rest as I thought we had. It took several further painful 4 a.m. to 8 a.m. presurgery searches through our sterilisation techniques only to prove that the culprit did not lie in this woodpile. The problem lay heavily on my mind, but I still could not accept the idea that "it was the tropics". That did not make sense. And then, one afternoon, I was walking from the wards to my office when I noticed nurses, sitting comfortably on the verandah near my office, making swabs by rolling them up in their bare hands and putting them in a bowl. These swabs looked mighty like the ones I was using in surgery.

"Yes," they said, " This is for surgery tomorrow morning."

No, they did not think that they normally went into the steriliser.

I called Matron. She confirmed my worst fears. "Doctor," she said, "These swabs are straight out of the original packets and are perfectly clean."

"Matron," I asked, "Are the nurses' hands straight out of original packets?" Matron blushed deeply, but the riddle of infected surgical wounds was solved. More importantly Matron was convinced about asepsis.

* * *

After Ron's operation, a surgical list of patients became routine and proper equipment was requisitioned to make surgical days routinely a pleasure for everyone. However, the surgical case load jumped to horrendous proportions. The surgically neglected population came to life and cases which had been in hiding, presented themselves at the hospital for treatment. With now over sixty patients in a hospital built for thirty two, the hospital was bulging at the seams with the usual proportions of medical, surgical, orthopaedic, maternity and paediatric cases. However, the surgical cases were making the heaviest demands.

Neglect of years had accumulated these cases and we were faced with the survivors who were numerous enough to cause an acute hospital accommodation problem. The outer islands presented no different a picture. Over the following months we worked our way through the problem. It would have been fine if this had been the only problem.

* * *

The economy had deteriorated as a result of the 1929 depression. The evidence of former good times were the ruins of the homes of better days visible everywhere. The kikau (coconut leaf thatch) shacks had returned. The settlements of the people from the outer islands on Rarotonga were now reminiscent of ghettos seen elsewhere in the world. The kikau shacks were not as good as their former traditional structures. Although the Polynesian three structure family unit compound was generally followed, one for living, one for sleeping and one for cooking and eating, the double walls were not.

The Southern Cook Islands are far enough south for there to be definite seasonal changes. Spring and Fall have the most erratic changes in temperature and humidity. At the change from the hot humid summer to the cool winter, erratic occurrences of cold early morning temperatures replaced the hot humid nights. Babies were often caught at these times with inadequate clothing. The seemingly Polynesian propensity for chest infections would result in a fulminating type of pneumonia. These caused deaths and in large part created the high infant mortality rate of those days.

The kikau shacks were inadequate to provide the necessary protection from these early morning sudden drops in temperature following a typically hot tropical night. When these "flash epidemics" occurred, heavy pressure was placed on our hospital accommodation and other activities had to be curtailed. Usually our working our way through the "Cold" surgical cases had to give way.

When tourists now complain that there are no more grass huts, I breathe a silent prayer of "Thank God". The relationship between a low standard of living and medical and social ills is unquestionable. By being alert for these sudden climatic changes and pressing the native medicine men into a watch-dog service, we were able to reduce infant mortality from 120 per 1000 live births to 66.

If one takes the time to examine the relationship between standard of living and medical ills, as I have, in the Tropics, in the Arctic, in the Third World and in the ghettos, it becomes evident that the pre-eminent factor is not climate. It is standard of living. Those in the poverty category have this and other ills.

Statistics for children to five years of age overwhelmingly determine the characteristic morbidity and mortality rates of a society. Once past the age of twelve the chances improve of living to the allotted three score and ten or more years. The diseases which affected morbidity and mortality among Eskimos and Athapascans in Alaska were no different from those that affected the statistics of the Cook Islands, India and other places with low economic standards of living. This is also true of fertility statistics. Fix up the economy and you'll fix up the social, medical and, I will add, the political ills of a society. We will get some new problems, but we can fix these in their turn. The new ones are not a direct substitution for the old ones. The benefits gained are very real. If you do not believe me try an imaginary swapping exercise with someone in your nearest lowest income area.

* * *

Routines and rosters had to be organised for all staff. The nursing staff was organised into three shifts a day. The largest shift was for the daytime working hours, a much smaller shift from 2 p.m. to 10 p.m. and a skeleton night shift from 10 p.m. to 6 a.m. The nurses fell into their routines easily and for all our years together, the hospital was kept clean by the co-operative efforts of the staff and ambulatory patients. It became routine for patients to bring their own ash trays. These were invariably paua, the smaller breed of the giant clam shells.

The Assistant Medical Practitioners were now almost fully into the work load of the different departments of medicine and were beginning to find their medical bents. As they did and I was sure they had, I shipped them overseas to various centres for as long as it was needed for them to osmotically infuse the benefits of an "on the job training" in the specialty they had naturally gravitated to with some jostling with one another for position.

A nursing school was started. The courses were given by both expatriate nurses, when we had some, and the AMPs. At the end of the three year period all our now trained nurses passed the New Zealand Trained Nurses' examination. Many of them from this first lot still form the backbone of our nursing profession today.

This was no mean feat for the girls. In the schooling system, it was mandatory that everybody had to leave school by the age of fourteen. Even if the teaching had been of the best quality, it would have been difficult to have gained much during this period. Regardless of this, our girls were able to absorb and comprehend the anatomy, physiology, principles of medical practice and practical nursing to mention only a few of the requirements for a fully Registered Nurse.

None of these steps was easy to achieve. The matter was complicated by the fact that I had fought and won increments for them as high as triple salary increases. It was and is still in the scheme of things in the Pacific islands that islanders are paid as low a wage as can possibly be manipulated. For this low wage, one is expected to work industriously for eight hours or more and make up enough for the living needs of their family by keeping chickens and pigs and planting food crops. This technique had been sold as being necessary to keep the economy in balance. God bless us, most everybody believed it, even the economists.

I was supposed to run a medical service and extract as much as I could from the staff who received a pittance and expected, after a full day's work, to go home and feed their animals and plant what land they had in order for their families to survive. To do it for pleasure, is not the same. That is recreation. To do it for survival while putting in a day's work is a different story. To make a long story short, my better salary arguments prevailed, not only for the AMPs, but also for the nurses and staff. We were on our way to a better medical service. We appointed a Chief for each of the newly created Departments of the Service and each was held accountable for providing a good service. These economic ideas permeated the rest of the Cook Islands, apparently with no economic ill effects. On the contrary it put the Cook Islanders at an advantage over islanders of other Pacific Islands States.

Along with Chiefs for the hospital services, positions filled by upgraded Assistant Medical Practitioners, we also developed one for Public Health. Except for a creditable volunteer Child Welfare organisation, started by my mother and her friends and supported in its volunteer efforts by the Health Department and my predecessor, the Public Health area was in bad shape.

Tuberculosis, leprosy, malnutrition, filariasis, yaws and the contagious diseases had the largest part of their control and prevention in the area of public health. There is a direct relationship between standard of living and the prevalence of these diseases. There is more to the control of disease than the availability of doctors, nurses and medications. To do an Albert Schweitzer act achieves temporary relief and not much more. The public health part of the medical profession should accept the fact that improving the economy is a potent part of their armamentarium against disease. To fight disease in the face of squalor and poverty is to win battles, but lose wars.

At this early time the medical profession was blessed with an effective array of vaccines and immunising agents and a programme to put these into effect was all that was needed and the programmes that we instituted in those days are, with additions, what we have in effect today.

With the help of Mr Amos from Fiji, we instituted a mosquito control programme. At that time filariasis and its long term effects, elephantiasis, was a serious problem. Filariasis is a worm that settles in the lymph nodes causing frequent attacks of secondary infection and fibrosis which eventually leads to a complete blockage of the lymphatic system in the affected area. Since the lymph cannot get back to where it can return into the circulation, swelling in the area drained by the affected lymphatic system occurs which eventually ends up in the condition called elephantiasis.

The vector mosquitos breed in water in small containers, staying always close to their breeding places and in sight of them. Therefore, if one keeps the village free of small containers, these mosquitoes disappear. If one combines this clean up with spraying with an insecticide and judicious medication with Hetrazan (an anti filarial drug) or its equivalent, one can eliminate filariasis and dengue fever. To assist the effectiveness of this and other programmes, we introduced a garbage collection system which has operated continuously to this day.[5]

Leprosy is transmitted by intimate and long term contact and, therefore, appears to behave like an hereditary disease. Polynesians are avid keepers of genealogies and this allowed us to zero in on families with a history of leprosy, check them out once a year and deal with the cases as they appear.

The Tuberculosis Sanatorium was, in a short time, operating fully with a full complement of patients. It was, however, too small to deal with the problem adequately and much home treatment of the less serious cases was resorted to. The jinx attached to the Sanatorium mentioned earlier was broken, again by finding a co-operative patient, willing to defy superstition. This brave person happened to be Geoffrey Henry, the father of my predecessor as Prime Minister, Albert Henry, and an uncle of the present Prime Minister, Geoffrey Henry.

* * *

Albert Henry returned to the Cook Islands in 1946 to try to institute a watersiders' union. He had strong affiliations in New Zealand with what passed there for a Communist Party and no doubt this had much to do with the purpose of his visit. However, I also like to believe that he was strongly motivated to do something for the Cook Islands and was doing the only thing he knew which might be of help to his people. He did create a strike and some troubles ensued and my friend the Resident Commissioner was hardly the person to handle this problem. In fact he made things worse.

My mother was in the forefront of the troubles and there is a photograph of her amongst the people lined up in front of the administration in an orderly manner, but nevertheless defying authority. I met Albert and his followers many times and attended his public meetings, at which I was always asked to speak. I always did, explaining that what we needed was not a waterside union, but a greater say in our own affairs. Albert was not too pleased with this approach because it diverted people from the planned objective of his mentors, for whom I felt he was a pawn. However, in personal meetings I was able to convince him that mine was a better objective than his one of disruption.

When he realised that his plan to form a watersiders' union along New Zealand lines was not getting off the ground and that people liked the idea of our having more say in our affairs, he left for New Zealand and never returned until 1965 to stand for the premiership after the Cook islands attained its self-governing status.

However, before he left, he formed the CIPA, the Cook Islands Progressive Association, an organisation dedicated to the uplifting of the Cook Islands economic, social and political status from the subordinate one it was then experiencing, I helped Albert in this, not only because I believed in these objectives, but also because it diverted Albert from his communistic type objectives.

Albert worked hard at doing things under this CIPA banner. Among them was an effort to put it into business as a co-operative movement to buy Cook Island products and sell them on the New Zealand market. He raised enough money for part payment of the purchase of a boat, the Lareta, a converted Fairmile subchaser which was quite unsuited to the islands trade.

It went the same way as many of his economic schemes, but not before achieving intense loyalty from a large number of the populace and an equally intense hatred from a not so large proportion of the populace which felt that it had been duped. This latter group were the ones who had put their hard earned pennies and labour into the enterprise and received none of the promised rewards. Albert's bid for political power in 1965 was based on the support of those in the former group. They had lost nothing, they also had gained nothing, but they had developed a loyalty to the idea, Albert and to a measure to me.

We both became recognised as upholders of the rights of self determination for our people. In our different ways we never relinquished our efforts and hope for the achievement of that objective. Our approaches to achieve it were very different, but we kept our respect for each other on the mutual recognition that our basic objectives were similar. This difference in approach kept us from ever becoming political partners. I knew very little about politics, but enough to know that expensive and non-productive socialism was not going to be the right thing for our resource-poor country.

CHAPTER FOUR

The Polynesians

Lacking in metals and maps, sailing only with the stars and a few lengths of sennit, some dried taro and a positive faith in their gods, these men accomplished miracles   JAMES A. MITCHENER

What men they must have been!

Courageous and adventuresome, yes. But they were master builders, peerless navigators, accomplished sailors and indefatigable explorers, as well. Whether driven by desperation (famine, war, pestilence?) or the pure spirit of adventure we know not. But driven they were, to chart routes to the farthest lands - and plumb the depths of their abilities   DILLINGHAM CORPORATION

Our men were very well received by the natives but it was not understood why they gave us a welcome and what was their intention. For we did not understand them, and to this may be attributed the evil thing that happened, which might have been avoided, if there had been someone to make us understand each other.   FERNANDEZ DE QUIROS

I was brought up in a Polynesian household. My first language was Rarotongan Polynesian. My step father was steeped in Polynesian folklore and tradition. He spent most of his time digging into our history, myths and legends. I was fascinated by it all and I learnt as much as I could from him and others. I gained an understanding of the way we were that I, along with others, believed in. Most of it was verbal. Some of it was written. On some I made notes. Some that were given to me in writing I carried with me all over the world. In my travels I lost several.

In the 1920s, Sir Peter Buck, Te Rangi Hiroa, visited my home and held long conversations with my stepfather and others. Afterwards, these conversations resulted in discussions between my step father, my mother and others about Sir Peter not believing a word of what they told him.

"He has come with pre-set ideas and does not believe anything that does not fit them," my step father used to complain.

Whether Sir Peter set the fashion or not, his attitude of doubt as to the veracity of first hand information from our people was the norm for almost all anthropologists who visited us. This attitude forced all of us to be wary of giving anthropologists traditional and historical information for fear of ridicule. We sat back and let them try to piece together our history from theories and a significant amount of misinformation.

Greg Dening in *Islands and Beaches* pointed out that anthropologists believed they could not really know those they observed unless they knew who they once were. So they began to elaborate schemes to discover some zero point. There could be no access to a zero point except by the historical method. The debates on whether myth and legend were history, whether traditional societies had a knowable past, whether the total histories of non-literate peoples could be written, overlooked what existed as fragments of history. Historians, long accustomed to formulating history out of a fragmented, limited knowledge of human events from marks on pieces of paper, were mystified by the purist qualms of anthropologists.

I continued my interest in the available fragments of the history of Polynesians. I have tried to interpret myth and legend where this is possible. I have looked at our maritime history through the eyes of a small boat sailor. I and others have done this in spite of the knowledge that presenting our view would probably raise a storm in academic circles. Maybe someday we can present our points of view and perhaps have them considered. My interest in this area has been an integral part of my personal life.

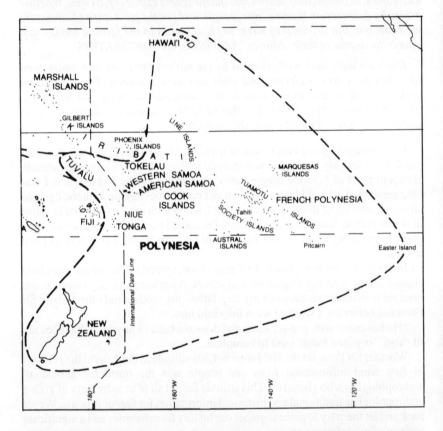

At one time, I seriously considered spending a goodly portion of my life in the formal study of Polynesians. When I examined the anthropological approach, I found it lacking. Anthropologists tended to formulate theories and then took to the field to prove them. When I became familiar with the debates of pros and cons, especially in the area of my love of ancient Polynesian seagoing canoes and navigation, I withdrew altogether. However, I have kept up with developments as best as I can. What follows in this and the next chapter are based on this personal interest. I am fully aware that they may be in direct conflict with current theories of academics who may have a view different from those held by Polynesians.

* * *

Polynesians occupy an area of the Pacific Ocean known as the Polynesian Triangle, bounded by a line drawn between New Zealand, Hawaii and Easter Island. The triangle includes land masses and their native people. The triangle bulges in its western boundary to include Tuvalu.

There are also pockets of Polynesians in parts of Melanesia and Micronesia. All of these speak languages so similar in basic words to those spoken in the Cook Islands that we are able to communicate with varying degrees of breadth and accuracy. This is remarkable when one considers that the people of these places have been, in several instances, separated from one another for centuries, in some cases for more than a thousand years.

At the South Pacific Forum Meeting held in Rotorua, New Zealand, in 1984, Mrs Mary Lini, the wife of the Prime Minister of Vanuatu understood what my wife and I were joking about in Rarotongan and joined our laughter. She comes from the island of Sikaiana off the Solomon Islands which is one of the Polynesian outliers. Likewise, Ati George Sokamanu and his wife come from Melanesian Vanuatu. George was the president of Vanuatu, but in 1989 he was deposed for an error of judgement in swearing in a new government without constitutional authority. In addition to 112 different Melanesian languages in Vanuatu, his village speaks a Polynesian language close enough to Rarotongan to permit considerable mutual understanding.

There are other isolated little islands in the midst of Melanesia such as Futuna in Vanuatu, Tikopia and Mungika in the Solomon Islands and Taku in Papua New Guinea which are inhabited by Polynesians, as are Kapingamarangi and Nukuoro in Micronesia.

Most of these are sufficiently "pure" Polynesians, who have lived in enough isolation from their immediate Melanesian neighbours to retain strong Polynesian characteristics of language and culture. In addition many Polynesians seem to have intermarried over the centuries with various peoples outside the Polynesian triangle and beyond these small "outliers".

Just before I sailed my yacht Miru from Wellington, New Zealand, to Peru on my way to Harvard in 1952, my own people in Rarotonga wished me to try to locate the descendants of our people who had sailed there on an historical expedition led by a legendary hero named Maui Marumamao. It was this expedition, Ua Turua of Pue Rarotonga told me, which on their return journey brought the kumara or sweet potato, a native of South America, to Polynesia.

* * *

Where do the Polynesians come from? When you ask this of a Polynesian, his answer will usually be, "From here," meaning here in the islands of the

Pacific Ocean (Moana Nui a Kiva). This frustrated the old time anthropologists who considered that the Polynesians had to come ready made from somewhere and Polynesians should know where. All they could get out of them was, "From 'Avaiki." Nobody seemed to know what that meant except that there were numerous 'Avaiki and its variants, Hawai'i, Havai'i, Hawaiki and Savai'i, scattered throughout the Polynesian triangle. Included among them are: Raiatea ('Avaiki), Rarotonga ('Avaiki Raro) and Nuku Hiva ('Avaiki Runga).

The best enlightenment that could be obtained was that Polynesians, who are away from their home island, would refer to it as their "'Avaiki", meaning the place where they originated. You can take it from there and make what you can of it. The anthropologists did and so did Thor Heyerdahl and others. Evidence points to the geographical origins of peoples ancestral to the Polynesians as being somewhere in the Malaysia to south China region.

Since all Polynesians refer to the place they were born or came from as 'Avaiki or its variants, these are the likely places first settled and from which succeeding steps of the settling process were taken. On that basis Savai'i is the likely place first settled in the Polynesian Triangle. From there Raiatea, Rarotonga and Nuku Hiva would be the next. Then would follow the islands to the east including Easter Island, Hawai'i to the north and New Zealand to the south. That is how the experts have seen it for a century or so.

Polynesians who migrated, quickly forgot their origins and transposed their myths and legends to their new home as though they originated there. The story of the overnight reconstitution of a tree cut down to make a canoe exists in nearly all islands which have trees. Therefore, to try to take history back to a zero point is not possible. But to reject the fragments is to throw away the very stuff from which history can be composed.

The progenitors were probably coastal or insular people with significant experience of the sea and confidence in using it to their advantage. The possibility of the introduction of an element from the people of South America as proposed by Thor Heyerdahl is not beyond the realm of conjecture, but the evidence for it is tenuous and its impact must have been small. The pig, the dog, the chicken and the numerous domesticated plants they brought with them is one of the strongest evidences that they came from somewhere in south-east Asia where the earliest and the most extensive domestication of animals and plants took place as early and even earlier than 7000 years ago.

Recent thinking has come closer to the Polynesians' way of thinking. Whatever the ultimate origins, evidence now leads the experts to believe that his claim to be "from here" seems valid in that Polynesians did not come ready made from anywhere. They developed physically, mentally, socially, economically and politically, into Polynesians right where they have been for the last three thousand years - in the oceanic islands of the Pacific.

At last there seems to be some agreement between Polynesians and anthropologists who had difficulty in believing what Polynesians told them if it differed from their own ideas. Some were led up garden paths of their own making. Once informants knew which garden path anthropologists wanted to take, they were not averse to leading them up that path with embellishments.

Informants, including my stepfather, often told me about this and thought it a great joke. "If they want lies," they used to say, " they will get lies."

The Polynesians love of allegory made things difficult. When Polynesians relate the myth that a canoe was reconstituted back into the tree each night, they had no greater purpose than to impress upon people to pay proper respect to conservation and the Gods and spirits of the forest. Polynesian historians, tumukorero, like the Priests of Christ throughout the dark ages, believed that ordinary people should not be privy to the sanctity of historical knowledge. The allegorical allusions and fanciful additions were added in conformity with this attitude. The ta'unga(s) of Ngatangiia in Rarotonga admitted as much to Stephen Savage in a yellowed, deteriorating and undated manuscript in my possession.[52]

Most historical manuscripts lie disintegrating or disintegrated with age because the purist mind had difficulty in accepting what they contained as being sufficient to form statements of history. Also these manuscripts, recorded by missionaries in many cases, are jealously guarded by families. Most have disappeared. The allegorical allusions in which history is clothed are sometimes appropriate as well as having proverbial meaning. It seems insensitive to throw them away along with the history that created them. It is a way of telling history that the Polynesians believed was in large part shaped by heroes, sometimes in co-operation and sometimes in strife with the Gods.

The practice of changing names of people, islands, places, canoes and discussing events a millennium apart as though they were contemporary, makes life difficult for anthropologists, historians and students alike. This, along with the missionaries' teaching that Polynesian history was best forgotten, as well as the disbelief of the mobility of Polynesians on the ocean of his home, is why the pre-contact history of Polynesia is generally lacking. With these distortions in communications and cultural gaps of understanding, Polynesians learned to be guarded about what they said for fear of ridicule.

The genealogy of my late wife and I and our relatives in eastern Polynesia is 116 generations. Multiply that by the formula of 25 years and we get 2900 years during which time seagoing Polynesian forebears had the great waters of the Pacific, Te Moana Nui a Kiva, stretched out before them, crying to be explored. Even if 25 years is too long for a generation, at least two millennia is likely. Once we accept the time frame that anthropologists and archaeologists are now accepting, it is not unlikely that much of the Pacific and its rim were known to the Polynesians before the birth of Christ.

Based on recent knowledge associated with the concept of an outrigger people and the dissemination of the culture associated with Lapita pottery, anthropologists now believe that Polynesians have been around the Pacific for at least three thousand years. Polynesians had entered and were exploring the Pacific about 2500 years before Columbus set off for America.

If, in the brief period between 1500 and 1800, Europeans in their relatively clumsy sailing vessels could discover the islands of the Pacific, how much more could sea going Polynesians in faster vessels discover over many more years. Most of the Pacific and much of its rim were probably known to the Polynesians well before any of them needed or decided or were forced to settle them.

Tradition says that Te'ira Panga (circa 500 AD) who preceded Iro (circa 1300 AD) by 21 generations was one of those who, tradition reports, went to Hawaii after he lost a war in south-eastern Polynesia.

Polynesians were from the beginning a people with a strong maritime flavour and all that goes with it in trading, communications, exploration, colonisation and navigation. Their origins must have been coastal and refuge for them was the sea and its isolated small land masses from early times. They seemed to have avoided settling continents like the plague.

They were also associated with the Lapita culture while they were in the Melanesian area and fabricated clay pots. As recently as 1990 a fragment was found on the island of Atiu by Earthwatch workers, the farthest east found so far. Where Polynesians did not manufacture them, they were valued as articles of trade. This further attests to their mobility on the ocean they chose to inhabit.

The fact that the Polynesians have integrated easily with Caucasians lends support to a Caucasian element in their origins. However, Langdon[46] reminds us not to ignore the fact that before Wallis, Bougainville and Cook, the Spanish had already been there. It is, however, unlikely that these earliest Spanish contacts would have made an impact in this area of Polynesia to the extent suggested.

Other similar contacts elsewhere in Polynesia did not. It is an historical fact that wherever the Spanish made contact with the peoples of the Pacific the shedding of blood was the invariable result rather than the engendering of friendly and influential relations. Langdon also claims that the great marae of Taputapuatea of Raiatea was a result of Spanish influence. This, in accordance with Rarotongan tradition, is also a mistake of time frame. Tangiia had the marae Taputapuatea built in Rarotonga (circa 1200) as a replica of the original in Raiatea. More recently Langdon has suggested that Iro (Hiro) was probably a Spaniard or a son of a Spaniard. Iro was more a contemporary of William the Conqueror than of de Quiros of the Bloody Sword. However, the suggestion that survivors of Spaniards wrecked in this area of Polynesia integrated with Polynesians is probably a fact, but no more of a fact than other Europeans who have been wrecked on islands elsewhere in the Pacific.

Various observers have considered particular aspects of Polynesian religion, myths and legends and some favourite sports as similar to those of the Greek, the Roman, with some claims of similarity to ancient Egyptian and Libyan cultures. The road of Toi, which circles Rarotonga from ancient times, was built to the width and using similar materials as those of Roman roads.

Still others have considered that the Polynesians were Israelites. Ra, the Polynesian word for the sun, was for them the manifestation of the Supreme God as is Ra who ruled over many lesser Gods in ancient Egypt. However, the evidence is as yet too fragmentary to know what relationships and contacts the Polynesians had outside the islands.

At contact, wrestling, boxing, archery, javelin throwing, running and others were traditional and favourite Polynesian sports. The travelling theatre and entertainment epitomised by the Are Kareoi of Rarotonga, the Areoi of Tahiti and the Ka'ioi of the Marquesas was an important feature of the Eastern

Polynesian culture as a means of employment for the common people. However, the presence of the theatre in this form in Western Polynesia has not been reported. Langdon[46], in his bid to ascribe features of Polynesian characteristics to outside influence, again attributes this to sixteenth century Spanish contacts.

The ability of Polynesians to learn to read quickly and their mathematics prompted early missionaries last century to consider that Polynesians must have come from a highly civilised people elsewhere. Throughout Polynesia the literacy rate quickly reached one of the highest in the world and has remained high. In the Cook Islands it is for all practical purposes 100 percent and has been so since before I was born. Other Polynesian states can boast no less a record. Their use of numbers was based on a ten system which is fully described by Reverend William Ellis.[32] This characteristic is so universal within Polynesia that it cannot be attributed to outside influence.

* * *

The genetic pool was kept well mixed by visits back and forth with neighbouring Polynesian islands by a cross section of the population, including persons of all classes, from the Ariki (King or High Chief) down to the meanest of the commoners. During these tere, as they were called in Eastern Polynesia and malaga in Samoa, formal and informal liaisons were made and marriages arranged at all social levels. Their common origin gave a base of common characteristics of Polynesian culture such that, with variations only, the languages, the social structure, and customs are similar, as are the people, the religious beliefs, myths and legends and ways of thinking. And most important of all, one's relatives are the same.

Within a very short time, wherever a Polynesian travels in his triangle, he will find or be found by persons to whom he can trace personal or cultural relationships and be royally treated. This practice of travelling to visit relatives and friends was in some measure confined to areas where they already had a relationship which helps explain the differences of detail between them. It still goes on today and, with air travel, maybe more than before. I have participated in the modern tere. They are expensive for the visitors, but often more so for the hosts.

Perhaps because of these extensive blood relationships, the extent of hospitality was unique in Polynesia. One cannot do better than to quote William Ellis to whom we are indebted for a number of contributions to our knowledge of Polynesians at or soon after contact. However, in their quest for funds to convert the "terrible heathen", they tended to exaggerate some of what they saw as unfavourable features of Polynesian life which are irreconcilable with their reports of favourable features.[32] With regard to hospitality he writes:

"Their Hospitality has, ever since their discovery, been proverbial, and cannot be exceeded. It is practised alike by all ranks, and is regulated only by the means of the individual by whom it is exercised. A poor man feels himself called upon when a friend from a distance visits his dwelling, to provide an entertainment for him, though he should thereby expend every article of food he possessed; and he would generally divide his fish or his breadfruit with anyone, even a stranger, who should be in need, or who should ask him for it."

Being Polynesian is not a matter of race or colour only. It is a state of mind. If you are brought up in the Polynesian way, it is unlikely that you will ever be anything else in your way of thinking and doing things. Europeans, Chinese or anybody brought up the Polynesian way, will recognisably be Polynesian to other Polynesians.

With stone, shells, wood and fibre they produced well finished seagoing vessels, woodwork and carving equal in finish and quality, attested to by the first contacts, to any produced by iron tools back in Europe.[31]

Agriculture, animal husbandry and fishing, was practised under the control of designated ta'unga (professionals) for purposes of conservation and regulation. The majority who did not have a profession, fished and farmed for themselves and contributed to community affairs. The aristocracy and the ta'unga were normally taken care of by the community in return for their administrative and other services. Commoner families who farmed the land of chiefs were obliged to supply the requirements, often onerous, of the title holder. The Ariki, the highest level of chief, in turn was often bled white by lesser title holders and hangers on. Especially was this the case if the Ariki wished to carry out a project or a war.[32,48]

Agriculture and animal husbandry along with fishing still form the basis of their economic life. To this has been added a high percentage of dependency on wages, salaries, business and, in places like New Zealand and Australia, the dole. Except for the last, all have been to the good and need to be more seriously considered by Polynesians and their leaders in places like New Zealand, Australia and Hawaii where modern technology is available.

Polynesians understood the value of nutrition and what it could do for mental and physical development. In all their migratory travels their important sources of food went with them. Except for coconut palms and a few non-fruiting trees, the Islands they populated may have been lush with forest, but contained few food plants.

Polynesians understood the value of protein, the main sources of which were the pig, the chicken, the dog and, of course, fish. While the rest of the world developed grain as the staple food, Polynesians developed a variety of leafy and tuberous root crops to meet their total nutritional needs.

When Europeans first contacted the Polynesians, they were astounded at their great size. The reason is now in part clear. There were interesting stories told us, when we were kids, of infants being selected to be warriors based on a set of criteria manifested in infancy. On selection they were fed the proper foods and given the proper training so that they would grow to a fearsome size and become great warriors. Most of those of the royal families who became Ariki were so nurtured, starting with a bevy of wet nurses. We could never get enough of the stories of the heroic feats of these warriors in both formal battles, single combat and the consequences of challenges made. So there was a clear understanding of what nutrition could and could not do and that it could be manipulated.

The socio-economic political system was typically that of a tribal/clan/extended family system with strong inter-tribal and inter-clan ties in a fairly successful attempt to maintain inter-tribal and inter-island harmony. The members of a clan traced descent from a common ancestor and to this extent a lord/serf relationship did not exist in the smaller communities. However, this was not always the case in the larger islands such as Hawaii, Samoa, Tonga and Tahiti, where personal relationships tended to be diluted. To say that Polynesians were not subject to the injustices that are generally found in a hierarchical society would be untrue.[32,48]

Marriage outside the clan was the rule. The Ariki of the tribes of different Polynesian islands were related to one another and chiefly marriages were often outside of one's own island. By this means inter-island harmony was insured to a fairly acceptable degree. Pa Tepaeru Ariki, Ariki of Takitumu, my late wife, had as strong traditional mana in the Islands of French Polynesia as in the Cook Islands through such relationships.

Tere party visits to other islands facilitated inter-island harmony. By this means inter-island tribal strife was minimised, the genetic pool widened, strong blood bonds established and a single language maintained. The social structure which also formed the basis of government was in many respects the same from one society to another. There were also significant differences. For example Tonga was a highly centralised state as was Tahiti under Pomare I at the time of Captain Cook's visit until the 1840s under the French at the time of Pomare V. The fleet that Captain Cook observed, from which he made an estimate of the population of Tahiti, was in preparation for a punitive expedition to Eimeo (Moorea) for rebellious behaviour. The influence of Pomare I extended into the Tuamotus and the Society Islands. In contrast, Samoa had a decentralised community for most of its history. In even greater contrast, the Marquesan society took democratic rights of the individual to proportions which threatened the existence of a cohesive society.

Though similarities were greatest in neighbouring clusters of islands, there was recognisable uniformity of practices throughout and even beyond the Polynesian triangle. For instance, the Fiji group is inhabited by a Melanesian people living under a Polynesian type of social structure through the influence of chiefs who are of Polynesian descent.

Chiefly and administrative titles in Polynesia, as opposed to more individually achieved leadership roles in Melanesia, are hereditary and held for life. Removal of a person from a title was by death, natural or otherwise, or by exile. In fact, for the 200 years before European contact in Tonga, for which good records exist, the highest chieftainship changed by murder more than by any other means. There were, however, other processes. For example, the Tahitian practice of passing on to the heir at his birth all the powers of the incumbent king may have evolved to avoid murder as a means of changing leadership. The incumbent king became in effect a regent.

Rivalry between members of the family for the top job was the cause of more strife in Polynesian life than any other cause. It was the most important impetus for leaving home and seeking a life elsewhere. Though such strife was rare between brothers, as their relative seniority was clear, seniority between half brothers, cousins and other relatives could be disputed as one might be senior on some criteria and junior on others (a younger claimant may be from a higher ranking mother). Jealousy of incumbents or of more proficient persons was the rule and only the strongest could hold his own under such circumstances. Besides these causes of strife from within the family circle, there was also the threat of rivalry between tribes with land and title acquisition heading the list of causes.

* * *

Ordinary individuals seeking refuge were accepted at the lowest level of the society. Something like the role of serf. Exiled persons of high rank might be installed with a rank title subordinate to that of the Ariki as the price for protection. Since exile was a common form of punishment, cases of this nature were common.

A responsibility of the Ariki and his leadership hierarchy was to ensure that there was always plenty of food, both to feed the resident population and for tere parties, visiting dignitaries and entertainment groups descending on them and not leaving until they had eaten their hosts out of house and home. An abundance of food was the mark of a well ordered and strong social unit which was not vulnerable and not subject to attack or diplomatic negotiations from positions of weakness. The rule in Polynesia is generous hospitable treatment for all strangers. Most Polynesians wish it were not so, but the custom goes on to this day.

* * *

The Gods and religious practices played a role in every aspect of Polynesian life. No activity, function or ceremony was performed without first calling on the assistance of the appropriate Gods. Using the God of the Christians, it is the same today, even in the most mundane of daily activities. Rongo, the God of War, as might be expected, was one of the most popular. The Hawaiian equivalent of the Cook Islands' Rongo is Lono and in Tahitian it is Ro'o, not Oro as appears in the literature.

* * *

Justice was achieved by a combination of religious belief and its accompanying sanctions, by social codes of conduct, and by the leadership hierarchy and ultimately the Ariki. It was a strong test of his leadership abilities. Control of all activities was reinforced by the tapu (taboo) system. Crime was by definition a breach of the tapu(s) set up by the leadership hierarchy. Crimes against persons were settled at personal levels.

Whereas western attitudes accept degrees of severity of crime with punishment fitting the crime, Polynesians view serious crime as punishable to the full extent, death or exile. Lesser infringements could be punished by haranguing, beating, destruction of property, burning of house or loss of land. Punishment for serious crime was dealt with by the Ariki himself or his heir apparent or by anybody designated by him. A test of an Ariki's ability to rule a people who were proud and often arrogant was that he could himself pronounce the death sentence and deliver the mortal blow. His mana was protected by a series of tapu surrounding his person. Infraction of them meant instant death, but that did not ensure security for an Ariki.

When an Ariki and his tribe made a decision to punish, the punishment applied to his relations as well, as they should not have let him go astray. The courteous way was to give the culprit or culprits time to find a solution satisfactory to all. Apology, submission and rendering of tribute was one way. Migration by sailing to find somewhere to resettle was another.

There was no formal judicial structure. The Ariki applied justice in the way he was trained and saw it. If a person appealed to an Ariki for redress about being treated unjustly by someone, he presented him with a pig and what might be done might not be due so much to justice, as to the pig.

* * *

The professional class in all fields of endeavour was an important element of Polynesian society. They were known as ta'unga in the Cook Islands, ta'ua in Tahiti, kahuna in Hawaii, tufuga in Samoa and tohunga in New Zealand and formed a class of their own. They resembled the guilds of former times in Europe. The professions ranged from navigation, agriculture, fishing, shipbuilding, carving, house building, medicine, history, tattooing, soothsaying and just about any of the services, arts and crafts needed by their society. Women were not excluded from some professions. However, due to the intense competition between practitioners in all the professions, they limited themselves mainly to weaving, raranga, the making of cloth, tapa, and decorating activities, akamanea, generally spurned by men.

The methods and techniques used in a profession were jealously guarded secrets. They were passed on only to members of the family. A community was judged by the quality of its ta'unga and a community which lacked a practitioner of one of the professions might beg, borrow or steal one and keep him and his family virtual, but very well treated, prisoners. This practice, when it occurred, was often a cause of wars and feuds. Navigators were no more and no less than one of these in a wide spectrum of professions.

A similar view of completeness of a social unit was taken in the matter of the socio-political structure. Whenever an island was settled by a lesser aristocracy or commoners only, the community so formed was considered incomplete and an Ariki from one of the Ariki families with the requisite high mana was also begged, borrowed or stolen to complete the structure.

Professional knowledge was not freely passed out as a person's mana or authority depended very much on it, so esoteric knowledge was revealed only to those within the family who would carry it on and maintain the family mana.

There were professions whose secrets were open books, but these, such as carving, house building, canoe building and others, were protected by excellence of implementation. The secrets of the profession of navigation were protected better than any other. This is why so little is known of the principles of navigation used by Polynesians. The awe with which navigators are regarded by the average person in our day gives some idea of the great mana with which ordinary Polynesians regarded famous navigators such as Iro Nui Ma Oata and the legends woven around them.

Those who followed the sea as seamen and navigators, did so as a profession and were classified as Ta'unga. They were good enough at it to give the world the impression that all Polynesians were navigators. A non-navigator Polynesian can be just as lost at sea as a non-navigator of any race.

The average Polynesian of the larger islands would rather toil in the field and feed his pigs, chickens and dogs than go fishing or travel the ocean for pleasure. Nevertheless, they were probably more sea minded than most peoples who live as close to the sea.

Ta'unga practised their professions to some extent outside of normal communal constraints. The quality of service was the price of this freedom. Ta'unga had had to serve a need. The alternative of making a living by working in the pa'i taro, the taro patch, in addition to fierce competition, spurred the ta'unga to maintain high standards.

* * *

The activities of this society took place in a context in which navigators and their seagoing vessels played a major role. In addition to the normal intercourse between islands for trade and social visits, there were those who were too proud to take a secondary or minor role in the society into which they were born. A new land and a new life was too tempting to ignore as possibilities for higher position, greater personal mana and greater fame. Exile or the promise of death were also strong stimuli to travel.

Karika, a famous ancestor of Rarotonga (circa 1300) was a Tui Manu'a or King of Manu'a island in eastern Samoa (American Samoa). He lost a challenge to his authority to a younger brother and took the honourable course - emigration. The stories about him and his contemporaries Tangiia, Tutapu and Iro might lead one to believe that Rarotongan history starts from that time. It would be like saying that the history of England started with William the Conqueror, who invaded England at about the same time. Rarotonga was already settled and the road of Toi had already been built long before.

* * *

The outrigger and double canoe was not forced on the Polynesians by the size of the trees available to them nor by their inability to build planked vessels with frames, and keels, modified as the latter may have been. Such planked vessels have existed throughout Polynesia from early times. They built them with outriggers because that is what one ends up with if one wants a vessel which, if rigged, manned and sailed properly, is fast, seaworthy and capable of long voyages. In terms of speed, seaworthiness and capability for long voyages, it is also the most cost-effective.

Their size was not inconsiderable. Captain James Cook measured the double naval "canoes" of King Pomare I of Tahiti and they averaged 108 feet in length.

It is said that some were so big and difficult to operate on a regular basis that they "perished ashore". The *Takitumu* was reported to be thirty roa (about six feet) or 180 feet long with a beam of 2 roa (twelve feet). For its size and speed, the Polynesian canoe expends the least initial, operating and maintenance costs of any sea-going vessel. If speed is secondary to cargo carrying capacity, two hulls can be joined side by side to obtain a less speedy, but serviceable cargo or general transport vessel. A very important consideration is that they are not only easily driven in a controllable manner by sail, but they are also relatively easily propelled at acceptable speeds by paddling, sculling or rowing, a point very much appreciated by other maritime peoples of yore and equally so by modern sailers using auxiliary power or motor sailers.

Many sailors today fear outrigger or multihulled vessels because of their likelihood to capsize when pressed suddenly by squalls or when sailed carelessly or recklessly. If we ignore some basic facts, this likelihood is real. Modern sailors build multihulls with a profile of sail plan proportionately like that on their ballasted monohulls. A conventional monohull, so rigged, has a power to weight ratio, as measured by square feet of sail area and pounds of displacement, of around 1 to 20, that is, 1 square foot of sail area to drive 20 pounds of boat displacement.

A similar profile of sail plan and overall length on a multihull will provide a power to weight ratio of around 1 to 4, or 1 square foot of sail area to drive only 4 pounds of boat. This results in a very high performance boat like the catamaran sailed by Dennis Connors in the America's Cup Challenge off San Diego or the trimaran, Steinlager 1, sailed spectacularly by Peter Blake in the Round Australia Race. Unless these are sailed with knowledge and care, they can capsize and are not a choice for round the world cruising sailors in this racing configuration.

At the other extreme, if one puts a sail plan on a multihull that will result in a power to weight ratio of 1 to 20, one will have a sail plan which looks small for the hull length. Its performance will be about equivalent to that of a monohull at practically no risk if normal care in sailing it is exercised. For a multihull, it will sail like a barge. If, however, one increases the sail plan on a multihull to obtain a power to weight ratio of around 1 to 10, like the New Zealand Tennent designed Turissimo catamaran, one will have a very much better performing multihull than a monohull of equivalent or longer length with only slightly increased risk when sailed with normal care.

The drawings of the Tahitian canoes by Webber in the journals of Cook's voyages, show relatively small sail area to hull length proportions. Yet Cook said these were able to sail rings around his ship and pinnaces. A sensible amount of sail on a multihull will result in a safe vessel. If one overpowers it, one must accept the risks. This is true for boats, automobiles, motor-cycles and aeroplanes.

Every multihull sailor must be acutely aware that the stability curve of a multihull is exactly opposite to that of a ballasted monohull. Where a ballasted monohull has its greatest righting moment when its spreaders are in the water

(90 degrees heel), the multihull has its greatest righting moment when its mast is straight up and down (0 degrees heel). From there on it is all loss of stability. In tropic waters a vessel can be hit by up to three squalls with sudden high winds in a night. If there is no sheet man on hand to let the sheet fly immediately and/or do the necessary procedures to avoid the effects of the squall, the worst that can happen to a monohull is a knockdown and torn sails. In a multihull before sails are torn, it will be upside down. Polynesians sailed their canoes with sheets tended at all times. The significant advantages of a multihull do not come without a price in vigilance and common sense sailoring.

Carrying a hunk of lead or a bilge full of rocks is a solution to capsizing, but it adds to initial cost of hull and rigging with higher wear and tear in use and, therefore, higher operating and maintenance costs and poor performance when compared with a multihull. And that is how the Polynesians seemed to have seen it.

* * *

The era for extensive Polynesian sea travel according to Rarotongan and Eastern Polynesian tradition took place before 1350 AD. It was also the time of maritime activity of the Vikings. References to earlier activity for the same reasons to Hawai'i and elsewhere is sufficient to indicate that the causes for migrating had existed for some time. Te'ira Panga, twenty one generations before Iro, about 550 AD, is reported to have sailed to Hawai'i as a result of losing a war. On the other hand, his son, Tuterangi (often spelt Tutarangi), whose title I carry, was an Ariki who preferred to range the oceans fighting than to administering his arikidom. His importance in the early history of Iti Nui (Fiji), Tonga and Samoa made up for his absence.

* * *

The migration to settle Aotearoa, New Zealand, (circa 1300) was the last of the migrations initiated by the famous ancestor Ka'ukura around 1200 AD. There is enough early post-contact evidence to show that although migrations stopped, voyaging did not. The stories of Polynesian voyagings are like Zane Grey's stories about cowboys who travelled a great deal on their horses, shooting up towns and each other. In the stories, they never lay a rope on a cow; only the exciting parts are recorded, not the mundane daily routine. No doubt the sailors of Polynesia and the cowboys of Texas accomplished useful ends.

* * *

There has been much controversy among anthropologists over whether the migration to New Zealand was a well planned migration, taking some months or longer to plan and organise, or was it the result of accidental drifting of lost canoes as claimed by Sharp.[54] There is no such controversy among Polynesians in the Cook Islands or Eastern Polynesia from where the migration started. Nor is there any confusion about it in the minds of the New Zealand Maoris. Nevertheless, we have stood aside and let the controversies take place between those who have the least reason to argue about it.

The need to migrate was often real. Strife that is common to all societies whose economy is based primarily on agriculture and land ownership was a prime cause. In such an economy only one can inherit with the same profitability as the father. Where others in the family exist, division of land with them very soon becomes unprofitable for all. An agriculturally based economy is a prescription for jealousy and strife within the family, spilling over to covetousness for the neighbouring lands of others resulting in territorial strife for their acquisition and protection. Where few other economic alternatives exist, warriorship to support offensive and defensive territorial wars, pillaging and colonisation of new lands become alternatives.

Colonisation of new lands, as the famous (to us his descendants) exponent of organised Polynesian migration, Ka'ukura Ariki, found is a stopgap solution. The cycle soon repeats itself. It was even so in his own lifetime. Later, other solutions were sought and included the limitation of population growth by infanticide also practised by Chinese and others faced with the same dilemma.

* * *

Polynesia has been blessed with early anthropologists who were almost one hundred percent landlubbers and disbelieved what Polynesians told them about their frequent travels between island communities of the Polynesian Triangle. Anthropologists could describe a beautiful pearl shell ornament and confirm that they were made no place else than Mangaia and not question the fact that the pearl shell had to be transported from at least 700 nautical miles away. Hawaiians and Marquesans travelled to Rarotonga (referred to by its old names, Nukutere and Avaiki Raro) to obtain the feathers of the Manu Kura or in Rarotongan the Kura Mo'omo'o (now extinct), highly valued for decorating royal clothing. In the face of such evidence, it is difficult to maintain that most long range Polynesian sea voyages were voyages of accident.

In the particular case of accidental drift voyages to New Zealand, 1400 nautical miles to the south-east, all factors of prevailing winds and currents are strongly against it. It would be unreasonable to believe that ten canoes from Eastern Polynesia would, together or separately, find the rare and unpredictable condition of an easterly wind below the level of the easterly Trades maintaining itself in the horse latitudes or in the area of the prevailing westerlies further south for many days to allow such drift voyages to take place from Eastern Polynesia to New Zealand.

Drift voyages did occur as they have occurred everywhere peoples have ventured on the open sea near their homes. From small Islands surrounded by a large ocean with a minimal lee protection, they can occur more frequently than anywhere else. In the Pacific, drift voyages have taken place for centuries and several have taken place during my lifetime interspersed with purposeful voyages.

It is only within my lifetime that peoples of elsewhere in the world have successfully challenged the large oceans in small boats in increasingly large numbers year by year. For many of them the challenge has been their first venture on to a boat or an ocean. Captain Voss, one of the first to circumnavigate the world in a small boat, did it in a canoe he modified. Disasters have occurred, but they are insignificant when compared to the large number of successes. Prior to this, most people elsewhere believed that it was unsafe to venture on the ocean in anything less than something resembling a floating island. Even narrow bodies of water such as the Bering straits, Torres straits and a few others were effective barriers to most peoples and many animals.

All the drift voyages as well as most of the purposeful ones that took place in my time did so in the belt of the easterly trade winds and were from east to west. The use of the large "steering paddle" as a leeboard referred to by William Ellis[32] has been experimented by me and is an effective measure for steering as well as preventing leeward drift in tacking to windward. The Hokule'a now sports one.

Parsonson[50] has dealt with the arguments on the issue of the weatherliness of Polynesian vessels and the capability of their navigators and concludes:

"The evidence thus shows that until quite recent times, Polynesian seamen were still making deliberate two-way voyages without benefit of intervening islands of from 720 to 1000 miles - the latter the distance from Taumako to Nukulaelae - and of 1270 miles with a single intermediate stop, from Sikaiana to Fiji, and 1400 miles from Niuatoputapu, sufficient, it might be thought, to have brought all the major island groups of the Pacific, the Chathams and New Zealand not excluded, within the range of their great double canoes. And in that same period, Micronesian proas were frequently going backwards and forwards over distances of at least 1000 miles between the Carolines and the Phillipines and the Marianas."

Some ask why the Polynesians stopped voyaging? They did not. They stopped migrating, but they did not stop voyaging. There were no more places to discover and exiles could find little respite by voyaging to places known to be already inhabited by Polynesians who, through population increase, had become highly territorial in outlook. In Rarotonga, exiles preferred seeking protection from one of the three tribes that inhabit it rather than seeking lands which they knew were inhabited and would pose as great, if not greater, difficulties of acceptance. One is very welcome to visit, but coming to stay in the numbers that are represented by extended families is another matter. The restrictions to exiles and other claimants to land use and occupation did not in any way affect visiting, intermarrying and exchanging gifts. Examples of such voyages are on record into the post contact era.

CHAPTER FIVE

Polynesian Navigation

... a literate society...must be able to set down on paper, in this case maps, charts and almanacs, what non-literate folk might easily read in the sky and carry in their heads. In the end it comes to imagine that the job can be done in no other way. G. S. PARSONSON

Swift, strong, seaworthy craft... European seaman marvelled at them. "Better could not have been made in Castille."

the Spanish explorer DE QUIROS in 1606.

"When we consider the imperfect tools which these people are possessed of, we can never sufficiently admire the patience and labour... " said Forster in 1777. "...our cabinet makers do not polish the more costly furniture better," said Cook. DILLINGHAM CORPORATION

The aspect of Polynesian culture that intrigued me most was navigation: the art based on the science of knowing where you are, where your destination is, how far apart they are in distance or time and what mean direction must be maintained to get there. Supplementary knowledge of hazards, as well as likely wind and current patterns are of fundamental assistance to the navigator.

It would be reasonable to presume that a high percentage of a Polynesian navigator's practice of his profession was carrying out voyages that he had carried out many times before in a sector of his ocean he knew well. He would know the direction of his destination, having taken it off the shore markers that exist on most islands. These indicated the rhumb line direction for every major destination he might seek. If these markers did not exist he would set up his own. One or two examples will suffice.

In Hawai'i there is a direction called, Ke Ala ki Kahiki, or The Way to Tahiti. This direction at the starting point gave the fundamental rhumb line around which navigational and judgemental considerations would be made. All islands of any importance had these direction range markers. When John Williams, the missionary, was in Atiu, he expressed a desire to go to Rarotonga. Rongomatane, an Ariki of Atiu, went aboard and gave John Williams directions how to manoeuvre his boat and, when it was spot on for Rarotonga, Rongomatane informed him. This is what John Williams wrote about the occasion:[58]

> "Knowing this we determined to adopt the native plan, and steered our vessel round to the starting point. Having arrived there, the chief was desired to look to the landmarks, while the vessel was being turned gradually around; and when his marks on the shore ranged with each other, he cried out 'That's it! That's it!' I looked immediately at the compass, and found the course to be SW by W and it proved to be as correct as if he had been an accomplished navigator."

John Williams sailed the course and is credited with the discovery of Rarotonga!

* * *

The Celestial Hemisphere and the celestial bodies in it are the bone and sinew of navigation. The world is round and every sailing master worth his salt throughout history has known this. Columbus knew it, but could say nothing about it for fear of the dungeons that Galileo suffered for demonstrating a simple truth of falling objects. How many times does a thinking sailor see islands and hulls with their shorelines and sails disappearing over the horizon to realise that the surface of the ocean is curved. Polynesian sailors worked within it as all who sail the oceans extensively must. Let the landlubbers of history speak for themselves.

The other important part of navigation is knowing and keeping track of the direction one is obliged to take to one's destination. Few voyages are made along the rhumb line. In non-instrument navigation, the stable ocean swells, the distance travelling ground swells, play a dominant role because stars are often obscured or they cannot be seen during the day. The seas which are caused by local wind effects, are secondary. They are subject to local wind change. Nevertheless, they are important in short term course keeping.

These are only some of the directional aids. A navigator is travelling in an upside-down bowl of the sky sitting on the sea. It is full of clues as to direction and the maintenance of that direction. The compass has blinded most of us to their existence and how they may be used.

* * *

As recently as the early part of this century, most sea captains used the sun declination tables in conjunction with a quadrant or sextant to perform "Sun Latitude Sailing", the simplest of navigational method using instruments. This is done by obtaining the altitude of the sun at noon, its highest point in the sky, and adding or subtracting the sun's declination obtained from the Nautical Almanac. Eventually the ship would reach a position which was on the Latitude of its destination. By maintaining this Latitude from noon to noon, a navigator "ran down" his destination. He need not bother about longitude. This is how the "Noon Sight" became a ritualistic part of navigation. They simply got on to the latitude of their destination with these noon sights, making sure they knew on which side of the destination they were, and "ran it down".

Captains did this in spite of the availability of Bowditch's sight reduction tables. Tables which are simpler to use have evolved, but even with these a longitude sight was laborious and needed an accurate chronometer. So, even the sea captains up to the early part of this century did not use a great deal more than their earlier Polynesian counterparts. The main thing extra they had was a sextant, which they used in a limited manner, and a compass.

Anyone can see that the sun moves north-south as well as east-west in a predictable manner. This predictability was, however, was of little use for navigation until the sun's declination tables came into being. Without a quadrant or sextant, Polynesian navigators had to do without the sun for navigation. It was, however, useful for steering a course by if one made adjustments for its movements by co-ordinating these with wind and wave directional movements. Not all of them will change at the same time.

The moon seems to move all over the sky without rhyme nor reason. Her quarterly periods vary from six to eight days. The constants the Polynesians recognised were that there was a new moon, a full moon and two phases when the moon was bisected into light and dark halves. With these they, as other peoples, divided the moon phases into quarters which vary in number of days from quarter to quarter and cycle to cycle. That is why the Polynesian moon calendar has extra names for the phases of the moon in each quarter to add or to subtract as demanded by the recognisable indicators of the quarters; the two half moons (Korekore Akaoti), the new moon, (Iro) and the full moon, (Marangi). Polynesians did not use the moon for navigation, except for steering a course on the same basis as the sun.

The planets were recognised as not behaving like stars. They did not, night after night or month after month, follow set tracks across the sky. However, Venus gives very acceptable east-west courses and can be followed well into daylight. Most planets were useful, if needed, because they are relatively slow in their wanderings. Being brighter than stars, some could be seen when stars were obscured or dimmed at the break of day or at dusk of night, the times for switching from a night to day, or day to night set of steering parameters.

The dome of the sky and its myriads of fixed stars presents, for all practical purposes, a constant picture every night. The only limitation is the optical acuity of the observer and the presence of obscuring clouds and other climatic phenomena. Legend has it that some Polynesians were able to distinguish the moons of Jupiter.

Being a constant picture, the position of the stars and the constellations are the most useful aids to a Polynesian navigator. The nightly picture it presents can be learned and seared into one's memory. For anybody as interested as a navigator must be, he will have noticed that this constant picture moves a set amount each night. Such an interested person would also note that each individual star, regardless of the time of night or time of year, follows the same east-west track night after night without any discernible north-south variation. In modern terms, its declination remains as constant as one needs it to be, night after night. The declinations of stars do change due to the earth's nutation or irregularity of movement on its axis, but this is too small to be of practical significance.

Every star track, therefore, stays in the same north-south relationship to any given point of reference on the Earth's surface. If this point is an island, that island always has the same north-south relationship with its east-west track to that star. Therefore, if one knew the track of the star, one also knew where that island was in relation to it. Conversely, if on that island, one could expect to find that star by keeping an eye on its east-west track. So a star (a zenith star) whose track runs directly over an island destination is a bonus. At any time during the night, the display of stars is a display of their east-west tracks in relation to as many places on the surface of Earth.

Although it is easiest with zenith stars, with practice any star close enough to its track can be used. A navigator who was skilled in judging how far a destination was north or south of a star track had a greater number of stars to work with than one who did not. A Polynesian navigator was not surveying the islands to plot their positions on an Admiralty Chart, he was simply trying to find his way, The accuracies needed for this are not as demanding.

All this means that since stars travel with the same constant declination, they are a reliable guide for "running down" an island by Star Latitude Sailing, simply by staying on or near the track of the selected star as judged when it is at or near the meridian of its zenith, a destination can be found. However, like Sun Latitude Sailing, the method gives no indication of Longitude except by 'dead' (DEDuced) reckoning.

With these limitations one can get around the destinations of any ocean pretty well. However, the Polynesians went one better and invented a sextant of their own for more reliable Star Latitude Sailing. This came to the attention of anthropologists during the early days when anthropologists roamed the South Seas with little knowledge of things nautical and disbelieved most things nautical that Polynesians told them. They assumed Polynesians wandered aimlessly about the ocean and populated the islands by accident.[52] They rejected the Polynesian sextant as a hoax.

* * *

When I returned to Rarotonga in 1945 to take up my medical duties, I came into intimate contact with it. First through my stepfather and then through my friend Temapare who was one of the last professional Tumukorero, or Polynesian historians. Their versions both recognisably described the same thing. Papa Raitia had made a diagram of it, a coconut shell cut across at a slanting angle with a hole at the low end and a notch at the top end. There were a number of holes encircling it. This was sitting above a wavy line representing the ocean and under an arch of ten stars equally spaced. It struck me that with a bit of work, the design would make an attractive coat of arms! We all tried to make some sense of the information before us. I was sceptical, but both swore that this was the "Titiro Etu" (literally, Star Peeker) used by Polynesian navigators. They informed me that it was filled with water to the ring of holes and, holding it so that the water was lined up with the ring of holes, one peered at one of the ten stars through the hole at the low end and lined up a star with the notch at the high end. Temapare's version was that a gourd with a hole instead of a notch was also used. All our thinking did not allow us to reach any enlightenment as to how the instrument could be used for navigation.

Polynesians were very secretive about professional knowledge and this could have been garbled to throw interested parties off track. The ten stars threw us all completely. Temapare was a little more scientific, while Papa kept reminding us of the supernatural powers of the ancestors. To him this was an instrument through which these supernatural powers could be mediated by a navigator.

Temapare kept looking for a more reasonable explanation. He remembered something about rubbing the inside of the coconut shell or gourd with coconut oil, and was disappointed that I, as a navigator, could not come up with a solution. That was why he had brought the matter to my attention.

We finally gave up the project. The theory of the anthropologist that the gourd sextant was a hoax was looking mighty good. But I gnawed at the problem off and on for some years. If the information we had was a deliberate attempt to confuse or an inaccurately remembered tradition, perhaps getting rid of what looked like garbage might help. I decided that the ten stars had to go as did the coconut oil and the wavy line representing the sea which, it was now apparent, had been added by Papa Raitia. The diagram had been his interpretation.

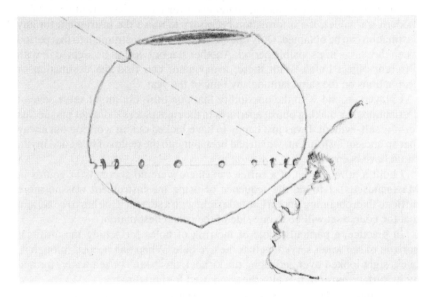

Having removed what I thought was garbage I was left with a coconut shell or a gourd with water in it to be lined up with holes through which water would not leak and with a means to line up a star. But what for? I then asked myself what kind of navigation can one do with an instrument that measures the altitude of a star or stars and does not need a chronometer, degrees of arc, sight reduction tables, a place called Greenwich, a nautical almanac or declination tables. This led me to perceive that the instrument could measure in a fixed sort of way the altitude of a star at one's meridian which could be the Latitude of a destination in relation to that star.

That was it! What the instrument could perform is a Star Latitude Sailing method to "run down" one's destination, which is the same as the Sun Latitude Sailing method. One did not need a chronometer, nor did one need a declination table because star declinations are fixed. Its degrees, conventional altitude or arc are irrelevant. All one has to know is that a particular altitude angle of a star obtained by the titiro etu puts one's canoe on the same east west track as one's destination. Keep the canoe on that track and one will run into one's destination. This had taken some years of intermittent and sometimes halfhearted spare time effort. Now it seemed to have paid off and to me it was exciting.

To work out how the instrument was used, we must go back to our trash can because we threw away the coconut oil as garbage. It wasn't. The instrument seems to have been made for a particular destination latitude and a particular star. When lined up with the eye hole and the object hole at the highest point of its passage across the sky, the east-west line upon which this happens will be the same Latitude as that of the destination. A star which subtends an angle of forty five degrees of arc will give the highest accuracy, but any star near enough will do. The star and the holes to be sighted through were probably made to fit the instrument on the destination island itself for future use in finding it. With modern star tables, the information necessary to make the instrument for any destination can be obtained. Only one star will limit the instrument to that period when the star is in its visible period. Another star or two can be sighted in with different object holes. With these, a navigator can find the destination or destinations on the same latitude any time of the year.

I played around with the possibility that one titiro etu might serve several destinations, by making object apertures in the right places. I did not pursue this for it is self-evident. I was just happy to have lucked out on working out a way that an ancient instrument, which had been put into the realm of hoax and myth, could have been used.

I built a titiro etu out of a coffee can (there were no coconuts or gourds in Massachusetts). I found the sequence of using the instrument was no more difficult than obtaining a noon Latitude sight with a sextant. One has to be certain that the course set will be to one side of the island destination.

In practice, a particular hole of the ring of holes for setting the artificial horizon of sea water served well as the eye hole. When one peeped through it, one's sight looked over and along the kiriatai, the "skin" of sea water, formed by its surface tension. It is also the word used for horizon.

As with a noon sight, wait until the star is near passing its highest point, the meridian we are on, oil the inside of the bowl and fill it to the ring of holes with sea water. Now one can see why the oil was needed. Being an anti wetting agent, it preserves the surface tension of the sea water and it will not leak out of the ring of holes as one tilts the instrument, within reason, to locate the star in the objective hole or notch.

What we have is an artificial horizon built into the instrument, just like a bubble sextant. Now peek through the eye hole to the object hole or notch higher up and on the other side of the instrument. Wiggle the instrument around until one sees the star in the object hole. Follow it by intermittent sightings as it ascends until it reaches it's highest point. This is easy to detect because it can be sensed as a broad, flat part of the curve of observations before they start to show that the star is descending.

Now look at the status of the artificial horizon. In our example, both the destination and the reference star is to the north. If the sea water of the artificial horizon is above that part of the ring of holes directly under the object hole, the canoe has not reached a point directly east (or west, as the case may be) of the destination and one must continue one's course. Alternatively, if the star is below the object hole when the sea water is in line with all the holes, we also have not reached the latitude of our destination.

When the star is in the object aperture and the water of the artificial horizon is in line with all the holes of the ring of holes, one has reached that point where the canoe can now be aimed directly east (or west, as the case may be) and the destination can be "run down". Since writing this I found a reference to the titiro etu by Jourdain who referred to it as the Sacred Calabash.[41]

One more piece of information is obtained from the titiro etu at the time the star is at this maximum meridian altitude. The line formed through the instrument and the star, or the line in the direction the user is looking through the instrument, is true north-south. He really does not need this information because, if the Southern cross is visible in the southern hemisphere, all he has to do is count five spans of the long arm of the cross in the downward direction and he will have due south or as near as one needs it to be. North of the equator, the Pole Star is due north or nearly so.

* * *

The Polynesian navigator's starting point was his reference point, which is just as valid as using a Mercator chart and expressing one's starting point in Latitude and Longitude from Greenwich. Where he wants to go to is a place in a direction he already knows from his range marks on the island where he is. If he knows that the island he wants to go to is around three sailing days away, all he has to do is sail on that course and in less than three days he will meet the signs that his destination is near by sea birds, a thermal cloud high over the island and a different pattern to the ocean waves. He does not have to know the exact patterns, but only to recognise that they are different. If circumstances are right, he might even get a whiff of the island.

How a Polynesian navigator keeps course can be illustrated by an example of a relatively short voyage. For the purposes of navigation, any island is thirty to fifty miles broader on every side than the land. An island ten miles wide presents to the navigator a front of a circle up to about 100 miles wide at best and up to 60 miles at worst. Not a difficult target.

Course is kept by noting the direction from the range markers and its relationship to the Southern Cross formula for obtaining south (tonga) or north (akarua) from the Pole Star. Either of these gives the direction he must steer, his Rhumb Line course. At night time, keeping course is not a problem. In the day time, the many clues include the wind in relation to the course when the voyage started, and each night with his north-south markers, the Pole star or the Southern Cross. If this wind had been steady for a day or so, there would also be waves (seas) travelling in the same direction. If the wind changed, he could hold his course by the old waves until new waves were formed. He would also note the direction of the more constant ground swell or swells (there can be several operating at the same time). He would note the position of the sun and the cloud formations and their inconstancy and use them to help him keep course.

At night, he could choose one star directly ahead to steer by, or one behind, or anything in any direction from his canoe that he could relate to his course as established by its relationship to his north-south markers.

He would keep other stars and the constellations in mind and their relationship to his course. If the stars he was steering by became obscured, he kept the others in the relationship with the course that he had noted and mentally reviewed from time to time.

If he integrated these things continuously, which the mind is quite capable of doing, he will have few problems in keeping on course. If he were interrupted by a storm, he would be able to reorient himself and carry on. The firmament of stars would be the most important single element that would put him back on track.

If forced to sail up wind, all he needed to do was sail on one tack for a set time, as judged by the movement of the sun and the stars, and do exactly the same thing on the other tack. This might take longer, but he would get there.

Polynesian navigators had as many as four selected relatives as apprentices, in various stages of training. They would work the shifts and give the Master the necessary rest and time to keep the mental integration of incoming information in proper order. This was the normal way a Polynesian navigator practised his profession. I have done it enough to know that it works.

* * *

The navigation discussed so far is Latitude navigation, which tells us only where we are on a line running east-west. That is all many of the captains of the clipper ships did for navigation in the Australian wool and wheat trade. The Spanish, the Dutch, the English and the whalers did the same to navigate to all parts of the world. Where travel is mainly in an east-west-east direction, this is essentially enough.

Travelling in a mainly north-south-north direction, especially in the Pacific, drifts east and west can be considerable. They had to be avoided or compensated for. Without a chronometer this was a tough assignment, but not impossible. A navigator who mastered both the Latitude and the Longitude problem would have a distinct advantage. Travelling to and from Hawaii out of Eastern Polynesia was where this skill was needed.

Preknowledge of the direction of one's destination was important. Having established this from the range markers, a navigator would study the sky and its stars to an extent dependent on how much of this skill he had already acquired. Some would not have followed the routine I am about to describe, but they would have to follow the principles involved.

Having established the direction of a distant destination, about 2,500 nautical miles between Hawaii and Tahiti, the navigator and his apprentices, would study the stars for several nights until they had the dome of the sky firmly in their minds. The movement of the stars is hardly perceptible from one night to the next, but perceptible after several nights (about 3 minutes and 56 seconds earlier each night or slightly less than 1 degrees of arc). In the time it takes to travel between Hawai'i and Tahiti, the stars could have moved up to 30 degrees of arc. That is a significant shift for a line of reference. Since it is consistent and predictable, it can be compensated for by being totally familiar with how much movement is taking place, to keep longitude mental computations in order.

The currents on these north-south voyages are as strong as 40 nautical miles or more per day and, if a navigator does not have a way of compensating for them, he can be in real trouble. The only way is to make allowance for the daily east to west movement of the stars, to compensate for the powerful, variable east to west currents and winds which are normal in this part of the Pacific Ocean.

Another problem is that the winds closer to Hawai'i are north-east trade winds with velocities normally between 18 to 25 knots. The winds closer to Tahiti are south-east trade winds with similar velocities. A rhumb line course obtained from his land markers, will not make Hawai'i going north or Tahiti going south. The winds are too far ahead to allow this. In addition the current is aiding and abetting the wind. Therefore, he must use the winds on the first part of the voyage to grab all the easting he can by travelling as far east of his rhumb line as he can, to beat the currents and winds forcing him to the west. When he is directly under Arcturus, he can run Hawai'i down.

* * *

What kind of vessels did the Polynesians use for these long voyages? Polynesians have ranged the main oceans of the world, except the Atlantic, for three thousand years or more. He did this in fast seagoing multihull vessels which could go up wind well enough to have explored and then populated a vast area of the world.[34], [39], [41], [42], [44], [45], [49] ,[50]

They were not in a great hurry and could afford to wait for favourable winds. One of the Society Islands canoes, "Wait for the West Wind", illustrates this sensible attitude. Also one has only to wait for an El Nino year to get winds blowing from the western quadrant with currents to match. in the El Nino year of 1972, my son Teremoana and I found ourselves bucking west to east currents up to 50 nautical miles per day near the equator, when sailing from the Panama Canal to Tahiti in our 42 foot cutter, Torea. We escaped by sailing south and making for Tahiti near 18 to 20 degrees south. We had intended to make for Tahiti via the Marquesas well to the north of the course we were forced to take.

* * *

Each type of double hulled vessel used by Polynesians for voyaging had different characteristics. The best known is the Hokule'a, the modern replica of the Hawai'ian voyaging canoe which has reproduced the voyages of the ancients without modern navigational instruments. It needs no further introduction in these pages. My good friend, Francis Cowan, did the same thing in 1986 from Raiatea to Rarotonga and on to New Zealand in a canoe, Havaiki Nui, he and his friends built along the lines of the Tahitian tipairua.

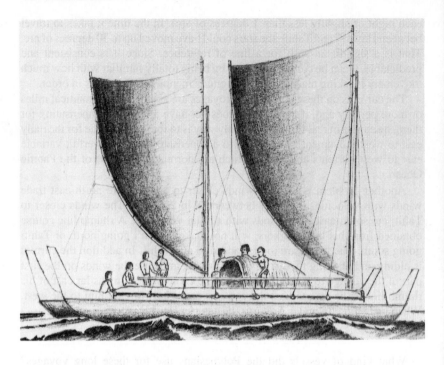

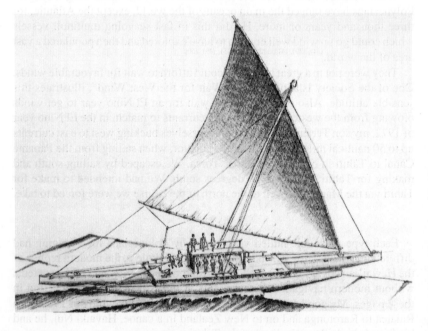

The Takitumu, which led The Fleet of seven canoes from Rarotonga was of the Samoan alia type. In this class we can include The Fijian ndrua and the Tongan kalia. The fact that some have thought her to be an outrigger confirms that she was not of the va'a tele or tongiaki type which have hulls of equal size. Whether one views an alia as an outrigger or a double hull is based on how one views the smaller hull. These we can categorise as the kalia class because they were developed by Tongans. They were outstanding examples of one of the highest developments of vessels in Oceania, if not the world. The ndrua of Fiji and the alia of Samoa are likely the resulting developments of the conquest and administration of Fiji and Samoa for a considerable time by the Tongans.[47] The ndrua were developed in Fiji, but most were built in the Lau group, inhabited by people of Tongan Polynesian extraction and not Fijian Melanesians. Elsewhere in Fiji, they were ordered for construction and owned in many cases by chiefs of Tongan extraction.

There is considerable confusion as to the characteristics of the Tongan tongiaki. It is no surprise that the descriptions of Tasman, Schouten and Cook disagree. It was their first experience with such vessels and differences between them and the later described kalia class may not be as remarkable as they have been made to seem.[39] The tongiaki of Tonga as described by Schouten, Tasman and Cook do not make sailing sense.

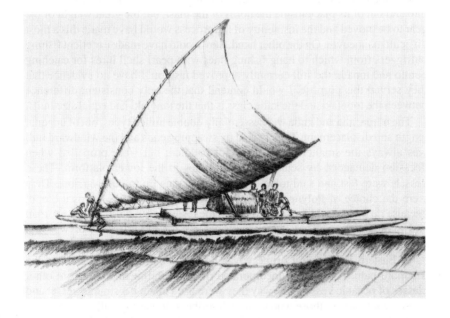

None of them seems to have seen a tongiaki change tack. Cook certainly did not, but thought that it came about through the eye of the wind. In that case, he said, the sail, while on one tack, had either to be unlaced from its spars and relaced to leeward of the mast or sailed with the sail pressing against the mast. The former would have created a good case for mutiny while the latter could be used as a reason for branding the Tongans as inept. However, in his drawing of the deck plan and in their separate descriptions, the mast was stepped well forward, but also leaning well forward and over one hull. The last two are earmarks of a vessel that comes about by swapping ends. Also there are never any drawings of the vessels with the sail pressed against the mast, a situation which must have occurred 50 percent of the time.

The artists' drawings are not compatible in some features with engineering principles. The mast set far forward with at least two thirds of the yard overhanging towards the stern would have produced high stress at the fulcrum formed by the mast crotch and an inordinate compression load on the mast, its step and their supporting timbers, especially if the sheet were hauled close.

Their insistence that the yard sat in the great horn of the mast, would be, with those heavy spars and mat sail, difficult to set in place without the assistance of a skyhook. This is not to impugn the veracity of such observers as Captain Cook, but the likely explanation is that the concepts evolved were quite new to European sailing technology and were thus misunderstood.

The long balancing spars described as sticking out on both sides "like great horns" could not have been for shrouds as the spring in them would have made them ineffective for this purpose. They may have been used for poking the yard into and out of its place inside the horns of the mast, but the great weight of the gear to be moved and the instability of the process would have made this a most difficult manoeuvre. On the other hand, they would have made excellent fishing outriggers from which to hang fishing lines with pearl shell lures for catching bonito and tuna in the still currently approved fashion. I have no evidence that they served this purpose. I would contend that the only consistent difference between the tongiaki and the kalia class is that the tongiaki had equal size hulls.

The ndrua, alia and kalia were essentially double hulled types, but of unequal length and displacement. They tacked by swapping ends and the windward hull was always the smaller. They were not paddled, but were propelled when occasion demanded by sculling through holes in the lower platform. These vessels were fast and said to be capable of carrying up to 200 warriors. They were the choice of Polynesian warrior kings and freebooters of royal blood, because no other could have commanded the resources to build, own, sail, man and maintain them. They were prime vessels for the purposes of war and migrating fleets.

In Eastern Polynesia a prime voyaging and migration candidate was the Tuamotu pahi. Although it incorporated much of the technology from other classes of oceanic vessels, the way they were used made it a strange vessel and caused confusion to those who tried to describe it. It was typically a catamaran type which ranged up to seventy five feet or more in length. Having been developed and built by the atoll dwelling Tuamotu inhabitants, where little timber was available, they were planked and framed using pieces of driftwood and whatever could be made to suit the purpose. Each hull was more substantial in beam dimensions than is usually credited to Pacific oceanic type vessels and had a deep vee in section.

Like the tongiaki, there is considerable confusion in the literature on exactly how the sails of the pahi were rigged. Like the western Polynesian canoes, it tacked by swapping ends, but did this in its own way by rehoisting the sail on the mast nearest the end that is to become the bow. By this fairly unique means for a large vessel, it satisfied the natural requirement that the centre of lateral effort of the sail or sails must be forward of the centre of lateral resistance of the hull.

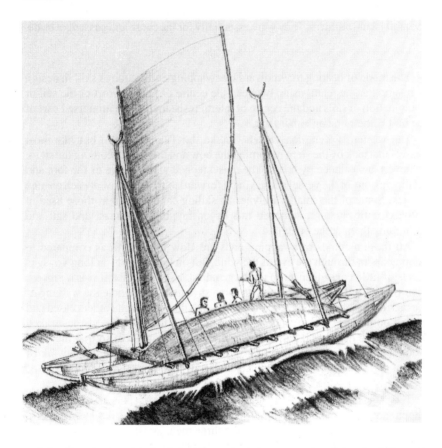

It is often depicted as having sails on both its masts. A quick calculation of the relationship of the centre of lateral effort to the centre of lateral resistance would show that, rigged in this manner, the centre of lateral effort would have been a long way aft of the centre of lateral resistance instead of forward of it. Rigged in this manner, she could not have sailed at all.

Confusion also arose in that often a biped mast was used and different sail types from a Spanish type lateen to a Hawaiian type Oceania rig have been depicted. Even the typical rig of the kalia class with one raking midship mast was described. From the performance point of view, it did not matter as long as the important relationship between sail pressure and hull resistance was obeyed.

The more lightly loaded windward hull had a raised shelter for passengers while the leeward hull carried cargo and stores. They were also used as a single hull with an outrigger which still maintained the swapping of ends for tacking purposes. The Tuamotu pahi ranked high as a voyaging vessel and were much favoured by kings of Tahiti and the Society Islands. At one time they were built in Tahiti and Raiatea by builders contracted from the Tuamotus to meet the demand. The availability of large timbers in quantity must have been a joy to the atoll island builders. They were essentially for the cargo and passenger trade.

* * *

The mode of beating to windward by swapping ends requires skill in design to insure that the relationship between the centre of lateral effort of the sail or combination of sails and the centre of lateral resistance of the immersed part of the hull is the same on either tack.

The western Polynesian vessels, unlike the Tuamotu pahi, but like most vessels that tack by the stern becoming the bow and the bow becoming the stern, achieved this balance by having the mast stepped at the centre of the fore and aft dimensions of the vessel and raking it forward to the new bow at each change of tack. Some of the smaller Polynesian sailing canoes, such as those used in Aitutaki until recently, achieved this by unshipping both mast and sail and reshipping them at the other end.

All these methods of swapping ends are slow to perform as compared to coming about through the eye of the wind, but on long boards on long voyages this is of little consequence. In the large ndrua, kalia and alia, it was a process requiring co-ordination of crew with three strong men to handle the walking of the tack ensemble from one end of the vessel to the other while others eased and hauled on the fore and aft running stays to swing the mast into its new raked position. The helmsman had to co-ordinate with all of them so that the wind would be in the right direction to give its substantial assistance to the work of all, but particularly the three on the tack. Let us look at the procedure in one of these great vessels.

The sheet is let fly and there is an almighty rattling of spars and thunderclap flapping of sails, shaking the ship from stem to stem or, if you like, stern to stern. The running forestay is eased while the three men, assisted by the pressure of the wind on sail and spars, lift the yard at the tack ensemble out of its socket. Still with the assistance of the wind, the hauling on the former backstay and easing of the former forestay is done in unison with the three sailors walking the tack via the lee of the mast, outside the lee shrouds and halyards, until they reach the socket for it in the new bow and thunk it in place. At the same time, the sheet and the heavy steering paddle is passed to its new position and the ship is sailed away on its new tack. Properly done, most of the effort of the procedure is performed by the wind and the operation takes less than a minute.

Throughout the procedure in a normal 18 to 22 knot trade wind, the sail continues to shake and flap with giant whip-cracking crashes while the mast and spars rattle their raucous complaint of an unstable condition. Chaos can reign and the three sailors who have the arduous job of carrying the shaking tack assembly from one end of the boat to the other, are sometimes thrown overboard by their thrashing, kicking charge. But, when the job is done and, as soon as the sail is sheeted in, there is hushed silence. Only the cracking creak and wrenching squeak of the heel of the mast in its step and the low moan of the wind in the rigging can be heard. Even the talk Polynesians indulge in to let others know that they are doing their assigned part of a co-ordinated effort, has ceased. This silence is quickly replaced by the rapidly increasing sounds of a ship thrashing its way to the next tack as the vessel accelerates at an astonishing rate from zero to its customary 9 to 12 knots on the wind. If the new board is a reach, she accelerates to speeds of 15 to 20 knots. When driven with everybody on all action stations and the sheet controlled by experienced sensitive hands to obtain the best out of sails and wind towards the edge of the limit of capsizing, she would do significantly more.

The big advantage of tacking by swapping ends is that the outrigger or the smaller hull or the more lightly loaded hull is always to windward and therefore lifted in large measure out of the water thus reducing the potentially destructive racking forces that take place between hulls. The windward hulls of these vessels were never flown out of the water.

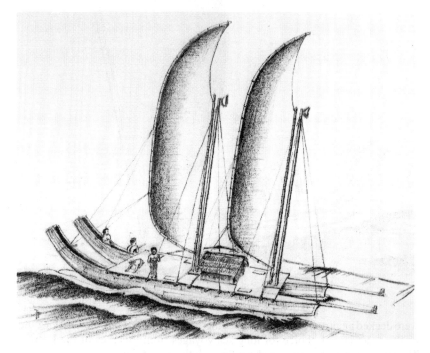

The other double hulled candidates for ocean voyaging are those vessels of Eastern Polynesia which tack through the eye of the wind. The tipairua is, to me, the most beautiful. Its dimensional proportions, hull lines and sail plan bespeak of a graceful and competent lady.

She could be as much as 90 feet in length, but most were 50 to 70 feet. She generally had two masts with the typical Tahitian sail with a rigidly supported curving leach that reached half as high again as the mast and curved over towards it. This arrangement leaves the top third of the luff unsupported which may have some as yet undetermined advantageous aerodynamic sail characteristics. Those who have used this sail speak of its superb windward properties, but they have difficult handling characteristics. Francis Cowan who owned and sailed a va'a motu rigged with such a sail, believes that they were developed for the conditions of the islands of Eastern Polynesia which require a great deal of windward sailing since they lie mainly east-west and not north-south as in Tonga, Tuvalu or the Caribbean.

Typically the sail area to hull displacement proportions of the tipairua were conservative. This should have made them handy, but not necessarily fast for multihulls. They would, therefore, have tended to be transports rather than escort or fighting type greyhounds. They normally had a shelter between the masts and

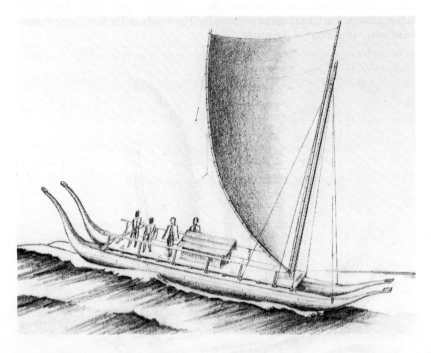

were decked against invading seas. For these reasons, if for no other, they would be the candidate of choice for long sea voyages from this area of the Pacific. The tipairua tacks by coming about through the eye of the wind.

The last Polynesian double canoe we will consider is the Marquesan vessel. In hull form and rig it closely resembles the Hawaiian canoe which was probably developed from it. It seems to have played its most important role in the first settlement of Hawaii. The later settlement of Hawai'i was by the Eastern Polynesians: Society Islanders, Tahitians and Rarotongans. A Rarotongan who went to Hawai'i was Naea Ariki from the Itiao and Naea clans of my family. His forebears came from the east in a single hulled vessel (vaka kumete), named Ao Re, World Beater, because of family discord, just after Tutapu gave chase to Tangiia.[53] Now another Naea Ariki was leaving Rarotonga for the same reason. Because of his rivalry with his cousin Ono Kura (Red Barracuda), he left for Tahiti and from there sailed for Hawai'i. My home and that of my sister Mary are on the family land, Aremango, Ngatangiia where they first landed in their canoe Ao Re. It is the only reference to a single hulled canoe that I know of.

These are the main candidates for voyaging and transport double hull vessels, though not a complete list. In the last migration to New Zealand from Rarotonga as the final rendezvous, it is generally believed that the tipairua was the choice of vessel used by those from Tahiti, Raiatea and the islands of the lower Cook group, but the Tuamotu Pahi cannot be ruled out. The same is believed for the settling of Hawaii by Eastern Polynesians (Circa 1300 AD) somewhat later than its settlement by Marquesans.

The Manihiki voyaging canoe has been described from models which are beautifully made and decorated, but, I fear, not accurately representing the real thing.[39] This is a peculiarity which seems common in models of vessels from

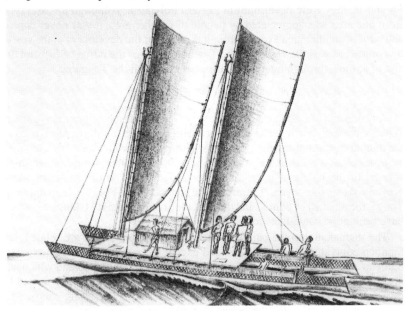

Oceania. The vessels were fine examples of craftsmanship and were lavishly decorated with inlaid pearl shell both inside and out and even in some places where their beauty and fine craftsmanship would be difficult to display to advantage.

In the illustration, I have tried to depict the extensive pearl shell inlay decoration of the bow and stern piece and the strake below the wash strake. I have also put the bow and stern configuration of the two hulls in the same direction which is the way I believe they were. As I think they came about through the eye of the wind, I have given it a sail configuration that would allow this to take place easily. Like the pahi, also built by atoll dwellers, this vessel had unique technological characteristics which, with only models to go by, cause some confusion.

The models, from which most of our knowledge of the vessel is derived, are built with definite bow and sterns in each hull which are identical, but they are put together in a head to stern manner which I believe is done as artistic license because, from a sailor's point of view, a vessel configured in this manner could not have sailed satisfactorily. The sails on the models are of the fore and aft kind and similar to those used in the Hawaiian voyaging canoe, which also tack by coming about through the wind. Several models of this canoe of one and two masted varieties were displayed in my home when I was a boy. I remember pondering over the problem of its sailing characteristics.

* * *

Although the ndrua, kalia, alia type was used both in Western and Eastern Polynesia, they were never built in Eastern Polynesia. Although a vessel type from one area was appreciated by people of another area, it was never copied and built in another area except through the aegis of the developers of the vessel by contract as was the case with the Tuamotu pahi, or the ndrua of Fiji and the alia of Samoa, through long colonial association with the Tongans.

* * *

Any one hull of a double canoe served very well as fast outriggered voyagers. When separated, outriggered and rigged with the same sail dimensions used in the double configuration, their power to weight ratios would have been reduced by as much as a third, giving them the type of performance required for high speeds. In the hands of intrepid warrior sailors, they would have been true greyhounds of the ocean. Therefore, the thamakau of Fiji, the hamatafua of Tonga, the amatasi of Samoa and the va'a motu of the Society Islands would all have been good candidates for high speed travel.

The thamakau and the hamatafua, like the ndrua and kalia are related. No Samoan equivalent has been described except by vague reference. I expect a Samoan equivalent existed and was supplanted by the sailing soatau which has often been wrongly referred to as the amatasi. Again models have tended to mislead. The sailing soatau is derived from the smaller paddling canoes, the paopao and the va'a alo (the bonito canoe). The amatasi was, I believe, the Samoan counterpart of the Tongan hamatafua and the Fijian thamakau, all derived from their bigger sisters of the kalia class. The outrigger hama, ama and thama prefix, common to all, indicate this relationship as well as the fact that they were outrigger canoes. The hamatafua class were not necessarily created

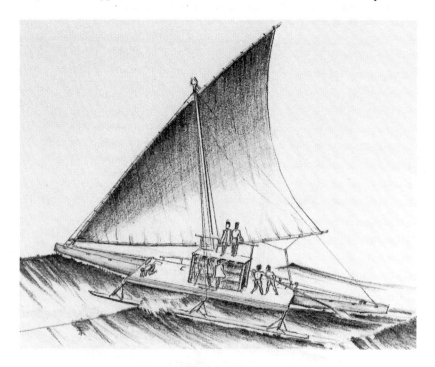

by separating the hulls of the kalia class. Although the derivations are clearly present, they were also built as a class from scratch. The influence of the Micronesian flying proa on the development of these western Polynesian canoes and those of Polynesian atolls across the equatorial Pacific cannot be denied.

The hamatafua class sail with the outrigger always to windward in the classic style. The va'a motu of Eastern Polynesia and the soatau of Samoa come about through the wind. Therefore, on one tack the outrigger is to windward and on the other it is to leeward. Although this may seem to be a problem, it is not. I have built and extensively sailed four va'a motu and, apart from a barely noticeable difference in helm characteristics, this is no problem in sailing, speed or handling on either tack. I have sailed them in the open ocean when conditions forced other boats to find shelter and an outboard speed boat sent to tell us to do the same could not catch us to give the message! We completed our planned trip.

According to William Ellis[32], the va'a motu was the vessel of choice on inter-island ocean passages because their design withstood the destructive racking forces better than double canoes. At high speeds in ocean conditions this would be significant. The va'a motu as opposed to the other vessels of

Eastern Polynesia has survived in basic concept to this day and the principles of its design characteristics should perhaps receive more attention by modern multihull sailors elsewhere. Having built and sailed four of them I have become an addicted aficionado of their sailing and seagoing qualities.

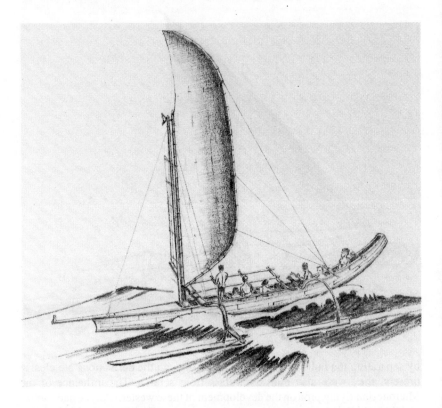

I know of no illustration from the time of the first contacts that depicted the va'a motu accurately. It seems that none of the artists understood the design and engineering concepts involved.

In its design nearly all the stresses of wind and waves are concentrated in one pivotal point where they are neutralised. That point is where the forward kiato (outrigger arm) is attached to the main hull. This point of attachment should be at or just forward of the centrepoint of the overall length. Then the weight of the outrigger when it is to windward, together with that of the crew on it to balance the vessel against the force of the wind, does not press the bow of the main hull into the sea. Most multihull sailors will know that this is an interesting event when it occurs and it never occurs except at high speeds. I have never been able to achieve this in a va'a motu, but have done so in a modern small high performance catamaran. It is a flipping of the catamaran over forwards and sideways.

The outrigger is attached to the main kiato just aft of its fore-aft centre of buoyancy. This is not critical but ensures that when the outrigger is depressed below the surface, it can continue moving forward in this submarine mode without being forced further under by forces acting on the top of the outrigger instead of on its bottom, tending to plane it upwards instead of downwards.

Outriggers of all Polynesian vessels are always on the left or port side because most people are right handed. Fishing and other activities are carried out over the side away from the outrigger and its potential for hindering. This is why Polynesians refer to the port side as ama (outrigger) and starboard as atea (clear). Throughout Polynesia aka'ama, come up to windward, and aka'atea, go off the wind, and their variants, are used regardless of whether the vessel tacks by swapping ends or by coming through the wind, indicating perhaps that the outrigger to windward mode of sailing was once basic throughout Oceania.

The curving up of the kiato on the starboard side away from the outrigger is to prevent this part of the kiato from digging into the ocean when the outrigger is flown too high, which it never should. The right flying position is when the outrigger is skipping the water. Often this extension was substituted for by a board attached separately to the hull, but in all respects in the same position in the hull and achieving the same purposes. Such boards, because of their slanting position, were often serrated for better footing. The use of these boards seemed to be the preferred method on large va'a motu and large soatau.

The outrigger is attached to the main kiato in a manner which allows it to pitch freely, but to be limited in its yaw (lateral) movements, The after kiato has a horizontal section long enough to allow of its attachment to the main hull and an upward looping section almost forming a semicircle attached to the outrigger at its outer end in a manner which allows a degree of universal movement. The design of this after kiato allows it to be flexible so that the outrigger can freely move in the pitch mode independently of the movements of the main hull. This removes the problems associated with the potentially destructive racking stresses common to other multihulls. The looping after kiato allows a wide freedom of this pitching movement and flexes to accommodate lateral and vertical changes of arc of the stern of the outrigger as it performs up and down movements in a single vertical plane.

The mast is stepped on deck a distance forward of the main kiato compatible with its need to be supported by shrouds from the hounds to the main kiato. It is stepped in a ball and socket arrangement to allow it free movement in any direction. This is necessary because the pull of the mast and sail on the windward shrouds bends the kiato upward and the mast leans to windward with slackened lee shrouds. Traditionally, the Tahitian rigid leach sail was used on the va'a motu. Nowadays any sail is used from the spritsail to the fully battened modern catamaran sail.

The modern va'a motu is built up to thirty five feet long, but there is no reason for a va'a motu not to be longer and the reported 50 to 60 footers would have posed no serious handling problems. Modern va'a motu, though degenerate examples of the original, reflect most of these characteristics, but are used almost exclusively for racing in Tahiti using hiking extensions like those now seen on the Australian open class 18 footers. These seem to also have been used traditionally. The sail area carried (spinnakers are not used) may be as large as those exploited by the 18 footers without their spinnakers.

Because of the high speeds the va'a motu (and the other high speed canoes) attains, it must be sailed on the same principles as an ice yacht which is mostly by the apparent wind and not the true wind. The sail is sheeted in on almost all tacks, a concept which many conventional monohull sailors find difficult to accept.

* * *

For the most part, high speed was not required, but when it was, it could be poured on and the destructive stresses imposed taken care of by the intelligent design and engineering concepts in these vessels, especially the va'a motu and vessels which sailed with outriggers always to windward. These were the ways of reducing racking forces and immersed surface frictional area.

When the period of migrations ceased, the need to travel in a group with an escort also ceased (circa 1300) and these vessels became vessels of trade and intercommunication between islands, warfare, freebooting, and for warrior kings hiring out their services as mercenaries. I believe that the favouring of the Tuamotu pahi by the kings of what is now French Polynesia until after European contact was because they made excellent trade and passenger vessels. Their role was taken over by the better bulk carrying characteristics of European vessels.

* * *

The ability of these vessels to go to windward has been questioned because they have no centre-boards or substantial keels. Much of the argument for drift voyages is based on this supposed lack of windward ability. This argument does not hold for the classical sailing outriggers of Micronesia, because the deep vee underwater part of the hull has been designed to overcome this. In the case of the Eastern Polynesian canoes, except for the pahi of the Tuamotus, there is validity to the argument because they are round bottomed and have less lateral resistance grip on the water. However, any sailor can solve leeward drift by sticking something into the water to increase lateral resistance. In some places this has been done by leeboards and in others, including the rafts of the Peruvians, by centre-boards. The ability of Polynesian vessels to sail to windward was better than the vessels of the Europeans who first came to the Pacific.[50] In Polynesia it was done by the large paddle doing double duty as a lee-board. William Ellis in his *Polynesian Researches*, volume 1, page 133, says of the va'a motu:

"In long voyages they have two or three steering paddles, including a large one, which they employ in stormy weather, to prevent the vessel from drifting to leeward."

After talking to Ben Finney of the Hokole'a about this, I later noticed that one was installed on her and there is precedence for its use.

CHAPTER SIX

Depart Rarotonga

I must go down to the sea again, To the lonely sea and the sky.
JOHN MASEFIELD

I suppose there comes a time in everybody's life when the challenges and goals of a job one has been in for some time comes to an end. This being my first professional job, it was my first experience of this completion of a cycle. It was devastating. In 1951 I had been five years in the job, first as Medical officer from late 1945 and then as Chief Medical Officer from 1948. I felt that I had done all that could be done. For some time now the Medical Department had been rolling along doing the job I wanted it to do with little help from me. This was as I had planned it, but it had occurred much earlier than I believed it could. New and uncomfortable emotions were now making themselves felt. I was confused.

I started to have unsettled feelings for which I had no explanation. I worried about them. The more I sought an explanation the more confused I became. After all, I was at the top of my profession in the area I had chosen to practice it and being well paid for it. Why all these unsettled feelings and a deep sense of lack of achievement? I should be happy and enjoying the high social status of my official position. I should be taking things easy and enjoying the leisure time that was now available for tennis, sailing, coaching in rugby and boxing, fishing and a variety of other activities I was now free to indulge in.

From what I had been taught and from what I had read of similar situations, I had expected it could take twenty years to put my medical goals into place. I had not counted on several things which shortened the time to reach these goals by many years. Among these were the intellectual capacity of the people in general and the medical, nursing and other staff's ability to grasp new concepts and abide by them. Then the very medically minded New Zealand people and their government gave me every support in achieving the goals. Because of these and other factors, I had been able to put my programmes into effect with little difficulty beyond some ineffective harassment from a few local expatriate officials.

As already described, when I first came into the job, conditions for providing a medical service to my people were indeed poor. Because of this I had sworn secretly to myself that I would try to provide the best service that I could so that, when it came time to hang up my stethoscope, my people would be able to tell the difference between a good and a poor medical service and would raise hell if what they got was not up to snuff.

Together we had cleaned up the general hospital and people were coming to it for all their medical requirements from practically all forms of surgery to good medical and paediatric care and a first class midwifery and maternity service. We had set up standing arrangements with the Auckland Public Hospital to give the specialist services that would have been foolish for us to have developed ourselves principally because of the insufficiency of such cases. These arrangements have lasted to this day, not without some abuse I must add.

We started a Nursing School which has continued to provide top training to world standards. We introduced a mosquito control programme which became the model for other medical services. We introduced a number of public health measures which included BCG vaccination for tuberculosis and standard vaccinations to control the common communicable diseases. We introduced needed food and beverage legislation. We established a garbage collection so necessary if one desires to control insect vectors of disease and other general health problems.

At the time that the unsettled feelings came over me, we had many students in training not only in Fiji, but also in New Zealand to provide future medical personnel, sanitation officers, public health nurses, laboratory technicians, maternity nurses, Xray technicians; all of which would give us some degree of self sufficiency and capability to handle the medical problems of Rarotonga and the outer Islands.

Some programmes we had set up for the future could not be implemented until our students overseas had completed their training and returned home. In the meantime, I was faced with the personal problem of having no more goals to achieve. That is what I later believed was causing my ephemeral emotional problems.

* * *

I requested the Dean of my Medical School, Sir Charles Hercus, to send a team to the Cook Islands over the long summer university vacations to do some research to define more clearly our medical problems so that they could be tackled with greater focus. He soon responded to my request. He himself would head the team, which arrived over the Christmas of 1950. It had been agreed that the best value could be derived in the time available by a health survey of Rarotonga as the most sophisticated community of the Cook Islands, and one of Pukapuka as the most isolated. These surveys have been the basis for many subsequent comparative studies and continue to hold interest as to the changes in the patterns of health over the years.

My close association with Sir Charles made him aware of my personal problems. He made the diagnosis and advised the cure. He said he had watched my career very closely over the years and was fully aware of my objectives.

"Tom," he said, "You have attained your goals. Frankly, it is time for you to move out and seek new ones. I know that you had planned to come back to the Cook Islands to stay, but that just will not do any more. There is no cure for what ails you, but to get out of the Cook Islands and find new fields to conquer."

His interest in the Cook Islands and my career in the past, in the present and for the future, he said, was related to the fact that he was the nephew of Reverend James Chalmers who had been a missionary to the Cook Islands as well as to Papua New Guinea. The stories his uncle had told him about the Cook Islands and the books written by and about Chalmers had always fascinated him. He had jumped at the idea of coming on this medical survey mission himself when he received my request.

Almost immediately my emotional symptoms disappeared. Life was all exciting again. I had no idea what this new life was going to be, but a step in the right direction had been made. This had given my spirits a great lift. The only thing that came immediately to mind was to find another place in dire medical straits, apply for a job there and see what I could do to provide a better medical service.

Somehow, this did not seem a feasible way for me to spend my life, but what else was I qualified to do. The gnawing desire to get into research to follow up my interest in the physiology of man exposed to hostile environments always sat at the back of my mind and often rose to consciousness for short but intensive periods. I always cut short these periods of desire, for I could not see any hope of ever being able to make this particular dream come true.

Although I had had unfailing support from the New Zealand government and my own people in achieving what I wanted, these goals had not been attained without problems, pain and anguish. Did I want this to be the pattern of my life? Moreover, I had no illusions about other administrations being anywhere near as supportive as the New Zealand administration had been to my particular ideas as to the quality of medical services a Pacific Island Territory should have. Quality did not come at bargain basement prices. Despite these negative thoughts, I made some enquiries of my friends in official circles in Wellington and the British Colonial Medical Service and their Australian equivalent.

These inquiries made me aware of several things, some of which I had already suspected. My reputation had gone before me and neither of these two services were keen for someone like me to come into their respective territories and stir up their respective medical pots. I also found that I was the highest paid public service medical officer in most of Oceania, Australia and New Zealand. To take any other job than the one I had would mean a substantial cut in salary and allowances. I was also made acutely aware of the fact that all I had to do was to hang on to my present job until 1958 and I could, at the age of 41, retire on a full pension. For employment purposes, the Cook Islands was categorised as a health risk assignment and time spent there counted as time and a half towards one's pension. By rights this should not have applied to me as a native of the Cook Islands, but my having been employed from New Zealand had waived this negative requirement. This new information was all very depressing to say the least. What had been a relatively simple decision to resolve my problem had now become much more complicated and financially unattractive.

* * *

It was now late 1951 and I was no nearer to a solution to my dilemma. All along I had discussed my problems with Lydia and she was all for a change, whatever this might be. The Cook Islands had already palled on her and any change I might contemplate would be OK by her. So I continued to pursue the matter, but without much success or satisfaction. In the mean time, I had resolved that satisfying pension requirements was not going to influence what I did with my life.

Then out of the blue, I received an invitation to spend time at Harvard University. This had come about through Harold Coolidge of the Pacific Science Board, an arm of the National Science Foundation based in Washington DC. I had met Harold at the Filariasis Conference in Papeete, Tahiti, early in 1951. Because of my work in public health and the content of my medical publications, people tended to think that public health was the primary area in which I worked. It was not.

The primary area in which I had worked was surgery. As a result of this misapprehension, Harold had arranged with the Harvard School of Public Health to have me attend there for a couple of years or so. Since I had put a fair amount of effort into Public Health, this was a reasonable assumption and I had learnt that what one does in life is not always according to one's choosing. Chance and opportunity play a far more important role than one would like to believe.

One can believe that one is master of one's fate and be stuck forever in the mud of it, or one can respond judiciously to the knockings of opportunity on the proverbial door and have an exciting time responding to them. You can be sure of plenty of moss in the former and plenty of rollicking adventure generously laced with knock backs in the latter. Each to his own. It was clear that making a move to new fields before 1958 might lose me my pension. It did just that. It was the first time, but not the last.

After my failure to find a suitable solution to my dilemma in the Pacific Region, Harold's offer as a heaven sent solution to my problem. I appreciated this as an honour and, at the very least, besides giving me an opportunity to be exposed to new and broader perspectives, it would give me respite and a chance to rearrange my priorities. I accepted with alacrity and completed the necessary paper work.

* * *

At the end of my first three year contract with the New Zealand Administration, I had successfully applied for a course in Tropical Medicine and Hygiene at the University of Sydney as a way of spending my six month's end of term furlough. The course required a full academic year of attendance and my application to the New Zealand Administration for an extra six month's leave without pay had been granted.

Since the Administration had most kindly given me this leave with half pay, it was not unreasonable of me to assume that they would give me leave of absence without pay for the period needed for me to complete my assignment to Harvard. There was enough time to make these arrangements. I had sincerely hoped to return to the region and ply my trade somewhere within the New Zealand colonial system.

My second three year term of office was up in March 1952. My hope that there would be no pension problems and no problems with a leave of absence of a year or so, was rudely dashed to pieces on some very hard administrative rocks. When I informed the Resident Commissioner of my good fortune, I immediately sensed that I had broken some very sacred taboo which for the moment was beyond my understanding.

I was told to wait while the Department of Island Territories was consulted. I was informed by my radio operator friends, many of whom were also Hams, that the wires to Wellington were burning hot. All messages were in code, but this did not stop the leaks. There was no particular secret about it all, but I had not voiced what I perceived as my good fortune until it was in the bag and until I had informed the authorities. This I was in the process of trying to do. Now the cat was out of the bag and, apart from some evidence of jealousy from some quarters, most were very happy for me.

In due time I was called to the Resident Commissioner's Office. The result of the burning up of the radio waves was most unexpected. I am sure the manner in which the message was delivered to me was not that which had been intended by its originators in Wellington. The Resident Commissioner was no more friendly towards me now than he had been at the beginning of our relationship and his contribution to the records in Rarotonga can attest to frank and uncomplimentary views on what kind of a person he thought I was.

The first part of the message, verbally conveyed to me, was that I was to give up ideas of going to Harvard and, instead, I could choose to attend any institution of medical learning in Great Britain for a similar period that was being contemplated for Harvard and the government would foot the bill.

I felt flattered. Then I was told the second part which in effect was that, if I insisted on pursuing my plans to go to Harvard, the Administration would sever all relations with me and I would never get a job in the Pacific again. I am sure that this was not part of the message from Wellington, but, at the time, I took the verbal message conveyed to me at its face value. If there had been one, I was not shown the original text of the actual message. At the time, it seemed pointless to think of it, let alone insist on it. I left the Resident Commissioner's office in stunned silence.

* * *

I continued my arrangements to end my term as Chief Medical Officer to the Cook Islands on the due date in March 1952 and thereafter to proceed to Harvard as expeditiously as I could with family consisting of wife Lydia, son John, son Tim and personal effects. Most of this fell on Lydia's capable shoulders. Our faithful servants were placed with friends who had always envied us of them. Our pets were also placed with friends who knew them well. Unnecessary impedimenta was distributed among a variety of friends in as satisfactory a manner as such a thing can be done.

* * *

Now I was faced with what everybody else thought was a new dilemma. I had acquired a 44 foot ketch rigged, ocean going yacht, the Soubrette, which I renamed the Miru, the mythical mother of the eight lines of the Polynesian race. For more than a year she had been hauled out and berthed in Wellington harbour for refit and had been pronounced fit and seaworthy to face the oceans of the world and any storms they might brew. Therefore, it was no dilemma for me, I had bought it to sail the Pacific Ocean. Now it had to do that and the Caribbean and the Atlantic as well. The Miru had been built for just such a purpose and after some twenty or so years, she was going to fulfil her destiny.

We were going to sail it to Boston and keep my appointment with Harvard. To sail the oceans was a dream I had always had as far back as I can remember. The opportunity to do this in a more substantial manner than had hitherto presented itself was now before me in a most fitting manner. There was purpose to it. Lydia had always known of this dream and was not a bit surprised that it was now time to face the reality of it. She did not like the sea any more than most women, but living with me over the years had exposed her to sailing and she had participated with me on relatively limited ocean voyages on several occasions.

Lydia's virtues at sea were not limited. She could cook in any weather and never got seasick. Anyone who does not appreciate these sailorly qualities has not been on an ocean voyage in a small boat. The art of sailing she wanted no part of even though she had crewed for me with great success in competitive outrigger canoe racing on the Lagoon of Muri in Rarotonga for several years. This, however, was to be the big one. About fourteen thousand nautical miles as the crow does not fly. It is a rare sailing route that follows the Rhumb Line.

* * *

There was still plenty of time to the month of March and I carried on my work as usual. This had become very little as far as medical work was concerned because the work of the staff had been going on smoothly for quite some time with little help from me. I was called upon only when difficult cases cropped up. Otherwise I purposely kept out of the way. Training had been an important part of my administration and to now interfere unnecessarily was to negate what training had achieved. However, I still had much non-medical work to perform.

The most time consuming of these consisted of dealing with my international duties. They had descended on me when the New Zealand Government appointed me as its International Representative for Pacific Affairs in 1949. This involved a great deal of paper work and decision making involving New Zealand's position on Pacific affairs as these pertained to the objectives, recommendations and questions raised within the purview of a number of international agencies of which the United Nations and its many arms were not the least. Any matter raised referable to the Pacific, regardless of origin or subject matter, was funnelled to me for response.

Since there was only one flight a fortnight into Rarotonga, the correspondence came in huge batches. Wellington was 1800 miles away and any help from that quarter required a cumbersome process to obtain. I carried on alone and must have done all right or nobody cared because no one made one murmur about any wrong recommendations and responses I might have made.

At first I was bewildered by the mass of material and I could not see how I could answer all of them, let alone make decisions when these were called for.

However, it became increasingly apparent that most of the mass of material was being generated by individuals most of whom had to do it to keep themselves busy. Or so it seemed. However, about three percent of the massive correspondence dealt with what I considered matters of importance.

Some were beyond my knowledge, some only time could resolve. Some seemed insoluble. Some were right up my alley and referred to matters I knew something about and had my own ideas how they should be dealt with. To these last I put some real effort into giving the best response that I could.

Eventually I worked out how to apply the three out-basket system. Into the first basket went the three percent of the correspondence I could really respond to with my very best effort. Into the second basket went that which, in my opinion, not even the Almighty could solve. These were promptly acknowledged and then filed, hopefully never to see the light of day again. The third basket contained correspondence on matters which time alone would clarify. They usually disappeared into limbo, never again to see the light of day. All correspondence was answered with a minimum of effort. I enjoyed this part of my work for the international perspectives that it opened up. I believe it played an important role in my overall view of things in certain areas of my subsequent personal and enforced interests.

* * *

It was getting near the end of this era of my life and, with about four weeks to go to departure day, the farewells began in earnest. These were, for the most part, private farewell functions which increased in crescendo from one or two a week to one or two a day and then to as many as four or five. Although, as in any society, goods, arts and crafts play an important role in the economic life of Polynesians, food plays a much more important role than in any other society I know.

Food was and still is the beginning and end of everything. It is the coin of the realm. As such it is also the way to express appreciation, love and gratitude. Food is the most important criterion of an individual's economic and social standing in his or her community. Therefore, the amount of food prepared and set out for a function or an occasion bears no relationship to the number of persons involved in it. Instead it has a direct relationship to the social, economic and personal mana (standing) of the individual or group instigating the occasion.

Whether or not the function involves one person or a host of people, the food prepared and set out always exceeds the guests by a factor of usually no less than two to one and often as high as ten to one. The ratio, as might be expected, also relates to the regard that the host has for the individual or group being honoured.

This Polynesian characteristic is one which always astonishes foreigners. They compare the amount of food to the number of guests and are struck by the disparity and apparent waste because the number of guests could not possibly consume the amount of food prepared and displayed. Even if they take into account the number of cooks, servers and helpers in attendance, the amount of food still exceeds that which could be consumed by them and the guests.

What they and everybody is seeing is not food to be eaten only, but also food to display the strength and unity of those providing it. Births, deaths, birthdays, releasing the souls of the dead, welcomes, farewells, honours, coming of age, supercisions, haircuttings, religious festivals and a few added modern additional reasons such as Twenty Firsts are all events taken advantage of, or even created, to display through the medium of food the economic strength and social unity of those holding the function and supplying the food.

Such feasts can be instigated by a nuclear family, an extended family, a clan or a tribe. Enjoying the food and filling one's stomach are secondary attributes of this medium of expression. As an example, death and releasing the soul (Kave Eva) is as common as death itself and is an important occasion for displaying and rebonding family ties in their most extended form. Missionaries and those who affect modern and more frugal ways have tried over the years to do away with sumptuous feasts at such occasions. These attempts have in all but rare cases failed and in the rare cases of success, time and pressure of the display incentive has seen to their eventual return.

Food is, therefore, the mortar that provides the bond to establish the strength and unity of a family, a clan and a tribe. Any weaknesses in the administration of any of these shows up in their inability to meet this social and economic fundamental cultural requirement. Especially in the olden days, a family, a clan and a tribe which was found wanting in this respect could be under threat of loss of its lands by a slow or a quick take-over by its neighbours.

That is one of the reasons why agriculture was the way it was when John Williams discovered Rarotonga. He described in detail the orderliness of the great variety of plantings on every square inch of available arable land. On an individual basis, Polynesians will often, on a casual basis, prefer to work for food than for money. Culturally food has greater meaning than money. This, of course, is changing rapidly as modern economics invade their societies.

This might lead one to believe that such a culture based on food would have been ideal for the health of the society as a whole. It might have been in the past, but in recent and leaner times, it did not prevent the evidence of widespread incipient malnutrition in infants and young children and even the infirm and the destitute. These it seemed were often sacrificed in leaner times to insure that the display and bonding effect of the symbol of economic wealth was not hindered on crucial occasions.

Where, as was the case in many of the feasts given to honour and farewell my small family, the food was obtained and prepared by the immediate family, only the host ate with the honoured guests while others served or entertained or joined in the topics of conversation under the general major domo control of the most senior or dominant female of the household. All of these ate after the host and the honoured guests had eaten.

When feasts were held for occasions involving a larger number of guests, members of the extended family were involved in direct proportion to the size of the guest list. A very large function would involve all of the extended family on the island where the function is to be held, as well as the extended family in other islands and even as far away as those living in New Zealand and Australia.

Typically a nuclear family feast given in honour of a guest and his immediate family such as mine consisted of a centre piece of a whole roast pig surrounded by a variety of other main dishes and side dishes. Immediately surrounding the whole pig would be the other main dishes of roast chicken, whole grilled or baked fish. Then there would be side dishes of marinated fish, shell fish au naturel as well as mixed into finely grated and fermented coconut. These would also be present in cooked and marinated preparations.

Interspersed among them would be the baked root vegetables and a variety of green vegetables cooked, sauced and in salad form. Amongst these there would be dishes of a variety of poke and poi prepared by pounding and mixing a variety of fruit with other ingredients to make a paste of sweet and pleasant tasting dessert type dishes. Always present will be dishes of mayonnaise, which is a type of Russian Salad.

If available there would be fresh prawns cooked in coconut sauce, broiled crayfish and coconut crab. The last is deemed by some visitors from New England to be more flavourful than Maine lobster. Green drinking coconuts would be at hand to wash it all down. The pattern of layout would be very similar to this for the large umukai, but there would just be more of it to match the number of guests. Always important ingredients of the umukai are the flowers, the ei or garlands and last but not least, the speeches.

What happens to the food the guests cannot consume, is not the mystery that it at first appears to be. Some goes to the guests to take home. Some goes to feed those helpers and servers who did not eat with the guests. Some is sent to people to whom the family is obligated for past favours. Some goes into the family freezer(s), accounted for as one of the most important possessions that a Polynesian family can own. In one way or another, what appears to strangers to be a waste, goes usefully into the economic and social pool so culturally important to a Polynesian.

In our last days in Rarotonga, we were indulged in this cultural enigma of food and what went with it. The feasts varied from group to group. Those of our more traditional hosts were sedate and subdued, accompanied only by opening and closing prayers, the ubiquitous speeches and the Imene Tuki or traditional and descanting religious tunes with the ancient words replaced by the biblical words of the new religion. The less formal groups turned our umukai into a rollicking fest of Cook Islands' Polynesian fast and languorous music accompanied by song and dance as only the Cook Islanders can produce and perform then and now. This was the pattern of the informal groups which usually consisted of both Europeans and Cook Islanders. The Cook Islands was already an integrated society.

* * *

I did not regard my leaving Rarotonga as a desertion of duty. In the more than seven years I had worked in the Cook Islands, I felt that I had laid a foundation that would be for the permanent good and this overcame any personal sentiments I had that I was abandoning my people. The Islanders commended my decision, but in the farewell speeches made in our honour I was distressed to detect again a note of uncertainty and lack of self- confidence.

"You have allowed us to play a part in your work, but, if you leave us, who will take care of us and see that things are done properly?"

The attitude of the Europeans to my leaving was little different from that of the Islanders. As the islanders had done, the Europeans pleaded, "What is the use of having built up a medical service? You must know as well as we that you will be scarcely out of sight of land when that service will start to fall apart again."

To both groups I tried to answer as honestly as I could. I explained that, if the service disintegrated, it would not go back to the way it was some years ago. "You all now know what modern medicine can give you, even in the partial isolation of the Cook Islands. I have no doubt," I said, "That in the knowledge of what you can expect, you yourselves will see that this is what you get."

It was now goodbye. I had reached most of the objectives I had set myself and the Department in the full knowledge that no one ever realises all one's dreams. For some time now there was only a very small effort necessary on my part to sustain momentum. Not much progress could now be made for at least five years when fresh personnel, now in training overseas, would be ready to return to the Cook Islands.

At the end of these last days, I was sitting in my office taking care of some final details and correspondence when one of my office staff knocked and entered, "Excuse me, Doctor," he said, "Would you mind coming down to the laundry. There's some trouble there."

I sighed. If there was one place that I did not take pride in, it was the laundry. All my periodic efforts in the past to upgrade this necessary adjunct to our service had met with official and in-house stubborn resistance. All our Hospital washing was still being done in the good old island way at the bottom of the hospital grounds. All day long and every day for many years before my time, a group of ancient ladies, their grandchildren, pet dogs and close friends, took turns in scrubbing, beating with sticks, rinsing and draping hospital linen and a variety of other personal looking male and female garments on available clothes lines, rocks and bushes in their area of the hospital grounds.

Each week there were different people to pay for these laundry services. The ancient ladies, most of whom had assisted in my upbringing, considered me to be their son and, therefore, very, very subject to their every wish and whim. So there was often trouble in the laundry. Usually I left these troubles to Matron. This time I hoped would be the last for me.

But what a surprise I had coming to me. No sooner had I put my head in the door of our washing premises than I was covered in ei. On a table was laid out food and a variety of bottled goods and an enormous tea kettle, a favourite means of surreptitiously dispensing home brew. The ancient ladies and their usual retinue and the groundsman all stood around wreathed in smiles while Mama Manu acted as spokeswoman.

"Our son," she began, "You are our guest. Last night all of us who have worked for you showed you and all the people of Rarotonga how much we have learned to love you. That is not enough. Our love is not for you just as a doctor, but as a man. Some of us here wiped your snotty nose and dirty bottom and in many ways took care of you when you were small. Today, we are joining together to show that love in the way we know you like best. Puia, bring out the guitars and ukuleles and fill the glasses."

CHAPTER SEVEN

Destination Boston

Our friends' kind thoughts seemed tinged with the colour of doom.

LYDIA DAVIS

In March 1952, my contract with the Cook Islands Administration was over. I had until September to be in Boston to be a full time student at Harvard for the course for Master of Public Health, to meet the US immigration requirements. On the face of it, we had plenty of time to meet this deadline. We got to Wellington, found lodgings and, as soon as I could, I went to check out my dream boat. My first sight of Miru was on the moorings, breasting a sharp harbour chop kicked up by a typical windy Wellington wind. She looked great and ready to meet whatever came her way. The workmanship of the work done on her was satisfactory, but nowhere near complete. My inability to be there for the fitting out had resulted in many things remaining to be done.

The Miru, formerly the Soubrette, had been designed and built to the ideas which designers of those days considered a good ocean voyaging yacht. Bruce Farr, Laurie Davidson, Ron Holland, Gary Mull, Lexcen and others have changed these ideas considerably since then to meet the needs of speed for the ever increasing ocean racing events of which the Whitbread Round the World Race and America's Cup are the most demanding.

The movements of their light displacement in a sea-way may not be as comfortable, but the gains in other ways may be significant compensations. Not the least of these is the high speeds attained in that part of the course through the Southern Ocean. We were going to travel the Pacific part of this ocean in the first part of our voyage to Boston. For comfortable ocean cruising, I still prefer boats like the Miru with some refinements in design.

The Miru was all wood, New Zealand kauri, of substantial scantlings. She was of three skin construction over substantial stringers supported by double skinned bulkheads. It seemed unlikely that any condition the oceans could dish out would harm her. I was relieved of any further anxieties on that score. She was going to keep her side of the bargain. It was up to us, her human partners, to keep ours. As it turned out we were all severely put to the test.

All we now needed was to get her victualled for the voyage, obtain the necessary charts and navigational instruments that I did not already have, install the radio equipment which as a Radio Ham I did have, check out the engine, generator and other mechanical and electrical equipment, insure that all sails and running gear were in order with spares and extras on hand, arrange the necessary papers, find two crew, obtain visas, say goodbye to friends and relations and set sail.

These steps take less time to say than to do. We did our part, but the US bureaucracy did not do theirs. To enter the United States we needed visas. In spite of a letter from a person at the highest level in the State Department in

Washington DC., informing all and sundry to give us any assistance we needed, we were unable to obtain them. After hanging around for six weeks with promises that they soon would be available, we could wait no longer and we set sail without them. Despite having tried to obtain visas in Lima, Balboa and Colon, we had to enter the United States without them. It was only in the United States that the letter from the high official carried weight. The Immigration Department demanded that we return to New Zealand as was normally required, but our high official was able to circumvent this requirement.

* * *

As a Radio Ham, ZK1AN, I decided that the best way to keep in communication with the world while at sea was to build myself a transmitter in as weather proof a box as I could. If I built it myself, I would be able to troubleshoot it and maintain it more easily myself. Since becoming a Ham in 1946, I had enjoyed building radio equipment and I doubt that any transmitter I built lasted more than a few months before it was torn down and replaced with a new one incorporating new concepts, different circuits and more effective physical layouts. I even built a double superheterodyne receiver which, surprise! surprise! worked the first time I turned it on. In all these efforts I was usually accompanied in advice and often outright unfavourable comments by my friend and mentor in these and other matters, Stuart Kingan, ZK1AA.

I installed this equipment on the Miru with due regard to the conditions we would meet in the Southern Ocean. It was important that the aerial was well insulated from the ocean for at least its lower part. It all tested out nicely and I was happy. However, while I was away from the boat for a day or so, some New Zealand Air Force radio technicians invaded Miru, examined my amateur efforts, threw their hands up in horror and installed very complicated, but beautiful equipment with through deck insulators for the aerials which unfortunately could be expected to be under water much of the time in the conditions we were going to meet.

I arrived on board to find the work completed with three smiling new friends in RNZAF uniforms happily sipping beer. Their beer I might add. After suitably toasting their achievements with numerous beers, they left in high good humour and I never saw them again.

I surveyed their very professional efforts, carefully packed away my own crude efforts and distastefully looked forward to the day I would have to replace their equipment with my own. That day never came. Apart from the loss of communications during the first critical days because of their aerial installation, their equipment worked beautifully throughout the voyage after I had reinstalled my own aerial. I wish again to thank them. For the beer too.

* * *

Even before leaving Rarotonga I, along with friends like Ron Powell, John Pratt, Captain Andy Thompson (a square rig Cape Horner) and Captain Boulton (also a square rig Cape Horner), had given considerable thought to what route we should take to reach Boston. Though there was, as we thought at that time, a comfortable margin of almost nine months to complete the voyage, the route to the west through the comfortable areas of the tropics and its easterly tradewinds for the most part would be cutting it too fine. It was several thousand miles longer, so we rejected it. All that was left was the route to the east using the westerly winds of the Roaring Forties.

I did not relish this route as it had a bad reputation from the clippership days and from the stories of my two Cape Horner friends. No small boat such as ours up to that time had braved its waters. I was even more discomfited by the fact that, if we did not leave soon, we would be into the winter fury of the Roaring Forties. A rough passage is bad enough but one does not take a rougher and a colder one by choice. There was no choice.

I had read just about everything I could on the Southern Ocean. It was exciting reading from the comfort and safety of an armchair. It was only after examining the Miru yet again that I felt that she was up to it. The question still was; were we, her crew, up to it?

* * *

The Southern Ocean is an interesting ocean. It is considered to start at forty degrees south Latitude. There is no land mass to speak of south of this to hinder the westerly winds which circle the globe in this region. These winds for the most part pass south of Cape of Good Hope, the Great Australian Bight and New Zealand, giving the winds free reign to build up speed and in turn build up waves of a size and force unequalled in any other ocean of Mother Earth. Cape Horn is the only land mass that juts significantly into it.

In the southern winter these conditions move north by about 10 to 20 degrees and markedly intensify their force. In Drake Passage where Cape Horn lies close to the Antarctic Peninsula of Graham Land, all the force and fury of the Southern Ocean is funnelled and concentrated into the hell it is known it can be. Cape Horn has its good days, but I was glad that Miru and her company did not have to gamble with its fickle and unpredictable moods on this voyage.

But the Southern Ocean is more than the Roaring Forties. To understand its anatomy and behaviour, we must think of it in relation to the oceans that adjoin it from the equator to the Antarctic. The wind, the principle actor in this region, has seven zones in which its characteristic behaviour varies markedly.

At the equator, the winds are zephyrs or absent and referred to as the Doldrums, made famous by Samuel Coleridge's "The Ancient Mariner". South of this, the south-east tradewinds typically blow constantly from around March to about the middle of December and extend south to about Latitude 25 degrees south with a typical velocity of 18 to 25 knots. South of this is another belt of calms that circle the Earth, known to sailors as the Horse Latitudes, why? I do not know. Typically it extends from about 25 degrees to 35 degrees Latitude south. From around 40 degrees on to about 50 degrees south is the Roaring Forties with typical wind velocities around 40 to 50 knots. From 50 degrees to 60 degrees south is the Furious Fifties. Its reputation is worse than the Roaring Forties, but it is doubtful that the conditions are very much worse. The Screaming Sixties may be worse from all accounts. At around 70 degrees S, we run into another encircling belt of calms and, abutting to the south of it, a second belt of south-east winds. Finally we have a blob of calms, frequently disturbed by high winds, sitting over the South Pole.

These conditions are typical, but can vary with the seasons and the effects of El Nino. Winds of over 100 mph have been reported from the South Pole as similar winds have been reported from the areas of calm. Calms have been reported from the Roaring Forties and the Furious Fifties. The seven regions shift in band width, latitude and intensity with passing barometric changes and the seasons. In the southern summer they shift to the south and in the winter to the north. The regions are so definite that one can be rollicking along before a fifty mile per hour wind of the Roaring Forties and a shift of course to the north will land one in the calms of the Horse Latitudes, as we were, for eleven frustrating days of absolute calm in our attempts to seek refuge from the cold.

This in brief is the anatomy of the ocean we planned to sail non-stop from Wellington to Callao, Peru. As usual the route could not be along a rhumb line. In this case, the rhumb line followed a great circle path that would have taken us too far south amongst the ice bergs and the very edge of Antarctica. Instead we planned a parallel latitude course which was considerably longer, but much safer from ice bergs and freezing temperatures.

Up to that time, our voyage in the Miru was the first west to east crossing of the South Pacific part of the Southern Ocean by a small yacht. We were now only five months to the September deadline and that was much too close. We were probably not going to make the deadline.

I figured that we would need two crew for the safe management of the ship and here I think Miru set another record. She arrived in Boston, five months after setting out on one of the hardest passages ever made in a small vessel, with the same ship's company she had in the beginning. More important, we were still on speaking terms. Choosing a suitable crew for small vessels is always difficult. Men who are willing and able to undertake a long, uncomfortable voyage are not usually the most stable individuals.

Stability is a most desirable quality on such ventures where lives are at stake. Experienced sailors who have the desirable qualities for such a voyage are usually weighed down with responsibilities of family, home and job. The crew-seeking skipper has, as a rule, only adventurers from whom to choose. There was no scarcity of applicants and Neil and Bill, the two I chose, proved to be better than the best I could have expected.

Those of us who have a yen for ocean cruising tend to learn as much about everything as we can because deep down we know that, some time, our very survival may depend upon it. These may go beyond the ordinary things a sailor might need to know. Some I have known who cannot tie a proper knot, but who somehow get by as yachtsmen. Some who can tie proper knots, know little else. Many know nothing about anything pertaining to the sea, but own a yacht and depend on everybody else to handle it. The owner is just along for the ride, the glory and the prestige and has the money to do his yachting this way.

However, serious sailors who contemplate ocean passages go out of their way to accumulate knowledge they believe might be useful if the opportunity to take to the sea in their own vessel ever arises. Some are so obsessed with this and the negative things that could happen on the high seas, they never realise their dream.

* * *

The media were on to our plans to cross the southern Pacific Ocean and gave us favourable write-ups, but pointed out the great dangers facing us and the hopes that we would overcome these by good seamanship and good luck. The luck part got more emphasis than the seamanship part! Nearly all releases praised our intrepid initiative. Some even used our example as a platform for ranting at the dying and dead spirit of adventure of modern New Zealanders.

Dinners were given in our honour and my newly acquired knowledge of the Southern Ocean was always welcomed as a conversation piece with questions being fired from all directions about possible facets and fantasies of what could happen during this long passage in the wildest ocean of our planet. Small boat voyaging was then in its relative infancy and the voyages of Captain Voss, Joshua Slocum, Erling and Julie Tambs and their kiddies, Johnny Wray, Alain Gerbault, Bill Robinson and others were still on the lips of yachtsman and the public. Our proposed voyage was viewed in heroic and epic proportions. Nevertheless, following these favourable releases, opposing views began to appear as Letters to the Editor.

This opposition, from the layman's point of view made a great deal of sense. I had not previously given the points of view expressed in these letters much serious thought. Most had not even entered my head. One does not seriously plan a project and then dwell unduly on its negative aspects, real or imagined. In effect these letters castigated me as an individual, and together with my wife as parents, for entertaining the thought of crossing this dangerous ocean with our children.

They made me have second thoughts. Perhaps I had entered this in a spirit of adventure with little regard for the comfort, welfare and safety of my children and those foolish enough to join me. However, the die was cast and there was no turning back. Alternative travel arrangements to Boston in the time available would have involved greater expense and the time involved in selling the Miru, a nigh impossible decision to make since she was a recent acquisition with barely a few hours of use since we acquired her.

The letters came mainly from religious groups of all denominations and the fierce attacks lasted for several weeks. Then suddenly they stopped and we were visited by each denomination in turn bringing gifts and tokens of best wishes and safety for our voyage. The Saint Christopher given us with great ceremony and blessings remained firmly attached to the bulkhead of the main cabin to the very end of Miru's life.

One denomination which had been particularly firm in its unfavourable opinions on our venture put a roster of two of its members round the clock to run messages and do our shopping for us day, night, rain or shine. Those who know the windy cold conditions of Wellington in June and July can appreciate the sacrifice this amounted to. Invitations to perform their vigil on board in the warmth of the cabin were consistently and firmly declined.

* * *

Eventually we could set a day for sailing, come hell or high water. We set sail at the appointed hour of near enough to 1 pm. in a blustery Sou'wester with warnings of worse to come. We cast off midst tears and best wishes of relatives, friends and many others we did not know personally. As Lydia later wrote, "Our friends' kind thoughts seemed to be tinged with the colour of doom."

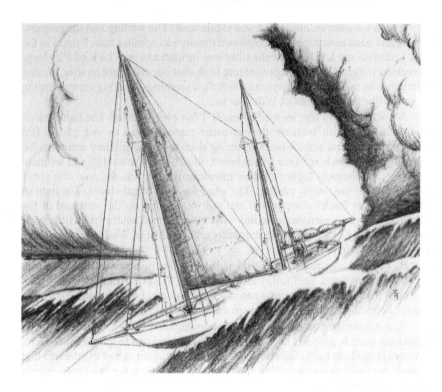

I had wanted to clear Cape Palliser before dark. We just managed to do so with a roar of enormous seas funnelling through Cook Strait and meeting the roll and twist of the cross swells sweeping up from along the Kaikoura coast of the South Island, urged on by the cold Sou'wester which by turns hummed, moaned and shrieked in the rigging. We were using the mainsail only on a broad reach on the starboard tack and it was more than enough to give us all the speed we needed.

The ancient three cylinder Ailsa Craig diesel for propulsion had been turned off as also had the 3 horse power diesel auxiliary which was for charging the batteries and keeping in operation the wonderful deep freeze which my sister

Mary and her husband, Ian, had bequeathed us. Tests had demonstrated that it could go over five days without needing a boost. Our 200 hundred pounds of meat seemed secure, provided we could keep everything in working order.

Before leaving the wharf, I asked Neil and Bill to check and top up the oil in both engines so that we would be free of this chore for a while. They topped up both engines right over the mark to make sure that the job was not needed for a long time to come. A foolish and nearly disastrous act which could have cost us our 200 pounds of meat.

* * *

At last we were on our way. I was exhilarated. The waiting and the preparations had been interminable. A boyhood dream was coming true. I stood in the cockpit with my left hand on the tiller and thrilled to every kick of it as huge breaking roller after breaking roller rose high over our starboard quarter, hissing their threats as they bore down on us with their seething, breaking crests hanging over us like predators about to devour us.

All of Miru's 44 feet seemed so small. I felt even smaller. The half dark of twilight seemed to increase their menace rushing upon us out of the fast gathering darkness and the black lowering skies to the stern. They seemed to be coming from nowhere. True to her breed, Miru's stern rose high and let them slip by, and the only legacy of their threatening mien was the cold wet spray and spume of their noisy passing. The wind was now at gale force. The light of Cape Palliser finally disappeared and we were alone on the vastness of the Southern Ocean, seven thousand miles from our planned landfall with little hope of successfully beating back to the safety and comfort of Wellington Harbour, now hard to windward.

By choice I was alone above deck in the first few hours of this long sea trek to our first planned land fall, Callao. I wanted to savour those hours. I was pleased that the rest of the crew had taken advantage of my obvious wish to be at the helm and all had gone below to the warmth and dryness.

With no noise of an engine, only the hum and hiss of wind and sea and the creaking stretch, give and take of sail, line, block and tackle shared my reverie. Alone, I could not help cogitating over the fact that again one of my dreams had come true and I again marvelled at the lack of effort on my part to consciously make them come true.

Providence always seemed to make the effort to make my smallest wish come true, usually in the best way possible, even if I did not at first see it that way. Up to this stormy night, it had always been so. From then until this time of writing, it has always been so. I am not seen by others as a praying man, but on this roaring, wild, dark night I let slip a prayer of thanks to the Power that controls our destinies. For similar reasons, I have let such prayers slip out before this night and I have had occasion to do so many times since.

It may seem incongruous to most that anyone should give thanks for having the good fortune to be blessed with being allowed to set out across so many thousands of miles on a hostile ocean, which would take at the very best 60 days to cross. It is not easy to explain, but I think Moses might have done the same thing, facing the desert with the children of Israel following blindly behind. Perhaps those of us who are given the opportunity to do these things are seeking a sort of freedom and personal challenge, some in the expanse of the sea, some in the barrenness of the desert, some in the grandeur of the mountains, some in the deathly white silence of the arctic wastes, some in the high speed of racers. And the most embarrassing thing anyone can do is ask why we do it.

* * *

The only obstruction of any significance to our passage to Callao was the Chatham Islands and one or two markings on the chart like "reef reported" or "breakers reported". The Chathams lay south of our course and for the moment somewhat to windward and not a threat if conditions stayed the way they were. So we rolled and rocked along with the wind blowing at about 45 knots from the south-west. Short experience of the weather cycle in the Cook Strait area had indicated that a Sou'wester of storm force was normally followed by a short period of calm and variable winds which in turn was followed by similarly intense winds from the north-west. So the Chathams could be a threat if we were forced to run a more southerly course than the easterly one we had been able to hold for the first two days after leaving Wellington.

But things were not to be as expected. The blustery gale conditions we had experienced since our departure worsened as had been intimated by the weather reports at the time of our departure. As predicted, the radio transmitting aerial and its through deck fitting was constantly awash and would not load from the transmitter. We were out of two way communications. The receiver was separate and that worked to perfection for weather reports, broadcast stations, short-wave stations and time signals from WWV for navigational purposes.

On the third day out, it started to really blow from the north-west. What had been promised for some days now was upon us. Reports from the Wellington radio stations confirmed that what we were getting and were in for was about the same as they were getting on the east coast of New Zealand. Winds were being reported with gusts over hurricane force, playing havoc with coastal shipping. We did not doubt it! We were getting our fair share.

The Miru had a set of storm sails to substitute for the staysail, the main and the mizzen. They were tanned and of a weight which made them stiff and difficult to handle, I referred to them as malleable iron, but their obvious strength gave us great confidence in them. In area, they were about the equivalent of Miru's double reefed normal livery. I decided to heave-to with the mizzen stormsail and tiller lashed to leeward. I had tried this combination off the Kaikouras on a shakedown trip from Wellington to Lyttelton and it had worked well in 50 knot winds using the standard mizzen with one reef in it. With the storm mizzen it worked well, at least in the beginning.

Before it got worse, I was able to indulge my own ideas of what a ship's company should do during a storm strong enough to cause the boat to be hove-to. My practice had always been to set the ship into its hove-to position and induce everybody and especially myself to have a quiet drink and then go to sleep until things got better.

Miru, like most vessels of her type, hove-to well and one could set a tumbler full of liquid on the cabin table without fearing for its safety and the safety of its contents. The three skinned hull and deck of the Miru were an effective insulation against the outside noise of the storm and the whistle of the wind in the rigging under normal storm and gale conditions. And this is how things were in the initial stages of this storm.

We had made the rule not to broach the liquor stores except for birthdays, anniversaries and special occasions. As Master, I tacitly reserved the right to change the rules. To indulge in that quiet drink before settling down to wait out a storm was one of these tacit reservations. So after putting Miru into her best hove-to position, I asked Lydia to break out the rum and for all to have a generous tot and go to sleep. But soon after we had our tot, things started to get interesting to the point that even Miru would not sit quietly as she had always done in the past.

She just would not remain hove-to on one tack or the other. Since being hove-to the way we were doing it required that the sail was to one side and the helm lashed to leeward, when she came on to the other tack she was all out of kilter and continued full circle. This meant that she could be caught by a breaking sea and be thrown on to her beam ends. Worse, she could be rolled through a full 360 degrees capsize.

* * *

I went below to start the generator to insure that the freezer would have enough cold to withstand the length of a storm. I wound the starting handle and came up solid against a brick wall. The same happened when we turned over the main engine. There was only one thing to do, sit and think. Finally I came to the conclusion that the upper cylinders were full of liquid and liquid does not compress. I questioned Neil and Bill and they admitted that they had with all good intention filled the sump with oil to far above the mark.

To cut a long story short, I tediously and with great difficulty took off the cylinder heads and did a valve job on both engines during the height of the storm. The valves, in trying to manage the burning heavy sump oil, had gunked up. The one cylinder Lister was relatively easy, but to do the main engine, I wedged myself in the available space with my backside supported by the bank of batteries, one knee against the engine, the other on the floor boards and my head hard against the structure that straddled the engine to support the mizzen mast stepped right over the engine. I was able to do the job, but at the expense of no skin on my knees and a large haematoma on my forehead. It was an exhausting job which left me limp as a rag and the storm still to be fought raging over my head. But the meat was saved and the main engine was on standby if it should be needed.

* * *

We went to work on alternatives. Running before with trailing warps was not a good idea because we would be heading for the Chathams with the approximately 50 mile broad stretch of its many islands lying almost directly in our path. We had a sea anchor, but from the beginning it never looked large enough to prevent our bows from being thrown around. We tried it anyway, but could not control the chafe of the warp through the chocks and we lost it along with some valuable spare line. We then tried old sails and bits of wood and anything we could tie on. These, each in their turn, helped for a little while, but in too short a time disintegrated and disappeared with loss of the gear tied to it and some more line.

In the end we just stood by and tended the sail and the tiller whenever she was thrown from one tack to the other. There were four days of this. We were all worn out. Only young John and Tim seemed unaffected by it all. They stayed in their bunks and somehow remained within the confines of their bunk boards. They played all sorts of games which kept them occupied.

Then there was a lull of confused seas on top of huge swells, more like tsunamis than waves, rolling in from the north-west. We rested as best as we could, thankful that what had seemed endless was at last all over. The barometer stood at a low 28.4 which told us that it was not all over. Within about 12 hours we were at it again. This time worse than before. Winds on the coast of New Zealand were now reported over 80 knots. Again, we had no doubts they were right. In the previous four days we had exhausted ourselves and run out of resources of trying to keep Miru in the best position to meet the storm. None had availed. We knew Miru could sit like a lady and let us sleep through storms up to 60 knots. What we were now experiencing, not even a lady like her could handle with aplomb in these unprecedented conditions. We were now in a full hurricane. Only the strength of Miru's timbers, the craftsmanship of her builders and the strength of her fastenings could now save her and us.

Thoroughly exhausted, we put up that storm mizzen of malleable iron, bolt-roped right around with one inch italian hemp. It disintegrated and disappeared like tissue paper in minutes. Only the bolt rope was left to show that there once had been a sail attached to it. It zipped and flailed in that uncompromising wind, screeching its anguish at the abuse it was receiving. There was none to hear it. There was too much screaming and screeching from the rest of the rigging; the stays, the shrouds, the halyards, the lifelines, the stanchions and the very masts and spars.

Miru was now a very naked lady fighting for her life and ours. Her hurricane deck was now clean and shiny with the stinging spume and scrubbing wash of the Southern Ocean for those endless days past and, as it turned out, for endless days to come. I stood for some time in the cockpit and saw that, with no help from us, Miru herself was keeping the desirable angle to the seas and was herself fore-reaching to maintain it whenever she was knocked off by a high breaking monster rearing out of the maelstrom to windward. I could not help thinking that if we had left her to herself from the beginning she would have done better. Occasionally a huge breaking wave would catch her when she was broadside on and roll her over until her spreaders were in the water. I wished I could have prevented this potentially dangerous happening, but I knew there was nothing more we could do. She was on her own. With difficulty, I lashed the tiller midships so that she could herself choose the tack she wanted to be on.

As reverently and as loudly as I could I yelled, "Its up to you, old girl." I then faced the teeth of the storm and as irreverently and, as loudly as I could, I cursed it with all the vehemence I could muster. I climbed below and battened down the main hatch behind me. None of the hatches were to be unbattened for the next three long days during which we hung on when hit broadside and rolled God knows how many degrees to leeward, time and time again. We soon learnt to anticipate by the roll to windward, when we were going to be thumped hard and rolled way over to leeward. Whoever got the first hint of this warning would yell, "Hang on." Mostly we would all call out at the same time. We all became experts at reading that telltale deep trough that preceded the big bad ones. In Wellington I had screwed heavy dowelling onto the overhead beams below decks as hand holds. Without them, I am sure we would have suffered greater injuries than the bruising we sustained. Whenever Miru was thrown on to the other tack we transferred the children to the equivalent lee bunk they occupied.

During these three days, the normally effective three skin insulation to outside noise had little effect on the noise of the storm. The scream of the wind in the rigging reached a pitch and intensity which was continuously piercing and did not vary as it normally does with the roll and pitch of the vessel. It was there and it stayed there, loud, high pitched and piercing. It penetrated the very bowels of Miru and its company huddled below decks. Only the firm, solid thump of the breaking waves on the hull could be sensed above the overall cacophony and violent movement that physically and mentally wore each of us down.

* * *

Throughout the seven days of these hurricane conditions we could, if we chose, see what went on outside through the portholes of the deckhouse. I spent hours watching the sea and its many extraordinary behavioural activities and imagined the type of vessel which would best meet them. A submarine well below the surface looked about the best bet. It was a fun exercise which helped while away the interminable duration of this storm and the enforced inactivity it imposed other than hanging on and constantly adjusting to the pitch, roll, yaw and kick of the vessel.

The most interesting to watch were the albatross and their lesser relatives who were our constant companions in the Southern Ocean. In stark contrast to ourselves they were in complete command of the situation and not once did I see any one of them discommoded for even the smallest instant by the huge breaking seas or the wind that screeched so violently in our rigging and dealt with us so harshly. Several times while watching them, I was jealously envious of their ability to handle so easily what we could not.

They sat on the sea when they wanted to as though they were taking a rest on a mill pond. In the air they zoomed over the waves, swooped rapidly to altitude, soared from one wave crest to another, ran down and up through the troughs of the waves, shooting high above them, diving down again to bank along the front or back of a wave with the tips of their wings barely clearing the ruffled surface of the ocean, all without the slightest flapping movement of their wings, hour after hour.

When the storm finally abated to gale force, which we learnt to accept as normal conditions, I rebuilt the radio transmitting aerial. Even in the normal conditions of the Southern Ocean, the neat through deck system installed by my RNZAF friends was never going to operate. Since leaving Wellington we had been out of contact with the world. This has never worried me, but in all my voyagings it has always worried the hell out of the world.

Because of this lack of radio contact, we had been presumed foundered in the storm with all lives lost. Word had been sent out to countries likely to find pieces of our wreckage to return these to the New Zealand government. I resurrected my amateur prepared aerial that had been packed away and put it back up again. We were now in two way communication with the world, loud and clear, only to be soundly blasted by all and sundry, officials and others, for having been off the air.

* * *

I reviewed our situation from the point of view of a ship's Master with full responsibility for the condition and safety of ship and company. We were a pitiful lot. Miru was pristine clean on deck. We had used very dirty unscoured sheep skin to fabricate her chafing gear. These were now as white as snow. All that might have been in any way loosely secured on deck was gone. Her strong rigging and solid masts were fully intact. The running rigging was frayed and chafed in many parts. The spare lines we had used up in the storm were not now available for replacement and long splices were going to be needed to put things right again. We ended up with fifty two of them in the running rigging.

Down below was a dank mess that would take some scrubbing, airing and sunshine to rectify. The crew were sure that we had capsized through 360 degrees. I was not sure, but neither was I prepared to argue against it having happened. There was evidence on the under side of the decking to indicate that we may have indeed capsized 360 degrees. Could we have done a 360 without my being sure of it? I don't know. The constant violent movement which ranged as much as, I believe, 90 degrees of arc, tended to disorient us as to our rolling status at any one time. I believe we did roll through 360 degrees, but I cannot be as certain of it as the rest of the crew.

The children, who at times had become my chief concern, came through the ordeal considerably better than the adults. After the storm, they were happily playing a noisy game with cards. What had been a dreadful ordeal for us had apparently passed over their heads as something ordinary. It is to the credit of the adults that we had not at any time throughout the storm conveyed our personal or collective concerns to the children, nor had we lessened to any degree their trust in us as their protectors.

Throughout it all the ship's company had behaved well. Lydia, after a short rebellious period at the very beginning of the voyage, never missed preparing a meal. This had much to do with the good morale of the crew throughout the voyage. The crew had promptly attended to many of the tasks above and below decks that were necessary to insure the safety of the ship and its company. We were physically and mentally exhausted, utterly drained of physical strength, moral fibre and human emotion.

* * *

We needed respite. Sailing on for what could seem like forever with cold gale force winds as normal weather conditions was not going to give us that respite. We should make for the nearest haven, take a well earned rest, pick ourselves up and carry on. The wind had now settled into its accustomed and chilly groove directly out of the west at 35 to 40 knots rising to 50 knots and over for no apparent reason. Throughout it all blue skies had rarely been absent and that was the case now.

The Chathams were just astern of us. Any thought of making for it was unattractive to me. Not only would it be a beat, but it was directly opposite to our destination and I knew of no safe harbours. Besides it was too close to New Zealand and the temptation to return might be too much. The nearest land that would be acceptable as a way-stop and in the general direction of our destination was Rapa Iti, the most southern island of French Polynesia, at about 28 degrees Latitude S and 144 degrees Longitude W. Going there would lose us time and significantly increase the total distance to be sailed. I did not discuss these possibilities with the crew until I had thought things out fully and come to a firm decision.

Rapa Iti was 2000 nautical miles from where we were now. If conditions held, we could make it in fairly good time. Like all sail boats, Miru did her best on a reach and a reach it would be if we turned for Rapa Iti. The decision was made and I passed it to the crew for comment. It was received with enthusiasm, but not without informing me that they were surprised that I would deviate from my original intention of doing the leg to South America non-stop. I mumbled something about what kind of an animal did they think I was. We reached Rapa Iti 22 days after leaving Wellington. For 17 of these days, Lydia and the kids were never able to come on deck and we, the crew, were never able to dispense with our safety harnesses while on deck. It was never below gale force the whole way.

We spent seven restful days in Rapa and we needed all of them to put ourselves together again. The Rapans spoke a Polynesian dialect so close to Rarotongan that I could converse with them freely and their kindness and hospitality were unstinting. We were worried about staying too long because this meant consumption of stores that we could not replace. Provisions were not available. The people were in greater need than we and we still had about 4500 nautical miles to sail to Callao. Rapa Iti is famous for the myth that there are two women to every man. A simple count showed that there were three more women than men. Another myth explodes.

At the end of our pleasant stay we set sail, heading south-west towards the Roaring Forties and its steady and reliable westerlies, even though these were more often than not gale force or stronger. From the day we left Wellington to the day we sighted the South American coast, we did not sight a single vessel.

After a while, for all we knew we, the sea and the sky was what the world was made of. Even the voices we communicated with by radio seemed to be from another planet.

We again quickly settled into the routine of life in a small boat at sea and each of us found deep solace in it to the extent that not one of us really wanted ever to reach land again. When we did, all without exception expressed the wish to be at sea again and to be rid of the land. This was a curious reaction that I have not seen or heard expressed elsewhere, but must have happened on the long hauls of the sailing ship days and might in part explain why sailors keep returning to sea.

* * *

Strong gale force winds was the dependable fare from Rapa iti to Callao, but mostly with sunny skies. There was some snow and some sleet and it was always cold. We met many whales on their way to the Bering Sea and the phosphorescence was often spectacular. For a day or so, huge isolated breaking seas roared at us from the south-west at intervals of about six hours. They inundated us each time. My only explanation was that they were the result of earthquake activity along the fault known to pass through the Antarctic. For twelve days Miru sailed herself in perfect conditions without anyone touching the tiller and averaging a nice 8 knots. Occasionally we made over 200 miles a day, but like all things, it is difficult to beat the law of averages in the long run. What the nice sailing days give you the calms and storms will take away.

I felt pangs of regret when we passed several hundred miles south of Pitcairn Island. My family had a long association with the descendants of the mutineers of the Bounty. My grandfather Captain Harries had performed a number of services for them and had helped move some of them to Norfolk Island. Much of this happened before I was born, but the association had left its mark of affection. Mary Anne McCoy took care of Mary and I as children and had lived with us until her death. My mother was named after her. Our home in Rarotonga was a home for any Pitcairn Islander who came by. Before we left Wellington, Fletcher Christian, a descendant of his namesake had visited us to wish us bon voyage and to ask me to call at Pitcairn Island to say hello to the folks. Time did not allow us to do so. It was a great disappointment to all of us that time had not allowed it.

After several days without seeing the sun, we sighted land only ten miles south of our destination and docked in Callao, out of food following lunch that day, all but out of fuel and water, but happy with having completed a long and arduous voyage that none had done before in a small yacht. That evening we dined well ashore, finishing off with peach melba, strong coffee and liqueurs. We not only felt satiated by the meal, we also felt deeply satisfied that we had accomplished what had been said to be impossible in a small boat. It felt strange to be on land again amongst people and the things that go with them.

The voyage from Callao, through the Panama Canal, the Yucatan channel, the East Coast, the Inland Waterway, Cape Cod and finally Boston are well worn tracks and any reference to this part of the voyage would be repetitious of many reports by other yachtsmen. However, the great welcome expressed by the whine of sirens, the whoop whoop whoop of ships of war, the squeak of small working vessels, the caaw caaw of mouth blown horns of sail boats, the deep throaty fhooomm of ocean liners and freighters whenever they sighted Miru gave us all a warm feeling which I am sure has remained with us and will be unforgettable to the end of our lives.

After having been met by friends in boats off the Boston Lighthouse, we were escorted up the harbour by a sizeable number of vessels. We docked at the private dock of the Science Museum on the Charles River and officially ended our voyage here with the keys to the city of Boston on a cold November 2 day in 1952 to start a new life in a civilisation strange to us.

* * *

Our arrival was mixed up with the arrivals of Mr Nixon and General Eisenhower and careering official Cadillacs and police sirens shared between us. The 1952 elections were imminent and on arriving at the Sheraton Plaza, I was mistaken for Richard Nixon and revelled in the applause from some and the heckling from others.

PART TWO

American Interlude

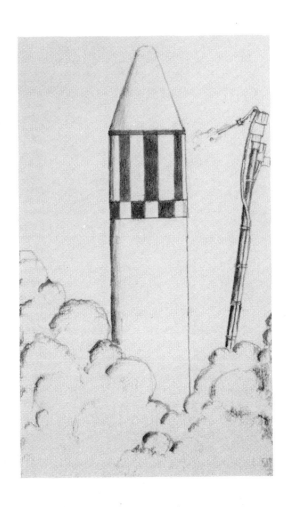

CHAPTER EIGHT

Harvard

God has given man the eye of investigation by which he may see and recognise truth. He has endowed man with ears that he may hear the message of reality and conferred upon him the gift of reason by which he may discover things for himself. This is his endowment and equipment for the investigation of reality. ABDU'L-BAHA

Whatever success Harvard graduates have is due to their own talents, honed by their experience at Harvard. Most people are judged, and have to be judged, on their own merits. CASPER W. WEINBERGER '38

Harvard School of Public Health personalities played a major role in the grand welcome we received on our arrival in Boston. I was soon facing the purpose of coming many thousands of miles. Six weeks late for class, I had to make up the time lost. Harvard does not accept excuses or give bouquets for late students. I joined the class of 52/53 with the understanding that I could not graduate until I had made up the time lost.

The Harvard School of Public Health had an interest in the public health problems of the world, especially of the Third World which had these problems in the extreme. Not that the United States did not have public health problems: it had them in abundance, but they were significantly different from those of the Third World of which the Cook Islands was a part. No country is ever free of such problems, but each stage of development is accompanied by new and different public health issues. The new ones can be as bad as the ones overcome, especially if they require new approaches and new technologies for both their recognition and their treatment.

For example the industrial pollution of water, not to mention that of air. Until the late sixties and early seventies, the extent of this problem had not been recognised in many industrially developed countries including the United States. Water standards were based on bacterial counts while many toxic and potentially mutagenic and carcinogenic substances in the water were unrecognised and untreated. Likewise in the food preparation and preservation industries, new technologies can affect more than just the nutritional value of the product. There are many other examples.

Dean Simmons of the Harvard School of Public Health was one of the few of his day, and even perhaps today, who realised the variety and universal depth of public health problems of the world and the role that his school could play in mitigating them. He therefore attempted to expand the teaching concepts of the School to include teachers and students from every part of the world and every aspect of medical care and knowledge which might impinge on public health. So it was no surprise that there were 26 countries represented in the student body of which I was a part, or that those who were from the United States represented all branches of the Armed Forces and the numerous departments of federal, state and local government. The great majority of students had already distinguished themselves in their respective fields of endeavour and each had much to contribute to their colleagues and, I must add, to the teaching staff.

The teaching staff were men of stature as they had to be to face a student body of such calibre. Their efforts were augmented by staff of the Harvard Medical School, some of whom were Nobel Prize winners. There was further assistance from outstanding experts from far and wide, within the United States and beyond. There was no reason for any of us not to be stimulated to assimilate the vast abundance of knowledge that surrounded us.

* * *

I was induced to stand for Class President and managed to win over other candidates. I considered it a great honour and privilege and it was a pleasure to hold this office with class mates who cooperated as only mature and caring people can. We identified the types of problems that we students might face and the type of functions and activities in which we wished to be involved academically, socially and culturally. The small committees we formed to organise and implement these tasks performed so well that the class achieved the highest academic records of any class before and since in that particular era, and had the highest proportion of class members who went on to achieve high honours in medicine in general and public health in particular. Moreover, they did so with social and cultural grace.

* * *

It was a busy year for me, and a hard one. Dean Simmons and his public relations staff were not going to let Lydia and me, who had achieved somewhat of a celebrity status, pass unexploited for raising money and enhancing the School's financial status by putting us to work giving talks to banks, insurance companies, affluent clubs and any organisation or group that seemed remotely likely to help the objectives of the School with generous donations. In addition, Lydia and I were invited to lecture to groups who paid us quite generously for these services. The money from these sources was a great help because, although we received assistance from the coffers of the Pacific Science Board and from the pharmaceutical company of Burroughs Wellcome, we needed all the money we could raise on our own. These lectures took up two or even three nights a week with sometimes considerable distances to travel. This took a heavy toll of my study time for Master of Public Health examinations, but, for the family to live in any kind of comfort, it was necessary to meet these demands.

Lydia did the donkey work on the book *Doctor to the Islands* that we were writing. Because of the fullness of my time, I would dictate my part of the book to her and to Ted Weeks, the editor of *Atlantic Monthly,* mostly on the run and more often than not over the telephone. I was to illustrate the book and the illustrations were often done at the oddest places, at the oddest times and with the oddest materials that happened to be readily to hand. Most were done with a fountain pen and often on hotel stationery and scraps of paper. But we managed to wend our way through these vicissitudes and were surprised that things were done and that other things just happened which included a pregnancy and a son and the loss of the Miru in the hurricane of November, 1954. On the bright side, I passed my exams with nothing less than a B and a high proportion of As and the book was completed, but yet to come out in print.

* * *

After graduation and as a medico who had done most of his work in surgery, I was well equipped in tropical medicine from the School of Tropical Medicine in Sydney, Australia, and now in Public Health from the Harvard School of Public Health. My wish to return to the Pacific prompted me to ask whether there would be a job if I returned. I received negative replies or no replies, but Professor Fred Stare of the Department of Nutrition had offered me a position as Research Associate in his department and that softened the blow that perhaps I was not welcome back home by the New Zealand colonial administration as had been indicated if I insisted on going to Harvard.

I was familiar with the Department of Nutrition and most of its personnel and was very happy to be counted in their number. My duties were to devote myself to teaching and research in whatever subjects I desired. It was a carte blanche situation which excited me no end. At last I could pursue one of my dreams which was to do research in cold physiology, prompted by those days so long ago at King's College and at Medical School with my pals on St. Clair Beach in Dunedin. However, this was in the realm of physiology more than in the realm of nutrition, so I was faced with a dilemma, a department wanted me and here I was wanting to do what may not be within the functions of the department.

There was a Department of Physiology within the School Of Public Health, but it had not shown an interest in me (there was no reason for them to have done so) and I hated the idea of having to leave a department which had shown a long term interest in me. Professor Jean Mayer was one of those who had accepted me into the department with enthusiasm. Of all the excellent people in the department I naturally and unconsciously developed closer relations with some than others. Jean was one of those I found easy to be with and talk with about all kinds of subjects. He had, in my view, a deeply academic, scholarly and open mind. He was quick to perceive the conceptual essence of things while others might flounder around perceiving them as bizarre and perhaps even dangerous sorties outside the pale. So I took my dilemma to Jean, though with some trepidation.

I had had too many experiences with others in similar academic positions who, when I expressed one of my ideas, would just stare at me as though I was from outer space. One professor in the Medical School in Dunedin, when I brought this same problem to him, embarked me on a totally fruitless task to prove that my results were not due to the changes in the temperature coefficient of the glass of the thermometers or to the compression of the anal muscles on the thermometers induced by cold water immersion. My results, which proved that neither pressure nor cold had an effect on thermometer readings, were received without interest, as were the preliminary results of those early experiments. This professor was a world famous researcher in his own area. My trepidation was born of a person once burned, twice shy.

I explained to Jean what I had experienced and done in cold research and what the meagre results of my sketchy experiments had led me to conclude. I explained my profound wish to investigate the phenomenon scientifically and definitively, but was inhibited by the fact that perhaps it did not fit into the objectives of the department. The last thing I wanted to do was disrupt the department by imposing my personal desires into its working philosophy.

Jean's reaction was explosively enthusiastic and highly favourable to my going ahead with my ideas and the research needed to elucidate them. He expressed understanding of the subject and said that, in spite of the fact that Alan Burton, Jim Hardy and Otto Edholm had put to rest the ghost of chemical thermogenesis, first propounded by Claude Bernard the famous eighteenth century French physiologist, he himself was of the opinion that Claude Bernard's thoughts should not be ignored and that he would put the resources of his laboratory at my disposal to pursue the matter with all haste.

I was flabbergasted that he knew so much about the subject which had been my personal secret for so many years and that he would put his laboratory complex at my disposal to work on it. That he knew so much about the subject became clearer later. As fate would have it, Jean had been plagued with the same ideas as myself through the inability of his hereditary obese-hyperglycemic mice to withstand cold.

The relevance of my proposed work still bothered me, but he pushed it aside stating firmly that, if Harvard bothered about where work was done, it would not have nurtured so many Nobel Prizes. I insisted that Fred Stare, the Chairman of the department be informed. Fred's enthusiasm for my interest was most comforting, and he said that a study of metabolism in the cold was a study of nutritional requirements under those conditions. I was happy. Once again an impossible dream was in the process of fulfilment and I gave my usual brief but heartfelt thanks to the Power that controls our destinies.

* * *

Happy as I was, I was scared. Just like the other times, but more so. While things were a dream, I had no fears. My recurring dreams had always been sources of womb-like comfort. They gave me a feeling of warmth and tranquillity whenever I dwelt on them. In fact, whenever I had problems in reality I would escape into whatever dream was foremost in my mind at the time and find deep comfort and personal security in it. Once my dreams became realities, they lost their tranquilizing effect.

The realisation of this particular dream brought serious problems. Unlike other dreams that had been fulfilled, I did not know anything about research. My dream had not included how to develop a research design, or how I was to go about doing the work, or what biological specimens could be used to measure whatever measurements I was going to make. My dream did not include a list of the instruments and odds and ends I would need and how to obtain them, let alone how to use them. Worse still, my dream did not include what data I was going to collect and what I was going to do with them after I had collected them. I was trained as a doctor of clinical medicine and few professions equip one worse for research than that. At heart we are still witch doctors.

Achieving the reality of my other dreams was not as scary. At least I knew, or thought I knew, what to do and how to do it in each case. The reality of this one left me numb and incapacitated. What my dreams had done in this case, which was quite unfair of them, was to put me in the position of seeing myself as a Newton, an Erhlich, a Koch, a Pasteur, a Rutherford, an Einstein, and all their ilk without the necessary trimmings, wherewithal or background to make it work.

* * *

I was given a desk in an office which I shared with a Scottish gentleman, also with a medical degree, who had also just joined the department with the same status as myself. He had not been a member of my class. While I sat at my desk nursing my state of numbness and incapacitation, Arthur was busy as a bee. He gave me and everybody else the most firm impression that he knew exactly what he was doing and the world was going to be shaken by the results. He had a bunch of white rats assigned to him in the basement three floors down and intimated to all that he was doing weird and wonderful things with them. But nobody quite knew what. The best communication we got out of Arthur was a knowing look. As office mates, we became good friends and did some confiding in each other. He learnt of my confusion and I learnt of his passions.

Before that, mostly I had sat at my desk contemplating the desktop and became intimately familiar with the different scars on its not so recently varnished surface. Alternately I just sat and stared blankly at the opposite wall. I don't even remember what colour it was. I dragged books from the library and read them in the hope that in the wisdom of their pages I would find the answer to overcome my numbed incapacitation, but this failed to generate any inspirational vision which fitted my particular needs for guidance. I came to the conclusion that perhaps creativity comes from within and has damn all to do with the written results of someone else's creative efforts. This is not true, at least not entirely, but that is how I felt. I had the creative concept in mind, but what was I going to do with it now that I had the wherewithal to do something about it, backed by the faith of Harvard in me.

* * *

Concerning my dilemma, Arthur suggested that I get a bunch of rats and, just by taking care of them and feeding them, I would appear to be just as busy as he and sooner or later something would turn up. My sincere confiding in him of my sacred research project, left him unperturbed and uninterested. On the other hand, my learning of his two passions perturbed and interested me tremendously. The first was golf. He was a scratch golfer and my mediocre golf found some improvement through the many games we played together and with our good friend, Stan Gershoff, whose golf was nearly on a par with mine, his being somewhat better.

His other passion which was much, much more interesting was planning how to rob banks. His current project was how to rob the main Boston Shawmut Bank. He would not tell me one way or the other whether any of his banking projects had ever come to fruition. Regardless, it was great therapy for me, as it must have been for him, to work together on this project. Somehow he had acquired plans of the Shawmut Bank and its environs. We spent hours poring over them and came up with numerous ways the bank could be robbed. None of them seemed very fool proof to me, but I was no expert. I never heard of the Shawmut Bank being robbed, so all our effort was nothing more than what it was, self prescribed psychiatric therapy.

* * *

My inability to come up with a satisfying research plan was beginning to become critical, as well as personally embarrassing. I was unaccustomed to not being able to get on with the job. At least Arthur was doing something. I knew that he was having the same problems as I and this was a great aid to salving my own conscience. However, besides the antics of Arthur, my conscience was also being salved by the activities of another newcomer to the department. He was from one of the Eastern countries. I never knew which. He was also busy as a bee, but there was little doubt in my mind that he was having the same problem as Arthur and I.

Chan had a laboratory to himself. Well, almost to himself. At least he was highly visible in it. He had the centre bench with its gas outlets, water faucets, sinks, centre consoles, and all they held, all to himself. Using these and the department stocks of glass tubing, rubber tubing, bunsen burners, glass and metal stopcocks, retorts, condensers, other departmental paraphernalia and whatever came to hand, he put together the most beautiful looking structures any of us had ever seen.

We were all fascinated as these grew and blossomed into their full beauty. The balance between glinting glass, red rubber, black rubber, light hued latex, aluminium scaffolding to hold it all together with its shiny stainless steel fixtures interspersed with black iron stands, more glass of differing contours and curves presented a picture that no one could deny was a work of avant garde sculpture. Into these structures, fluids of different colours ran hither and thither. As each structure was completed, it was, after a suitable display period, dissembled and another grew in its place, more beautiful than the one it replaced. No one dared ask what they were supposed to do. They were so sculpturally beautiful it seemed superfluous, if not sacrilegious, to do so. Chan's laboratory was the first place that Fred Stare took visitors. He showed off Chan's current work of art with a wry smile and pleaded ignorance as to its function on the basis that he was only the Chairman of the Department.

* * *

What I have said about my early days in the department might give the impression that the Department of Nutrition was replete with people who did not know what was up and what was down. This was, of course, far from the truth. There were those who joined the Nutrition Department and other Departments from my class who seemed to find their feet with no difficulty.

The behavioural activities of Arthur, Chan and myself demonstrated the difficulties some of us were experiencing in adapting to a work situation in which you were given the facilities and absolutely nothing else. What you did with them was up to you and absolutely nobody else. Until you came up with what you were going to do with the facilities, you were on your own. It illustrated that Harvard gives people like Arthur, Chan and myself opportunities, but not all of us are able to make immediate or eventual use of them. Until we solved our respective adaptation problems we were, in different degrees and forms, exhibiting the biological phenomenon of "displacement activity". Being unable immediately to meet the demands of our new situation, we were doing things that in some way resembled what each of us was expected to be doing. Arthur fed and took care of rats assigned to him, but not much else. Chan built structures that looked like those that analyse chemical compounds in biochemical reactions. I assumed the role of thinker and scholar using Rodin's chin on hand, staring into space attitude as my model, and poring over books. I never knew Chan's background. Arthur had been a competent editor of medically and scientifically oriented publications. Each in our own way eventually came out of our respective morbid states. We were not in them for as long as it seems to take to tell about them, but for me it was long enough.

My dilemma was due to the fact that I still thought like a clinician and considered working on my research problem using human subjects as I had up to that time in a somewhat desultory manner. Using human subjects in my present situation was not even a remote possibility although I had a go at it. During the time spent cogitating over how to approach my research problem, I had become closer to the works of Jean, Stan, Peter, Mark, George, Martha, Margaret, Steve, Bob and many others and had begun to realise that the animal model allowed one a greater latitude of effort to examine biological mysteries. When I looked back to my simple efforts of long ago using humans, the truth of this struck home. My friends were most supportive of my efforts to come to grips with my problem, but Jean had shown a scientific understanding of it beyond anything I could have hoped for. Not only had he allowed me free use of what space and equipment was available in his own laboratory complex, but he was also, in more ways than one, instrumental in getting me started. This included setting up the experiments, collecting the data, organising them, applying the proper statistical analyses and writing the reports for publication.

* * *

It was natural that our first efforts together should have involved the use of Jean's beloved hereditary obese-hyperglycemic mice. Jean had already shown that these mice were extremely sensitive to cold and died if inadvertently left exposed to cold which their non-obese siblings withstand indefinitely. We had come to the conclusion that these mice were dying not because of the failure of normal heat loss mechanisms, but because of their inability to produce the extra necessary heat to survive in the cold. Therefore, it was probable that the chemical heat production postulated by Claude Bernard was real. We were certain in our own minds that what was missing in these mice was the chemical thermogenesis that Jean and I, in almost antipodal parts of the world, had become interested in independently. It seemed that providence was again playing a hand. It also seemed that, if I had tried, I could not have found another person as interested as myself in the same problem, or a better model than Jean's mice to begin working to obtain the understanding needed to begin demonstrating our hypothesis.

The mice were obese because they were unable to use their fat under normal circumstances. In the cold they were still unable to use their fat as fuel for the production of the extra heat needed for their survival. A great indication that we were right would be if these mice shivered when they were in the cold. As soon as I could, I put several of them in the cold room at about 3 degrees celsius to satisfy myself on this point. Sure enough they shivered like crazy.

We felt that we were well on the way to establishing the scientific truth that, in addition to the production of heat by voluntary muscular activity (exercise for instance) and involuntary muscular activity (shivering), there was another type of heat production which was produced by a non-muscular activity type of heat production which Claude Bernard had called chemical thermogenesis. Claude Bernard did not know that this was really chemical in nature and neither did we. So I began calling it "Nonshivering Thermogenesis". This hypothesis, if correct was not going to sit well with Alan Burton, Jim Hardy, Otto Edholm and others.

Our first study on the subject was a kind of stage setting for what was yet to come.[6] It was based on experiments in the cold with three groups of mice, namely, mice with the Hereditary Obese-hyperglycemic Syndrome, their normal siblings and thirdly, mice made obese by the administration of goldthioglucose. This compound causes obesity by increasing food intake. Once used for the treatment of arthritic conditions in humans, it caused obesity as a side effect. The obesity so caused does not affect the normal metabolism of fat as does obesity in the Obese-Hyperglycemic mice. The experiment showed that all the three groups exhibited the normal responses to cold such as shivering and piloerection (fluffing up of the fur). The non-obese and goldthioglucose treated siblings in addition increased their heat production, as measured by oxygen consumption, and withstood the cold for more than three days. On the other hand, the Obese-Hyperglycemic mice lost body temperature, failed to increase their oxygen consumption and became moribund on exposure to 3 degrees celsius after only 2.2 hours.

As a result of this first study we were able to conclude that the extreme sensitivity of the Obese-Hyperglycemic mice to cold was not due to obesity itself, nor was it due to their inability to shiver or piloerect. It was, in fact, due to their inability to increase their metabolism to produce the heat required to combat the effects of cold.

At this point I must diverge and talk about animals used in the manner I am describing, not to try to justify what I and other researchers do with animals or even humans in the interest of knowledge, as that would be fruitless. I and most colleagues in research always did everything we could to avoid having to use animals in research, but we had no choice unless we were to forego our duty to seek the truth of our inspirations. So we went ahead in the most humane way possible and used animals whose biological mechanisms are similar to our own.

Animals, like all biological beings, respond to kind treatment and try to cooperate with what you are trying to work out with them. Rats and mice are no different. Those that I worked with were not comfortable in the situations I put them. Apart from the cold they had to put up with a little discomfort from the electrodes and thermocouples I attached to them once every two or three days for as long as four weeks in my acclimatisation experiments. If they became upset, they could ruin a session of measurements. This was true to a degree for most measurements and certainly for electromyographic measurements of their shivering activity. With careful handling and explanations of what was needed of them, their seemingly active co-operation gave me what I needed. You might doubt my veracity, but I swear they knew what was wanted of them. The rats and mice that we used were bred for experimental purposes. Except for occasional experimental purposes, they lived very well indeed. If it were not for our research need of them they would not exist at all.

However, there are some exceptions to this co-operative response. I have never had any problems with any animals except monkeys. I have never worked with apes so I must exclude them. Monkeys can be tame. This was true for the time they were left to adapt to their new surroundings. As soon as we put them to work in programs I was using in the study of the behavioural effects of psychoactive drugs, they became resentful, uncooperative and had to be handled so that they could not take a piece out of you.

Suppliers of monkeys, unless otherwise requested, remove their canine teeth. So I cannot be the only one with this problem. But I have friends who get along with them famously, canine teeth and all, but I do not recall seeing these monkeys in a work situation. Maybe I have been influenced by one of my favourite books, the Mowgli stories from the *"Jungle Book"* by Rudyard Kipling where he tells about the Banda Log or the monkey people. His stories about them may have prejudiced my views about monkeys. Anyway, I work with them badly. It is always an armed truce between us. In this respect they remind me of a number of people I do not seem to be able to get along with. This was a pity because I worked with monkeys (Rhesus, Green and Squirrel) off and on for much of my research life. I have had a good relationship with all other animals I have worked with. My dogs cooperated so well that when it came time to draw blood from them they would hold out their paws and wag their tails. Horses, rats, mice, dogs, many others, even skunks, I have no problems with. But monkeys were another thing.

The next set of studies was to call upon my knowledge of electronics as a Radio Amateur (usually referred to as a "Ham".) I knew that radio frequency waves are a form of high frequency electromagnetic wave energy which can produce heat in materials in indirect proportion to their dieletric constant. In the simplest terms it is how a microwave oven works. At that time we did not have commercial microwave ovens and physiologists encountered problems trying to understand what I and my home built apparatus was doing. My little, low powered microwave oven, because of the nature of the experiment, was open so that whatever was in it was open to the cold environment in which it was to be used with a mouse or rat between the radiating elements.

The rationale was to show that at the right energy levels in the cold, my little microwave oven could substitute for the missing chemical thermogenesis of the Obese-Hyperglycemic mice and could keep them alive indefinitely in the same cold to which it otherwise was so sensitive. The results of this experiment were as expected. The micro oven, at levels which did not affect shivering or raised skin temperature, substituted for the missing thermogenesis in the genetically obese mice and replaced half of the requirements for heat production usually provided by increased oxidation in normal animals exposed to cold. The microwave oven, therefore, could be used for physiologic dissection of the reaction of homeotherms (warm blooded animals) to cold.[7,8]

I had already observed the disappearance of shivering with apparent acclimatisation in my own case at King's and in the case of my friends on the beach of St. Clair. So we needed to pin-point this mechanism as far as possible. Our review of the literature, with which we were already becoming quite familiar, showed that the elucidation of the nature of the stimulus for shivering was already a classic physiological problem.

The earliest workers, around 1895, had concluded that shivering could be induced either through reflex effect of cold on the skin or, in animals recovering from the hypothermia of deep anaesthesia, because of the drop in central body temperature. More recently, other hypotheses have been proposed. Some, including most text books, have emphasised exclusively the role of drop in body temperature. A fall in skin temperature was considered by many as the main stimulus, but definitive experiments were on the whole missing. My preliminary observations on human subjects, myself and my friends in New Zealand, had shown clearly that shivering was present when the body temperature was higher than normal, but in the presence of a lowered skin temperature. Confusion seems to have reigned because observations had been made under a variety of circumstances including recovery from hypothermia. Our interest was the stimulus for the response within normal physiological limits.

* * *

This time, I again brought my Ham Radio skills into play, but in a different way. Jean and I were both adamant that we needed a way of quantitatively measuring shivering. It was not very difficult for us to settle on a myograpgh which records the activity of muscles through electrodes placed in electrical contact with the skin. However, what one gets from such an arrangement is a line of squiggles of wave forms on paper or oscilloscope with widely varying amplitudes and frequencies. There was little doubt in my mind that these were true instantaneous representations of the activity of muscle. But they were not quantitative. I needed something that would give me a product of the frequency and amplitude of the squiggles and accumulate these over a set period, to represent the activity of muscle per unit of time as measured by its electrical activity. It did not matter whether the units were absolute as long as they were relative.

I knew what was needed electronically and was willing to build it if the worst came to the worst. Far better and quicker would be that such an instrument existed and that I could lay my hands on one. My friend Gerry Letvin, across the Charles River at MIT, was doing wonderful things in elucidating the neurological pathways of the spinal nervous system. Believe it or not, his research was being supported out of Chicago by the remnants of the old Al Capone gang. While visiting him one day, I mentioned my problem. Gerry's work involved electronics and we often swapped know-how.

When I apprised Gerry of my need, he told me that Tony Philbrick, over in Downtown Boston was putting together such an instrument which Gerry needed to do the same thing with EEG recordings. He indicated, but I am not really sure that he did, that he was in no hurry for the instrument! I left Gerry as politely and as unhurriedly as I could and hotfooted it over to Tony's workshop.

I happened to know Tony, so with no great fanfare of hi, hello, how are you, I went straight to the heart of things. My contact with Tony had not in any way resembled my present visit. It was to do with hypnotism, which he and his friends were investigating. My invitation to the group was to come up with a research design to prove that hypnotism was the cat's pyjamas as a therapeutic agent in certain situations. As an anaesthetic I believe the application was. I came up with a research design, but heard nothing more about it. I think the design was too rigid.

What Tony had put together was pretty, as all functional things are. Its proportions to my mind vied with those of Venus de Milo. It was about twenty inches long, six inches high and six inches wide. It was crackle black in its metal protective parts and shiny black bakerlite on the top where its dials, meters, toggle switches and female sockets, into which male plugs were to be pushed, formed a pattern of functional beauty. It took only one look at it and a cursory examination of the circuit diagram to know that I had struck pay dirt.

It was just a black box to everybody else, but to me it was manna from heaven. In no uncertain terms I said, "Tony this is mine." He looked a little upset and replied, "Tom, this is a prototype and Gerry has first call on it." I explained that I had just come from Gerry's and he had informed me he was in no particular hurry. We wrangled some more, but I was able to convince him that my need was greater than anything he could imagine and I walked out with it. When I got it set up, I invited both Gerry and Tony to come and see it in operation. After seeing what it was doing, all was forgiven.[10]

Jean and I did some further work using the tools I have just described which allowed us to dissect the two types of thermogenesis involved in the mechanisms by which hot blooded animals combat the effects of acute exposure to cold.[11] In addition we showed that after acclimatisation to cold for a period of exposure of three weeks, the animals lost their need to shiver and withstood the cold with only about half the heat production needed when they were in the unacclimatised state, but I was unable to complete this series of experiments until much later.[15]

To summarise, the work we did together proved conclusively to ourselves that there were two mechanisms involved, but to most of our other colleagues and those who had worked hard and long in the field, we had shown nothing. As a result, some of the papers we presented for publication were turned down by the readers. But as luck would have it, the Editor of the *American Journal of Physiology* was a friend of Jean's and being convinced that we were on the right track, he published them. The controversy that was to rage for the next few years forced me to do a great deal of experimental work in both animals and humans which now, in the light of final scientific acceptance, seems to have been unnecessary and time consuming.

* * *

I am a medical doctor. I cannot change what in me as a person made me one. Neither can I change what my training made of me. However, I am also by nature scientifically minded. This made me choose medicine as a career, but medicine in practice was not a scientific discipline at the time of my choosing it. It has come a long way since, but still not enough to be classified as a profession of the sciences. The practise of medicine is very pragmatic. We are faced with real people with real medical problems that need real treatment and right now. To face up to this, we have no recourse but to use the armamentarium available to us and get the job done as expediently as possible.

Although I was now as deeply into basic research as anyone could be, I was faced with a schizoid type of situation. I, the pragmatic Doctor of Medicine, asked myself what did it matter if people believed that there was no such thing as nonshivering thermogenesis? The world would not come to an end. But I also asked myself, as a scientist, about the worth of a truth. Truth is not related to its worth as an item of daily usage. Truth has an inherent value of its own. As such it must be established and declared. Its value will become evident in its own time. The judgement of its worth is not necessarily ours to make.

Our pragmatic approach to dealing with medical problems could only have been possible through the bringing together of a great many unrelated and independent truths each established and declared separately. Our use of them in the treatment of the sick does not make us scientists. However, they do make artists of us, for the doctor who does not use what is available to him with sensitivity and skill cannot be a good healer.

By 1955, I realised that I could not go on just working with animals. As a medical man I must show the mechanism in man and resort to animals for the finer definitions as these became necessary. The work that Jean and I had done with animals had convinced us that we were right in so far as we had gone. What became important to me was to demonstrate this in man. My own observations in man in New Zealand were desultory and of no great scientific conviction except to me in the form of obtaining some insight into the problem.

* * *

One day Dr Kaare Rodahl, a dapper Norwegian, came into the department. He was a Doctor of Medicine with a background of interest and research into the effects of cold on man. His work was more with survival than mechanisms. He had come to see if I was interested in being a part of a laboratory that had just been built on Ladd Air Force Base, now Fort Wainwright, near Fairbanks, Alaska, known as the Arctic Aeromedical Laboratory. I told him I would be most interested, but only if human subjects were available to me in order to pursue my research interests. His assurance that this was no problem made his offer irresistible. As it turned out there was a problem, but there were also compensations. My quest was again held up, but this time for, relatively speaking, a little while only.

* * *

Leaving Boston was not easy. The friends we had made, my colleagues at the school of Public Health, the Medical School and its teaching hospitals as well as those at other teaching institutions, my sailing friends and so many more were all going to be difficult to leave.

We had developed an affection for Boston, its environs, Massachusetts and New England. Physically Boston is a mixture of the old and the new, put together in a higgledy piggledy manner which for me added greatly to its charm. At the time, there were few tall buildings and its streets had grown from cow paths, therefore, following no pattern that a city designer might have planned. This also contributed to its charm. When the Prudential Building went streaking into the sky, it stuck out like a sore thumb, but not too objectionably. It served a purpose and was a forerunner of things to come. Now the Prudential no longer looks aloof and lonely and what has joined it has not changed Boston's basic character and charm. I was there to visit Jean and Stan and other friends in 1988 and found Boston to be still Boston.

The Department of Nutrition was particularly difficult to leave, but Fred Stare, always solicitous of our welfare, put me on leave of absence with an open invitation to return to the fold when I came to my senses. He and the staff had made it plain that I was making a mistake and had succumbed to the blandishments of "that fast talking Norwegian".

* * *

Harvard had expanded my horizons enormously and painlessly. In its environs one learns without knowing that one is learning. It all seems to be done with mirrors and osmosis. This fact became clear when Sir Douglas Robb, my mentor from my hospital days in New Zealand, visited Boston and spent some time with me. At the "Merry Go Round" restaurant (no longer in existence) of the Sheraton Plaza Hotel, he put this method to the test. Even before we ordered our meal, Sir Douglas said firmly, "Tom, bring me up to date on the latest in all branches of medicine." I realised this was no social luncheon. I was going to have to earn my lunch. I was nonplussed because I felt I was not going to be of much help to him. He had put his lunch money on the wrong horse and I said so. He was not to be put off. "Come on, Tom, you must have learnt something all the years you've spent here, so go ahead. Teach me."

I had great personal respect for Sir Douglas and the last thing I wanted to do was let him down. I do not remember eating or what I ate, but I reached deep into my mind and surprised myself. I talked and I talked. Words came welling out on one subject after another. I talked about new thoughts and research on techniques in heart surgery which I knew was of particular interest to him; about what we had been doing on intravenous feeding and the attendant problems; about the latest thinking in aspects of dentistry including fluoridation of water which was very new and the arguments for and against it were at their hottest; about the new thoughts on immunisation against poliomyelitis and the work Enders and Webber were doing on it. They were given the Nobel Prize for it. And so it went on till dinner time. He paid for the dinner also and we did not finish what he started until 9 pm.

I was not conscious that I knew these things. In retrospect I realised that some I had picked up in the Staff Luncheon Room where we swapped our findings and thoughts in an informal but nevertheless serious manner. Whenever I got bored doing my own thing, I used to visit different research colleagues in their research laboratories or medical colleagues in their teaching hospitals and just shoot the bull about what we were up to, what we were finding and how our conclusions were shaping. It was a painless, effective and pleasant way to keep in touch with things. Leaving it all was painful, but the next step in the search for my particular "Holy Grail" had to be taken.

CHAPTER NINE

Alaska

The people of the Southern ice, they trade with the whalers crew.

Their women have many ribbons, but their tents are torn and few.

But the people of the Elder Ice, beyond the white man's ken-

Their spears are made of the narwhal horn, and they are the last of the men.

RUDYARD KIPLING

We decided that going to Alaska would be a good opportunity to see as much as we could of America and Canada. We picked the interstate road at the top of the US, then we would turn up into Canada towards Calgary and Edmonton, join the Alcan Highway to White Horse and on to Fairbanks, our final destination.

Our preparations were relatively simple compared with what we had been used to. Our goods and chattels were now reduced to personal effects and some unpartable, but mobile, impedimenta. I am an addict of fast, pretty cars and it was with sorrow that I had to turn in my sporty 1954 Loewe designed Studebaker sedan for a Studebaker station wagon.

In June 1955, after saying goodbye to our friends over the past two or three weeks, we left Marblehead, our home town for the past three years or so and set off across the US and beyond. Apart from the lure of my "Holy Grail", the itchy feet of my Polynesian and other sea-going ancestry probably had something to do with my ready willingness to pack up and take off. I do not think it was much different from others who have found a good reason for doing the same, Ulysses and Jason not excepted. I differ only in that I dragged my family along with me. This time the family had grown with our third son, Robert Teremoana Harries Davis, now just turned 12 months old.

We followed our planned route and camped in the open when we could and used motels when we could not. We kept away from the cities as we wanted to get some feel for the vast country and its hospitable inhabitants and their changing accents as we moved westward.

* * *

The Alcan Highway was the roughest road I have ever travelled, before or since. Our Studebaker station wagon was a marvel to have come through it all with only limited damage to her under parts, none of which held us up. The dust pervaded every part of the car and all items within it, including ourselves. A vehicle in front was the worst that could happen. For miles its dust would hang over the road. There was no escape except to race past it, if the road would allow it, and get away from it as far as possible. By doing this we became the offending party. The road was constructed of gravel straight from the creeks and river beds with no processing. I was curious, so I measured the size of this gravel and the larger units ranged up to 9 inches in diameter. Many of the travellers gave up and some abandoned their trailers which were particularly vulnerable on this type of road. I am told that things are better now.

We passed through some very beautiful country in the Rocky Mountains of Canada, but through Alaska to Fairbanks was most unattractive, especially as we neared Fairbanks where the sides of the highway was littered with beer cans and empty samples of every kind of container devised by the packaging industry. I could not help suppressing the momentary feeling of despair at having decided to venture into this area of seeming desolation. But as it turned out there were compensations of all kinds. Not the least of these was the enormous camaraderie of the people of Alaska, the transition of this countryside into the beauty of winter. The snow covered all things that marred it in summer. The breathtaking beauty of other parts of Alaska not far away and the numerous opportunities to be close to unadulterated nature and the wild life it supported were tremendous compensations.

* * *

The camaraderie in Alaska is said to result from everyone being dependent on others for survival and security. The failure of one's heating system can cause death from cold, and a fire from an overworked heating system can also be disastrous. In a breakdown on the highway, if other drivers pass you by, as they do elsewhere, you could die. If you are lost in the wilderness, there is little time for planning and cogitation and the intense efforts of everybody give the best hope of rescue. This Samaritan requirement, consciously caring for one another's safety, engenders good human qualities which permeate the society.

* * *

I revelled in the arctic wild flowers and the mushrooms of which Alaska has every variety. I ended up with two varieties more than the acknowledged champion of photography of arctic flowers, Doug Prescott, the then Mayor of Fairbanks. This was because I had been to St. Lawrence Island and he had not. I photographed and ate all the mushrooms I could after, of course, checking them out for spore patterns and physical characteristics. I was tempted to experiment with the known psychoactive effects of some of them, but did not have the stomach for it.

I fished whenever and wherever opportunity arose. The hunting instinct has always been as strong in me as it must be in most men. I am happy to say the other instincts of preserving nature and its wild life have been stronger. While in the abundance of this wildlife, I shot only one caribou, which kept us in meat for that winter. I also shot some ptarmigan for the table.

* * *

We were given comfortable family quarters on the Base close to the town of Fairbanks. As most ordinary goods and services were totally catered for on Base at bargain Post Exchange (PX) prices, Fairbanks thrived on the supply of entertainment, female company, off-base restaurant food and bar drinks at off-base prices. It was a "tourist" trade composed of almost one hundred percent Air Force personnel, hungry for the fleshly aspects of tourism. The large number of bars and entertainment establishments attested to the success of the industry that fulfilled these needs. That art form, strip-tease dancing, was very much in evidence, but there were few of the performers that I would judge as very good. Nobody seemed to care whether they danced well or not!

These off-base services attracted those in the entertainment world from many of the large cities of the United States. Many came to escape their problems back home, many of which were of a criminal nature. Lydia and I got to know a number of them and they were always solicitous of our welfare and our enjoyment when we were having a night on the town. We did not allow their background nor their occupation to interfere with our personal friendship. At no time did any of them take advantage of this.

* * *

Fairbanks was a frontier town in the best tradition of frontier towns in what was then a territory of the United States. The freedom from restraint that one has come to associate with frontier towns of the wild west was its chief characteristic. One could start a pub crawl at 5 pm. and by midnight one would not have covered half of the available bars in Fairbanks, without touching the night spots and strip joints that prevailed in the heart of town.

The wearing of pistols slung on hips, especially during the hunting season, was usual. On rare occasions they were used to settle drunken arguments. The shooting was not of the reputed calibre of Wild Bill Hickock and damage was rare. On one occasion during our time there, an innocent bystander who had just arrived and was having his first outing, had the heel of his boot shot away. That is pretty bad shooting.

On another occasion, damage was caused when two lovely ladies of the night squared off on Second Ave to settle an argument over a man equally desired by both. It would probably not have come to much if one of them had not let off a shot that went through the windscreen and out the rear window of her opponent's brand new "Push Button" Plymouth. This so angered the owner, she emptied her six gun into her adversary. At the trial the defence based its argument on who shot "first" and the prosecution based its argument on who shot the "mostest". From the reports in the *Daily News Miner*, I was not sure whether the defendant was acquitted because of justifiable homicide or self-defence or both, but acquitted she was.

* * *

Fairbanks is set out in square blocks with numbers denoting streets one way and letters or names denoting streets the other way. There were few buildings with more than two stories. the town seemed to bustle at all hours, especially during the long nights of winter when on 22 December, the sun peeped over the horizon for about twenty to thirty minutes in twenty four hours and snow lay everywhere, unmarred in most places, but packed tight on the roads for easier travel than in summer.

That winter the snowfall was much greater than usual. It gave the wild animals a bad time covering their hunting territories. They were forced to use the cleared highways which gave everybody a good opportunity to view them almost daily. It was good that the hunting laws were strict because the animals became easy targets. There were some uncomfortable incidents as a result of this heavy snowfall. Some people took advantage of it and many animals, which might have escaped molestation, were shot. I mention only a few of these. It was reported that a 180 pound wolf was killed on the highway in the Big Delta area. A big bull buffalo bison took on a motor vehicle and immobilised it. The passengers were not injured. A beautiful silver wolf and its black mate in the Fort Yukon area were ambushed and killed. As a result of the heavy snowfall, they had been forced to feed off the husky teams chained in the backyard of almost every household. Contrary to popular belief, wolves do not kill for pleasure. This pair killed one husky about every five days for food. The residents became unnecessarily nervous about this for their own lives. I say unnecessarily because there is no verified account of wolves (or whales I might add) having made an unprovoked direct attack on man. During my visits to Fort Yukon for hospital duty during the period of this incident, I was advised to carry a weapon, but it was not necessary in my opinion. I acquired the pelt of the silver male and bequeathed it to a friend.

* * *

The Arctic Aeromedical Laboratory, on Ladd Air Force Base, now called Fort Wainwright, had not been occupied for very long. Much equipment was still wanting and some building was still in progress. I was Director of the Department of Arctic Medicine, in charge of bacteriological research, veterinary research, Arctic medicine, epidemiology, field biology and any medically related problems that might come our way.

It became obvious that there was not going to be any opportunity to pursue my "Holy Grail". I had been "fast talked", but my contract was for only a year and there was much that could be done that could be exciting because most of what I was given responsibility for had qualified staff to carry out the work and they were in areas with which I was familiar. Most of the staff had been sitting around waiting for something to happen and needed only a little spark to set them going. I tried to get some physiology on human subjects going, but I just could not get anything in this area off the ground beyond the type of work that could not be treated in any manner other than anecdotal.

There was a Department of Physiology, but its Director and staff was not interested in my problem. So I temporarily put aside the pursuit of my Holy Grail and put my efforts into support of the bacteriological, parasitological, field biological work with my personal efforts oriented towards epidemiology and medical services. The last was wished on me in part by the Alaskan Department of Health and the Episcopalian Church in Fort Yukon where it had a hospital.

The Air Force was most supportive of our interests and made a Beaver, a small single engined aircraft, with pilot, available for my use. Although I was a civilian, the US armed forces gives its civilian employees equivalent military ranks which are honoured by them and the Public Service in every way. At this time my equivalent rank was Brigadier General and this was of great assistance in carrying out my projects and other responsibilities which fell to my lot. My pilot was also a keen fisherman and we carried our rods in the fuselage of the Beaver. When opportunity arose and we were on floats, we would land on a lake and fish for land-locked salmon or whatever was offering. This we did by taxiing up wind and drifting down wind the length of the lake casting or trolling our lines behind.

With the assistance of this plane, much was done. I was able to medically service the Episcopalian Mission hospital, the Frank Starbuck Hospital, in Fort Yukon. It was about 110 miles north of Fairbanks and sat directly on the Arctic Circle. The hospital had a matron and nurses, but lost its doctor a short time after my arrival in the area. I could not refuse their plea for me to fill the void. This would have been difficult without the little Beaver to fly me to and from Fort Yukon on weekends and whenever emergencies arose.

At Fort Yukon the work load was not always heavy. A part Indian woman of indeterminate age who had heard I was a keen fisherman would wake me in the early mornings and take me fishing for northern pike. Sometimes this would be a rude and cold awakening and the trip on her outboard powered flat bottomed John boat was often miserably cold. She had favourite spots for these which were backwaters off the Yukon River. Once there any discomforts disappeared. There was always fish and the pike fought well with spectacular aerial displays on 8 pound test line. Avoiding the weed during these battles added to the challenge these fish presented. In true Indian fashion few words were spoken. Our relationship was a tacit one and in this manner we enjoyed our friendship and mutual enjoyment of fishing.

* * *

The patients I saw at the hospital and at out-patients were mostly Athapascan Indians with an occasional white trader, trapper or Eskimo. At first I was surprised that tuberculosis was here in the Arctic at about the same level of prevalence as in the Pacific. This was true all over the Arctic. It was a misnomer to call tuberculosis the "scourge of the Pacific". In truth it was the scourge of the economically underprivileged, no matter where or who they were.

I am sure that we dealt with only a small percentage of the ailments of the people of Fort Yukon and its environs. On the hit and run assistance basis I was able to give to the service, I was not able to delve into the depth of what ailments might have lain under the surface. As in the Cook Islands, there must have been many. The Arctic also had its share of medicine men and shamans. Most times that was all that was available.

The Indians did not handle alcohol well. For some reason, perhaps because of cost, they preferred and were able to get wine. The drinking of it was accompanied by the usual outbreaks of fights and domestic strife and some ended up in the hospital for treatment. Eskimos seemed to handle this problem in a more satisfactory manner. The Indian population tended to be concentrated more in the central areas while the Eskimos were concentrated more on the coast, but with a sprinkling all over Alaska. For all practical purposes Fort Yukon was Indian territory.

* * *

I was also able to do some mercy work. One of these involved Arctic Village, an Athapascan Indian village of around 100 souls, about one hundred and fifty miles north of Fort Yukon as the crow flies. This village was experiencing infant deaths and one of its men had travelled a tortuous 200 miles or so by dog sled to Fort Yukon to plead for medical help. The Department of Health requested the Air Force for my services to fly to the rescue.

It was January at the height of winter. I was made aware of the hazards of the flight. The Air Force was very conscious of these. It had just lost some personnel who had been forced down somewhere north of Fort Yukon near enough to the area I was asked to go. The search had revealed they had made no attempt to light a fire or use the emergency rations and equipment with which the aircraft had been routinely supplied. One of the crew had been found some distance from the aircraft naked. They all died of cold exposure. Panic may have played the major role in this tragedy. There was no other obvious reason for it.

The village had no airstrip but a landing could be made on the ice of the nearby river using skis. The Air Force made it plain to the Department of Health that they would not risk its little Beaver or its pilot. They told me that, as a civilian, I could go if I wanted to, but they would not be responsible for whatever might happen. I could not refuse, so I told the Health Department that I would go if they could find a bush pilot to fly me there. I vaguely entertained the idea that no bush pilot would volunteer for the job. This was a vain hope because bush pilots I knew were made of sterner stuff.

The bush pilots of Alaska are legendary, a breed unto themselves. They will fly anywhere and land on any kind of airstrip or, if necessary, on no airstrip at all. They were responsible for opening up Alaska as their equivalents were responsible for opening up Canada and the northern US. Accidents occurred, but these were so rare that it was not a matter for great concern. The Laboratory used their services frequently and the places they would land their planes were unbelievable. Many times the landings were hair raising to say the least. Flying is boring to me and I think to most who do it hour after hour. Some bush pilots overcame this by handing over the controls to a passenger, giving course instructions and requesting that they be woken at a certain time or when a certain landmark was observed. In this way I put in many hours of flying time.

The Health Department put the word out to all bush pilots who might be in the area. I do not know how many responded, but the one selected said he would pick me up at Fort Yukon, the nearest fuelling place to our destination. The little Beaver was allowed to take me that far. My heart sank when I saw the plane that was to take me. I had imagined that, with all the talk of hazards, it would at least be a two engined aircraft. Instead it was a one-engined plane equipped with skis. The pilot looked at me with my 200 pounds plus and remarked that he hoped I was not taking along everything and the kitchen sink because fuel was going to be touch and go. I told him I did not have much more than I was wearing, some change of clothes, antibiotics, palliatives and some intravenous fluids. He asked me how long he would have to wait for me. I told him about a week to ten days should be about right to get the job done properly.

"Well, Chum," He said, "You'll be staying on your own, "I'll be flying back and will come for you in 10 days time." I had not expected anything else.

After stowing my gear, he sighed and told me to hop in and away we went. It was a clear sunny day and the view was breathtaking winter scene of undisturbed snow and ice. If there had been wild life about, there was no evidence of it. The snow was unriven. We flew into the eastern part of the Brook's Range of mountains. The soaring peaks and snow fields of midwinter were a sight to behold, a vast, desolate, rugged land where, it was easy to believe that no man had ventured.

I find conversation on a small plane difficult and I usually make little attempt to start or pursue one. That's how it was this time. So I never got to know the pilot on a personal basis. Our on-ground contact was minimal. I would like to acknowledge his part in this mission. He was typical of the breed and that is saying a great deal.

I could not help thinking of the great difficulties we would encounter if our plane was forced down. I had brought my own survival equipment: a well-honed hunting knife, a small compass, some C rations, my 357 magnum pistol and my medical bag. Looking down on this wild, beautiful, expansive and lonely desolation made me and my survival gear seem puny and hopelessly inadequate.

I had not seen anything that resembled survival equipment on the plane when I stowed my gear, but it must have been there. For a moment, I thought he might have had the same views as Cape Horn sailors who refused to learn to swim because that would ensure a quick end if they went overboard. That seemed to be the attitude of the crew of the Air Force plane which came down in this area a little while earlier. I have had enough experience of survival incidents to reject this attitude altogether and know of many occasions where lives would have been saved if simple rules had been followed.

The Air Force crew mentioned were found within three days. This was unusually long but, if they had half tried, they could have survived those three days and several more easily. All they had to do was stay with the plane, light a fire, use their survival equipment and rations and wait for rescue. It will come, as it did. An aeroplane, its crew, a shelter of any kind and a simple display of signals in the snow are easier to find than crew wandering around in the wasteland. If the weather turns into a blizzard, digging a snow cave in the nearest snow drift and sitting it out is the best course of action.

Similar rules apply to survival at sea. As long as the boat floats, stay with it. It is easier to spot than a life-raft or a bobbing head in the water. Masterly inactivity gives one a much better chance than active efforts indulged in only because one feels that one must do something. There are many cases of vessels found abandoned but the crew lost. The Hokule'a capsize was another prime example; the crew member who set out to find help was lost while those who stayed with the capsized Hokule'a were saved. The examples are numerous. After reviewing the survival possibilities that I knew while flying over this desolation I was left in no doubt as to what would be the best course to follow if we came down: sit tight, stay alive and wait. Where we were going was no secret and it would only be a matter of time before we would be found. Too much emphasis is put on food in survival conditions. Its great if you have it, but not having it is of less consequence than most people believe. Water is much more important. If you have water, you can survive without food for up to three weeks or more. Without water, however, one cannot survive much longer than three days.

After making my emergency survival plans, I felt much better. In other circumstances I would have just sat back, relaxed and fallen asleep. This was not possible because we were flying low enough for me to marvel at the spectacular vistas of the Arctic that kept unfolding below.

Finally we spotted Arctic Village lying about half a mile from the bank of the upper reaches of the East Fork river, a tributary of the Chandalar river which in turn flows into the Yukon. The people also spotted us and were already starting on their way to the river's edge. The river was a frozen sheet of ice lightly covered with snow. But it was not flat. There were pressure ridges all over it, caused by the expansion of water as it turns into ice. I looked at the pilot, but he ignored me and continued circling, I presumed looking for a likely place to land. None of it looked good to me and thoughts of flying back with mission unaccomplished passed through my head.

In the end the pilot made his decision and we were on our approach to a landing. It still did not look too good to me and kept looking worse the closer we came. It flashed through my mind that we were on skis and skis have no brakes. I held on tight, but, before I could worry any further, we were on ice and dodging the pressure ridges like a race car around the chicanes. Through it all I held my breath and it was only after we stopped and were taxiing towards the waiting crowd that I let out my breath with a shuddering sigh. The pilot looked at me and smiled. I don't remember returning his smile.

Stiffly, I got out of the plane. The pilot helped me out with my things and said, "Good luck, chum, see you in ten days." I said my thanks and wished him luck also. He got back into the plane and in a moment was whirling away in the direction of Fort Yukon and for what passed as civilisation in these parts.

The people of the village stood where they had stopped at the edge of the ice. I stood where the pilot had left me on the sheet of ice of the river. We stared at one another, neither making the first move. There were no means of communication between Arctic Village and the outside world and my arrival was not heralded and for all they knew I was just another stranger. Finally I walked towards them and one of them detached himself from the crowd and came towards me. As we shook hands I told him who I was and that I had come to try to solve their medical problem. He took my medical bag and signalled others to pick up the rest of my gear. He informed me that he was the headman of the village. I had hoped he would be "Big Chief Something Or Other", but they seemed to have run out of these. We made our way towards the village in the brisk, windless cold of about minus 50 degrees F (-45.56C) in the dull steel light of the chilly Arctic twilight.

The village consisted of small houses lined up on either side of what passed for a road with smoke coming out of the galvanised piping smokestacks sticking out of the tin roofs. They were much alike in size and of simple foursquare design of one room with an outside pit latrine and the usual sled huskies chained to posts just out of reach of one another. They were of variegated wood construction, probably hand sawn. Climatically the village was still in the taiga (tree belt), but edging towards the tundra (treeless, wind-packed snow belt), the two regions that broadly characterise the Arctic. I was shown to my quarters which was a house just like the others. A fire was started. The inside of the house was still as cold as the outside, but it warmed up quickly. Most houses in the Arctic and subarctic are small, so that they are easy to heat. In every house I entered, and in the end I was a guest of most, the measured temperature was never below 80 degrees F (26.67C) and some were above this.

After I had installed myself in my quarters, I asked the headman to take me to see the patients. There were ten of them left. Some had succumbed. On examination they appeared to be suffering from a fulminating type of pneumonia, not unlike that which used to afflict our Cook Islands infants and the main cause of the high infant mortality. I could not ascertain any circumstances which might have brought the condition about. Except for an odd plane to bring in some supplies during the summer, there had been no contact with the outside world. If it were intrinsically caused by their own bugs, it could be caused by the pneumococcus bug normally in the throat of man waiting for the right conditions to blossom forth. If this were so, the condition should respond well to antibiotics. I treated the patients with penicillin, still the best of the antibiotics. They all recovered without incident. However, I needed the extra days to insure that there were no new cases and no relapses. As it happened there were none and those extra days turned into almost three weeks. I began to wonder whether the outside world had forgotten me.

* * *

As was my custom when I visited isolated villages or islands, I gave everybody a physical examination and found no serious medical problems needing further attention than I was able to provide. So there was much time on my hands. The headman and many of his cronies and I became close friends. I learnt that they had created Arctic Village some years before to escape the evils of civilisation of Fort Yukon from where they had originated. They told me that the evil life their youth were exposed to in Fort Yukon forced them to emigrate and settle here. Their numbers were just over one hundred and they felt that those responsible for them being here had done the right thing. They were happy, they explained. However, the house I occupied was one which was empty because its owners had returned to the evils of Fort Yukon. Happiness is relative.

Their needs were few and the occasional flights that came during the summer brought their few outside needs. My lack of knowledge of their needs, the weight restriction and the speed with which things happened had precluded my bringing any goods with me except the few cans of C Rations. I chose to eat what they ate. They lived on caribou meat which they told me had to include the brown back fat, the partially digested lichen of the intestines and the offal.

About every three days some of the young men would harness their huskies to sleds and hunt caribou for the whole village. Three to four caribou seemed to suffice the whole village for this period. Any extra was stored in the frozen state. This diet made nutritional sense and I found no difficulty in conforming to it. I was used to strange foods and never refrained from eating the foods of the many societies with which I came into contact. I did this on the assumption that what did them no harm, would do me no harm. I cannot remember this practise ever causing me problems.

Finally, some three weeks after my arrival, we heard the motor of the plane. It was time to leave. Suddenly an indefinable air of gloom fell on the village. I was not fully conscious of it at first, but, in retrospect, it seemed to have started at the sound of the plane. At that time I was only conscious of the fact that at last I could return to home and family. It seemed that everybody was in my little house helping me get ready, but with gloom and in quiet silence. I gradually began to recognise it as something serious. It then dawned on me that they were unhappy I was leaving. I was embarrassed and did not know how to handle it. This had happened to me before. I had been marooned on the island of Mauke for a similar period. I could not handle it that time either. I had never been able to handle similar occasions involving Polynesian welcomes and farewells.

I continued my preparations, by now infected by the emotions behind this display of silence and gloom. I could not avoid becoming silent and gloomy myself, and even more embarrassed. I cursed myself for not being able to master the situation. In the pervading silence and gloom we made our way to the plane waiting on the sheet of ice of the river with the pilot standing by and the engine still idling. To have stopped the engine in the sub-zero temperature would have jeopardised its ability to restart without warm-up facilities.

As we moved down the road, the tears and the wailing began and increased in crescendo as we neared the departure point. The headman clung to my right arm while his weeping wife clung to the other and others clung to them as though forming a chain of contact with each other and me. Others walked sobbing closely behind. It seemed that most, if not all, the village was my farewell retinue. It made me feel worse than ever. In such situations I have managed to control my emotions knowing full well that, if I once gave in to them, I would become a blubbering idiot. As before, I managed it this time, but only by occupying my thoughts in making a scientific objective observation of this scene and comparing it to the old familiar scenes of farewells back home. I had used this ruse of objective scientific observation to control my emotions several times before. Somehow we made it to the plane without my breaking down.

The pilot, who had been watching, said, "What the hell have you been up to, Chum ?" I gave him a knowing smile which seemed to satisfy him and away we flew from my Arctic Paradise. I did not even bother to ask him what had delayed him. His answer, I am sure, would have been a knowing smile. And it would have meant nothing more than mine.

* * *

Our research covered a variety of subjects. We did a good deal of protective clothing and equipment testing which brought out some fundamentals which we thought were important.[12] Most of the clothing designed by the armed forces and the clothing industry was for protection against cold and wind only. These did not take into account what would happen[5] when the wearer was physically active and thereby generating a great deal of heat and sweat of his own. Armed forces personnel do this in carrying out their usual military functions. Once this condition is generated and the physical activity ceases, you have a potentially dangerous condition of losing heat rapidly through evaporation and even becoming encased in your own frozen sweat-laden clothing.

The Eskimo had solved this problem by evolving the loosely fitting parka which, apart from its heat conserving qualities, could be adjusted to ventilate any developing overheating and high humidity caused by sweating when physical exertion was required. This was done by a drawstring around the hood opening and another around the waist or bottom hem of the parka. Draw these tight when you want to conserve body heat and loosen them to dissipate excess body heat and humidity when these were increased during physical activity. This worked on the principle that hot moist air rises and is known as the "chimney effect". The adjustments of the Eskimo Parka to deal with this varying problem are infinite.

The higher military personnel seemed to be immune to these niceties of Arctic clothing design. However, in low physical activity conditions the military clothing was very good. The Arctic sleeping bag protected me from freezing for two nights in the open at minus 67 degrees F (+19.44C). There was a fire. Of course, it must have helped, but fire or not I doubt that I would have survived with any other sleeping bag.

Another project we thought was important was the finding that field mice (oeconomus oeconomus, or voles) and other small animals live happily in the Arctic in temperatures ranging down to minus 70 degrees F (about -57C) and lower. The physics of surface area to mass ratio clearly indicated that they should not be surviving in these temperatures. So Bill Pruitt our field biologist, set out to unravel the mystery. He found that these "little critters", as he referred to them, were able to live happily at these temperatures because they were never exposed to the low air temperatures except on the very limited occasions they came to the surface. Their world was under the snow in the spaces created by the ground cover where the temperatures were never much below freezing. Bill with much effort characterised the temperature gradients of this world and showed that all over the taiga and the tundra, undersnow and underground temperatures were just below freezing. This is very much warmer than minus 70 degrees F or about minus 57 degrees Celsius.

Eskimos were fully aware of this. It is the reason they build (or used to build) their winter quarters almost fully underground. This precluded their need to heat their quarters from minus 70 degrees F to a comfortable temperature. They needed to do this only from plus 30 degrees F (-1.11C). When the spring thaw came and threatened to flood their winter homes, they abandoned them for skin tents until winter came around again.

It was, therefore, natural that we would try to apply this knowledge to Arctic survival situations. So some of us went igloo building. The idea was that, in order to use this ground heat, one needed to remove the snow, thus exposing the source of heat, and build an insulated shelter over the top to capture and retain the heat so released. No doubt there are several ways this can be done. But our idea was to assist the military in survival situations using materials at hand. No better insulating material was universally available in the Arctic than snow, we thought, and an igloo-like structure made of snow seemed the best way to use it. Eskimos had thought so too from the earliest of times.

Igloo building can only be easily done with wind packed tundra snow. In this state it is composed of tiny air cells and conforms to the thermodynamic principles of a perfect insulator next to a vacuum. Therefore on the tundra, if you are able to cut your blocks down to ground surface and build your igloo over this, it will be heated up to an inside temperature just below freezing without much assistance. The use of one candle will do it quicker, about a half hour. An inside temperature above freezing must not be allowed for this will destroy the insulating properties of the igloo.

An eight foot diameter igloo can comfortably serve four to six people and protect them from cold, wind and blizzard conditions. The taiga snow is quite unsuitable for igloo building and our attempts to adapt the igloo to it to capture and conserve the exposed ground heat were not inconsiderable. Our team tried packing the snow by stamping it down with snow shoes and skis and cutting the blocks from the resulting packed snow. The results were generally unsatisfactory. Using a blown up weather balloon over which snow was shovelled, and then removing the balloon by deflating it and modifying the inside space by digging out the snow, proved to be a poor best effort. We simplified everything down to scraping the snow down to ground level and making a structure over this with any materials at hand and covering this with say a parachute and piling snow over that. This proved to be the best bet in survival situations.

Disappointingly, the Survival Group of the Air Force and the higher ups, were immune to our efforts or failed to recognise the principles involved. They were stuck with their makeshift tents made out of parachutes, which had no insulating properties. They were raised over the surface of the snow, which Bill had shown was the coldest area of the temperature gradient. They continued to ignore the free heat available to them a few inches below the snow surface. It would seem that regardless of whose military forces it is, they continue to disregard these simple measures and the fine insulating properties of the snow surrounding them.

* * *

Also through Bill Pruitt, the Laboratory became involved in saving the wolf from the extermination efforts of the Fish and Wildlife Service which had brought its own stateside brand of prejudices into Alaska. In the US proper, the wolf and the coyote preyed on cattle and sheep as these invaded their territory. Although the coyote has managed to survive in small numbers, the wolf has been successfully eliminated on the basis that they were pests. Despite the fact that Alaska supports no cattle or sheep, the Fish and Wildlife Service still applied the same thinking to the wolf and the most extraordinary measures were taken to eliminate them from this refuge. Because there were no cattle and sheep, the wolf's useful and age-old purpose in culling out the weak and the sick from the caribou herds was used as the excuse. Some of the methods used were bizarre. None were as bizarre as the dropping of poisoned meat indiscriminately into the wild life territory. The wolf is not by nature a scavenger, therefore, this practise affected other animals such as the bear, the fox, the wolverine and many other creatures as harmless as the wolf in this natural wildlife territory.

Bill was a pioneer of those who took up the cudgels to save the wolf. After several years of unpopular effort he along with a few others convinced the world that the wolf is not as depicted by Red Riding Hood and the many fiction stories maligning his noble qualities. As mentioned earlier, there is no authenticated unprovoked attack on man by a wolf. Except in rare cases, animals of the wild do everything they can to avoid man. They know that man is their worst enemy.

Animals are smarter than we give them credit. They soon learn what is safe and what is not. They very quickly learn the boundaries of sanctuaries. How often have hunters on an unarmed survey reported an abundance of game which became invisible when they went forth with guns to hunt them. How often have fishermen reported that a successful lure soon becomes unsuccessful. Wild animal photographers go amongst them with reports of abortive charges only, while armed hunters are regularly reported killed. In Alaska, no one was allowed to hunt within a quarter mile on either side of any highway and every animal clearly knew this rule.

Once I had an opportunity to test it. I had driven to a favourite spot of mine on the Chatanika River when I spotted a black bear not far from the road. I thought I would have a game with him. I got out of the car with my shot-gun which I often carried in the hope of some ptarmigan. He took absolutely no notice except to stare at me. I walked towards him and he bounded off a hundred yards or so and sat on his haunches. He waited till I came closer and repeated the manoeuvre with a playful toss of his head. I tried to edge him towards the quarter mile boundary, but he knew what I was trying to do and continued taunting me. We must have done this for about 2 miles before I returned to my vehicle quite sure that we both knew the rules.

* * *

I became fascinated with the tapeworm of hydatid disease (echinococcosis) in Alaska, having had some contact with it in New Zealand where the dog is the host and the sheep the intermediate host.[13] Man is an accidental intermediate host. In Alaska there are two types of the hydatid disease tapeworm. The host of Echinococcus Granulosus is the wolf and the host of Echinococcus Alveolars is the fox. The dog can be host to both. The intermediate host is the moose for the former and the vole for the latter. Man can be an accidental host to either by infection with the eggs through contact with any of the three hosts, the dog, the wolf or the fox, with the dog playing the more important role by having closer contact with man.

The disease in man produces cysts in every part of the body with the liver being the most common site. The military personnel stationed at Gambell on St. Lawrence Island as determined by blood tests had about half the rate found in the natives of Gambell. Studies indicated that the disease was widespread in the Alaskan Mainland and the Bering Sea islands.

* * *

The Alaskan Health Department prevailed on me to fly to Kotzebue on the west coast of Alaska on the Bering Sea and the village of Kiana on the Kobuk river not too far from Kotzebue to investigate a reported outbreak of infectious hepatitis.[14] So off I went with an assistant and what paraphernalia we thought we needed. I did not use the Beaver because there were fairly regular milk run flights to the Kotzebue area. I flew the plane most of the way while the pilot slept. I enjoyed doing that and the pilot's need for sleep seemed greater than mine. My assistant and I put up at the only hotel in Kotzebue. It was not the Ritz, but it served our purpose.

There had been a dry spell and the sources of water, collected from the roof in 50 US gallon drums or purchased from a vendor at $2 per 50 gallons, was at a premium. The village is strung along the seaside and looks out over the Bering Sea in a north-westerly direction. On the shore side of the village, undulating grassy and marshy land reaches about a half mile to the edge of several ponds which played an important part in the causation of the outbreak.

Kotzebue had a population of about 1000 permanent residents. Ninety five percent of them were Eskimo and the rest were Civil Aeronautics Administration (CAA) personnel housed about a quarter of a mile to the south of the village. In addition there were a few traders, school teachers, hospital personnel and the clergy. It was August and, at this time of the year, the population increased by some two hundred people due to an influx of Eskimos from nearby villages. These people lived in tents in two camps, one at the northern end and the other at the southern end of Kotzebue proper. There was little in the way of hygiene facilities. Annually they came to Kotzebue to complete their hunting and fishing for winter food and clothing - an important activity as their winter survival depended on it. As transients and for other reasons, the water supply arrangements to the permanent residents were not readily available to them.

Generally, infectious hepatitis appears in a population in a sporadic manner with cases here and there, separated fairly widely both in time of appearance and geographic location, with no apparent relationship to one another. In Kotzebue the cases occurred between August 4 to 29 and over two thirds of them in South Camp. This was quite uncharacteristic of infectious hepatitis and most characteristic of a waterborne transmitted disease. So we looked for water as the source and it did not take long to pin this down. Of the seven ponds, the edges of North Pond and South Pond which were closest to the temporary camps, were littered with faeces. These ponds had banks which were high enough to provide some degree of seclusion and privacy. However, North Camp had access to a well and its use by them was sufficient reason why cases in this camp were minimal.

Bacterial counts made on the water from these ponds and other sources of water ranged up to 5000 per millilitre. Of the nine sources only three were negative for human contamination. The commercial and the CAA sources were amongst these. Once the epidemiology of the outbreak was clarified we advised the people how to avoid further infection and in addition we gave household contacts Gamma Globulin. No further cases developed.

Cases were also occurring in other villages nearby, but transport limitations precluded visiting them except the village of Kiana where, as was probably the case in other villages, the distribution of cases was within the incubation period indicating a common source of infection which we were never able to track down. With difficulty we advised all villages in the area how to avoid further cases, but could do little else.

There was ample evidence that the inhabitants of Alaska, both Eskimo and Indian and, by association others, were demonstrating the public health problems of a Third World. There was no doubt in my mind that the conditions which prevailed in Kotzebue and Kiana prevailed throughout Alaska and that the conditions we saw that summer took place every summer causing epidemic or endemic situations involving one or another of the infectious diseases. A study we carried out on enteric pathogens in Barrow, the most northern settlement in Alaska, further confirmed this probability.[4]

* * *

In my medical travels throughout Alaska, I had opportunities to examine the population and treat the sick. I was struck with the similarity of chest complaints between its indigenous inhabitants and those of Polynesia. The prime complaints that came to my attention were the pneumonias and tuberculosis. In most instances these went untreated and I felt that those I treated in passing were a drop in the proverbial bucket of those needing treatment. Poor economic circumstances, poor communications and isolation from medical services were taking their toll.

My willingness to respond to their call through the Alaskan Health Department seemed a puny effort in comparison to the magnitude of the problem. It gave pitiful hope which could not be sustained or increased to have sufficient and useful impact. Because of the little I could do and the false hope it gave, I felt exasperated and often thought that I made things worse than better. I gave hope, but could not sustain it. But I had already learnt that one does what one can to improve our human lot without worrying about whether it can be sustained or not. Sadly I am informed things have not improved significantly.

There had been no light at the end of the tunnel in the search for my "Holy Grail". My contract with the Air Force was nearing its end and I thought I might as well return to the Pacific and give my attention to the medical problems of my own region. Then one day a medical Army Colonel, Tim Timmerman, from Army Headquarters in Washington, turned up and without much ado offered me the post of Chief Research Physician at the United States Army Medical Research Laboratory in Fort Knox Kentucky. I was to take charge of the human research programme. I could not believe my ears that there was a place that was using human subjects and I was to take charge of it totally.

Suddenly, at the end of the tunnel there was now a blinding, blaze of light. But it faded as suddenly as it had appeared. It was being dampened by the emotions of caution that rose inside me. I had been fast talked before. I indicated my doubts. Tim reassured me and, on second thoughts, I said to myself, "What the hell, it's a better chance towards my purpose than what I have here." So I agreed and on the very day after my contract with the Air Force ended, we were on the other road out of Alaska which headed south along the Mighty Fraser River towards Seattle, through the Western States, across the Bible Belt, into Kentucky and Fort Knox just south of Louisville.

* * *

Soon after we arrived in Alaska, we acquired a blue eyed husky whose father as well as his mother were half wolf, the father being the most recently bred from the wolf. The mother, Jenny, had a big litter and the breeder, Libby, well known for her dog sled racing abilities, decided that she would get rid of all but six of the litter so that Jenny could look after the remainder properly.

I asked Libby to allow me to hand raise those assigned to be "put down". Libby told me that it was impossible to raise a wolf bred husky by hand feeding. I begged her to let me try and I spent the next three days trying my best to keep them alive by three hour feedings. Within three days I had lost a great deal of sleep and they all died. It was not easy to believe that these bundles of hard strong muscle which felt like cricket balls or baseballs, not at all like fluffy soft puppies, should survive only with the tender care of their mother. But I learnt the hard way. Prior to this we had picked out Kiona, the Polynesian word for snow, and called him Ki for short and awaited the eight weeks that Jenny was needed to take care of him and not some damn fool human being like me.

Ki became part of the family, but had to be taught some manners. Growling, he grabbed and wolfed his food. In time he was convinced to desist from these bad habits. I had to stop him from guarding the home and its boundaries. I tried to make him realise his great strength and to be gentle. The first two he learnt quickly, but in a stubborn kind of way. The last he learnt only after he broke the hind leg of his close friend, a neighbour's cocker spaniel while playing with him. He was genuinely upset by this incident. Fortunately, I was able to take care of the break and kept the patient at my home until the fracture healed. Thereafter, Ki learnt his strength and took care never to harm another creature, man or beast.

For all practical purposes Ki was all wolf. He was a stickler for a code of ethics. Life was made up of routine, cleanliness of person and habits and the importance of the pack of which we as a family became. However, we, in his opinion, did not suffice to satisfy his leadership qualities. In Fairbanks, he left us for a period of three weeks and led a pack of huskies until caught and impounded. The photograph in the Daily News Miner of the pack and later the impoundment with his photo as the leader, alerted us of his whereabouts. The whole family immediately paid a visit to the pound and claimed him. In the meantime he had befriended the pound keeper who spoke highly of his virtues. We scolded and teased Ki about his escapade and he did not repeat it again in quite this way.

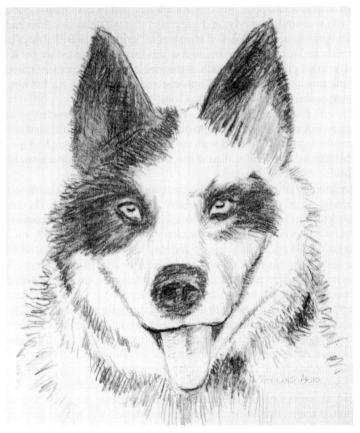

His qualities of leadership constantly showed through and became well known. Bill Pruitt had a team of huskies and I asked him if he would put Ki in the team. Bill said that he would harness him as right wheel, which is the position immediately in front of the sled, so that we could keep an eye on him. I rode the sled while Bill stood on the back to do all the mushing, heeing and hawing bit. In real life mushing is not done, but heeing and hawing for right and left is.

Huskies are always raring to go once they are in harness and there is no need for mushing at all. We took off. That is all of us except Ki. He decided that this was not for him. I yelled at him. Bill yelled at him. The leader way up front looked back and yipped at him. The husky next to him in the harness bit him. But Ki lay in a foetal position skating along on his back. We stopped and Bill's lead dog swung back to look at things. I bent down and talked to Ki and he stood up unperturbed. I was mortified. Obviously this story was not going to stay hidden in the wilderness.

Since Ki was now standing up and staring fixedly ahead, I gaily said to Bill, "He's OK now. Let's go." More mortification. Ki lay on his back forming a sled runner of it and was again towed, yelled at, yipped at and bitten until blood flowed. Again we stopped. My mortification turned to desperation. I looked at Bill, who was smiling wryly, and suggested that we unharness him and that I get him home as best I could. Bill is a lover of "critters", as Bill always referred to animals, and it was perhaps because of this that he suggested we put Ki in the lead. By now I did not think much of the idea of further experimentation. I did not think much of Ki either. Bill unharnessed my bloodied Ki, led him to the front and exchanged him with his lead dog.

I thought I was imagining things, but Ki seemed to be standing up straight and taking notice. Bill and I got into our respective places on the sled and when he gave the signal, Ki took off with the high yips of a team dog and the rest of the team behind him. Bill smiled at me and I smiled back with a heart bursting with pride.

The strength of Ki was something not easily believed. His neck was thick and strong. A collar other than a choke chain would not stay on. He could tow me and kids on a sled using the choke chain as a harness. He could break a normal husky chain by extending the chain to its limit and snapping his head. I had to have a plough chain made up and ring bolted to the house foundation.

He never used his teeth on any animal or human. His disciplinary method was to strike with his paw and bowl the offending dog over. That was all that was necessary and that is how he broke his friend's leg. He used his paws like a cat and manipulated things with them. After disciplining another dog, that dog no longer existed. If any disciplined dog inadvertently got in his way, he simply walked over him as though he were part of the ground. To Ki, that dog simply did not exist. After knowing Ki, I appreciated the Mowgli stories more than ever and the perspicacity of Rudyard Kipling in portraying the wolf.

Working huskies of Alaska, Canada and Greenland are bred back to the wolf as often as necessary to give strength and endurance for work. In the work situation, it seems that ownership can be transferred without problems. In my experience, this is not true when they become involved in an intimate relationship with a human or a family. A wolf mates for life and stays with the same pack, usually siblings, for life.

The wolf, like the wild goose, when the mate dies, life is ended. While in Alaska and Greenland, I witnessed instance after instance of huskies left behind by military personnel after their tour of duty ended. Within a short time after separation, as little as three weeks, their loving pets have become totally recalcitrant towards their new owners and the animals have had to be destroyed. In particular this was the case for Satan, Ki's full brother. They were entirely unable to transfer their affections or loyalties to their new owners. When it came time to leave Alaska, I was determined that this was not going to happen to Ki, so we took him to Kentucky. We prepared to leave Fairbanks in a storm of Letters to the Editor that we were taking out of Alaska one of the greatest dogs that Alaska has bred and we should not be allowed to do so. Only Libby and perhaps one or two others understood my motives.

It was only during our first days back in civilisation that we realised that we had what looked like and in some other, but harmless, ways acted as a wild animal. Ki in his best humour looked the most savage of beasts. When people saw him, they froze in their tracks. Constantly I had to kick Ki playfully, pull his ear or tail to convey the impression that his look was worse than his bite.

The dogs of civilisation would take one look at Ki and take off in the opposite direction. When I took him to the vet for his injections the vet froze. At my request Ki got on the table for his injections while I unfroze the vet. I assured him that it would be all right for him to give the injection. From that moment on the vet loved him nearly as much as we did and would drop by just to say hello to Ki.

In civilisation, owning Ki was not all a bed of roses. Strangers kept freezing at the sight of him and a few had to be helped out of this state. Ki loved beagles, they could take food from him and sleep with him in his big kennel. When loose he formed an all beagle pack which roamed the environs of Elizabethtown, quite harmlessly I tried to assure everybody.

Once we showed him as a siberian husky. We bathed and made him beautiful every way we could. The fact that we had to do it twice because he rolled in the dirt was beside the point. In the ring with son Tim as handler, he was beautiful. His guard hairs shone like silver strands under the fluorescent lights and he stood and walked like the king that he was. The judge refused to get in the ring with him and gave him first prize from outside it.

After three years in civilisation, he contracted canine weils disease to which he had no resistance. After nearly a week, bleeding from every orifice and with the close professional attention of his friend the vet and myself, there was no hope. Then, in the early morning while I was attending him, he rose from a prostrate state to his full four square height, raised his head and let out the most horrendous wolf howl, sprang high in the air and fell on his back dead. That day a Wolf died.

* * *

Our stay in Alaska had been packed with action. The whole family seemed to enjoy it. Lydia, unlike myself, seemed to enjoy the military aspects of living on Base and having contacts with military personnel. Perhaps it had something to do with the Duke of Wellington, an ancestor of hers by marriage. The kids and I enjoyed the fishing and I particularly enjoyed fishing for pike on spinning reel gear and fly fishing for grayling, a great fighter for its size. I enjoyed the nearness of the wild life.

My medical work had brought me close to the Indians and the Eskimos and I hoped that they enjoyed knowing me as much as I enjoyed knowing them. My research work and that of my colleagues had been fruitful and I would like to believe useful. As a South Pacific Island boy, the Arctic was fascinating, beautiful and spectacular in its own way, but I did not feel that a steady diet of it was for me. The camaraderie of the people reminded me of home and it would do the world good to borrow some of it.

CHAPTER TEN

Feet on the Ground, Head in Space

Looking at the stars always makes me dream, as simply as I dream over the black dots representing towns and villages on a map. Why, I ask myself, shouldn't the shining dots of the sky be as accessible as the black dots on the map of France? VINCENT VAN GOGH

In Kentucky, we settled in Elizabethtown. The United States Army Medical Research Laboratory (USAMRL) at Fort Knox, where I was going to work, was under the command of Colonel Reece Blair, commonly known to many as Joe. Reece, a medical doctor himself, had done a good deal of research in the environmental field of cold and heat research. The Civilian Director was Dr Floyd Odel who had a PhD in physics and had done some definitive work using high speed photography in the study of the destructive effects of bullets and missiles. Reece and Floyd, like me, had both been recently assigned to USAMRL. We were all new on the job so it could have been a situation of the blind leading the blind. The three of us became good friends and worked well together.

Lydia and the kids settled in without difficulty. The school was as they were elsewhere in the United States and the children had few problems with it. They made friends easily. As she had in the Alaska, Lydia seemed to like the military way of life at Fort Knox. In particular she enjoyed the company of the family of our commanding officer and we became good friends.

USAMRL was a prestigious research facility with four main Divisions (Physiology, Psychology, Chemistry and Medicine). Some of its research was classified. That which was not, was published in the general literature or by the laboratory itself. At the time of my arrival, human subjects were used in the Psychology Division which took the main responsibility for research requiring human subjects from all Divisions. The research was carried out by PhDs under the safety direction of Doctors of Medicine who were doing their two years of required military service.

As Chief Research Physician, I had overall responsibility for the research on human beings as well as any medical research performed by the Laboratory. These included ensuring that the research had no ill effects on the human subjects, that the practices used by the researchers were medically acceptable, and that the research had useful objectives.

The doctors assigned to the laboratory were unhappy. They saw their job as merely standing by in case anything went wrong without having any real responsibilties for the design and conduct of the research programmes. They had applied to be assigned to USAMRL because they had an interest in research, but in practice they were fall guys for a group of PhDs who were having all the fun. In retrospect, most of them were sorry they had not requested a posting to one of the many military clinical hospitals. This was a pity because much of the important work which had come out of this research facility in the past had been carried out by medical doctors doing their compulsory military service.

The practices being used in carrying out this research did not, in my opinion, conform to the accepted norms between doctor and patient let alone between a non-medical researcher and a human subject. The Laboratory's use of human subjects was one of my responsibilities. I felt that, for research to be productive in this area, the responsibility for the research objectives should remain within the departments where the research was initiated and carried out. What was needed was a clarification of the procedural practises, proper placement of professional responsibilities and protection of the welfare of the subjects.

Sometime earlier, someone had produced a form to be signed by the subjects. This in effect said they understood what was going to be done to them, they agreed to it and could pull out of the programme at any time. This signed statement was believed by PhDs and MDs alike, to absolve them from responsibility if anything went wrong. I instinctively knew this could not be so. People just cannot sign away their welfare in this manner as was fondly being believed. There must be something in law or medical ethics dealing with it.

I felt that I could not start using human subjects in my own   research until I clarified the matter. So I began the search. I delved into the legalities pertaining to what a Doctor of Medicine can and cannot do to patients as these might apply to the research situation, and wrote a document which was eventually, with modifications, applied to the use of human subjects in all US government facilities. In essence it stated that doctors cannot do anything to a patient without the patient's actual or implied consent. In the law a medical procedure is an invasion of personality. Implied consent is when the patient, by an act of compliance to a medical procedure, agrees that the doctor may proceed. A simple example is a patient rolling up his sleeve for the taking of a blood pressure reading or a blood sample.

An implied or actual consent, written or otherwise, does not absolve a doctor or investigator from responsibility if something should go wrong. At no time does the welfare of the patient or, in our case, the subject, fall outside the responsibility of the doctor or the investigator. A written consent only ensures that the investigator has taken steps to be certain that the subject understands the purpose of the investigation, has agreed to the procedures pertaining to it, understands any side effects or hazards associated with the investigation, knows that he can pull out of the programme at will. Such a signed statement should also ensure that it does not in any way release the investigator from full responsibility for the welfare of the human subject.

The document upset the investigators who felt that the authority they deemed necessary for the successful performance of their investigations had been undermined. It was explained that there really was no change in the performance of their investigations except a need to alter their attitude towards it. The power they thought they had and thought was necessary was never there and was never necessary.

I asked the principal investigators to consider involving the medical doctors in their investigations as colleagues. This worked, not so much because I had requested it, but because there was a new realisation that the medical doctors had greater authority than before and could seriously affect the course of their investigations.

* * *

In time and with a better understanding all round, the post of Chief Research Physician became almost redundant, but I still kept an eye on it. I was now able to turn my attention to pursuing my own research. By coming to Fort Knox, I had struck a most favourable climate within which to carry out my own research. Because of Colonel Reece Blair's background, he was already familiar with my published works. He was most supportive when I informed him what my research programme was going to be. To facilitate it further, he and Floyd put me in charge of the Medical Research Division where all the facilities were available to do both heat and cold research.

* * *

Because the climatic rooms had not been used for a long time, they were in a poor state of repair. The heating mechanisms were workable, but the cooling systems were not. In a way this was a blessing because we were able to install the latest state of the art cooling equipment.

We had none of the measurement and recording equipment we needed. There was no difficulty in obtaining human subjects and, after a two year hiatus, I was into my personal research again. I was happy, my staff were happy, the subjects, after briefings and a first taste of being exposed to a cold of +5 Celsius in shorts only, were happy. The subjects indicated it was far better than tramping the hills and listening to sergeants bawling them out. Some of the subjects wrote home and gave their families a run down on what they were doing.

Letters from parents went screaming to Congress about the tortures their boys in service were going through. When their boys received word what their innocent remarks had incited, they were flabbergasted. They came to my office to express their regrets at what had taken place. One of them was in tears and all refused the demands of their parents to leave the program.

Three Generals of the Army turned up soon after. With a cursory introduction, they walked into the cold room in which the boys were being exposed. They stayed in the cold room for about ten minutes and talked with the subjects. They came out, examined the measuring and recording equipment, consulted each other, introduced themselves and said, "Carry on, Doctor Davis," and left. I never heard anymore.

* * *

In contrast with my first experience with research at Harvard, I was in no doubts as to my research plans. I knew what instruments I needed, the data I was going to collect, what I was going to do with it. I also knew how I was going to write up my findings and conclusions. The two years since circumstances had forced me to put my own research aside, made me itch to get started again. It took no time to get the climatic rooms operating, even less time for my military technicians to "acquire" all the equipment I needed and to talk "soldiers" into becoming human subjects.

There is a communication and fellowship link which threads through the Armed Forces at the Master Sergeant and NCO Level. If one was in tune with it, the impossible could be achieved. I was first keenly aware of this in Alaska. There was nothing we wanted done that could not be accomplished. Most anything we needed was obtained through this system that seemed to weave itself through the very fabric of the Armed Forces. If I had depended on conventional channels, it is doubtful that what we needed would have arrived before my contract in Alaska was over. So within one month of being free to get on with our research programme, my Division at Fort Knox was fully equipped and ready to work. One of the rules of the system is that you don't question how it was done. Just be grateful.

* * *

Elizabethtown, commonly known as E-Town, was about 12 miles south of Fort Knox and was the main town of Hardin county. It had a population of about 20,000 and despite it being a north-south border state, it was recognisably southern in character. It was a good town. Its people were polite, but viewed those of us working at Fort Knox with some diffidence. We made friends with the permanent residents and gradually became part of the scenery and the community.

It had a country club and its share of illicit goings on including the brewing of varying qualities of "white lightning", most of which were unpalatable to me, but relished by the locals at all social levels.

E-town, unlike Fairbanks in Alaska, had escaped the infection of providing services to the large population of Fort Knox which was second only to that of Louisville the capital of the State of Kentucky. Whether this was by design or accident was not clear to me. Distance from Fort Knox may have had much to do with it, but apathy, lack of enterprise and perhaps deliberate planning may have played their respective roles. Its location in Hardin County, an alcohol dry County, also probably had something to do with it. I was glad it was the way it was. The area on the main drag that passed by Ft. Knox had its share of bars and entertainment establishments which served the off-base activities of the military.

Wes Hardin, the famous outlaw and gunslinger of the wild west came from the Hardins of this area. Hardin County did not give the impression of being a breeding place for desperadoes, but it did have its occasions of blood and guts. One of my children's friends and, therefore, a frequent visitor to our home, had lost his father because he failed to move a boundary fence the three feet that his neighbour thought it ought to have been. In another incident, a downtown retailer considered it his southern gentlemanly duty to dispose of a persistent and supposedly unwelcome suitor of his secretary. It was believed by some that the secretary was only being feminine and her noes were really yesses. In each case a shot-gun at close range was used.

Hardin County had more than its share of mentally handicapped persons whose needs and difficulties Lydia and I, but more particularly Lydia, did much to overcome. Most of these were children up to late teenage. They were given a place to receive care and instruction in a church basement. It was provided with an untrained volunteer teacher who did her best without remuneration. We looked into the matter as thoroughly as we could at the local, state and national level.

All that could be done at the local level was being done. It was not much and our attempts to induce the local government to pay the teacher failed. We had no greater success with the state government. At the federal level we were referred to the United Fund and the Red Feather Fund which were non-government organisations which assisted community projects.

The main constraint was that a visible, local, organised effort must be in existence with evidence of tangible achievements. As there had never been any such organised effort, all appeals to these national organisations had failed. It became evident that we needed to initiate a local organisation and for it to raise funds and start something.

The immediate need was a building and paid qualified personnel for the care and education of mentally handicapped persons. The forming of an organisation was not difficult. Some despondency due to past failures to obtain help from national organisations was overcome with assurances that they would help if we showed evidence that we were willing to help ourselves.

In the meantime, I had acquired a sports car, a license to race it which I did with gusto at every opportunity at the nearby race circuits in Illinois, Indiana, Ohio, Alabama and Kansas. I was made President of the Kentucky Chapter of the Sports Car Club of America and this gave me access to some influential people in the Louisville area. My research into the mysteries of the physiological responses to hostile environments and my active role in the early space programme had started to hit the media and given me some local 'mana'. So I was able to get help from my friends in Louisville to augment what Lydia and I could do at the local level.

The net result of our efforts was to mount a country fair with all the goodies that go with it including a full blown carnival. Another was a beauty contest in which my sports car friends displayed the contestants riding slowly through the town dressed in flowing evening gowns. They were deliciously draped in various provocative attitudes on the trunks or bonnets of the sports and racing cars. Apart from overheating problems of some of our race tuned cars, it was a great way to show off the beauties for which the State of Kentucky is well known.

Freddie Chapman organised a horse show with show horses coming from as far away as Texas. The fair ran for a week in fine weather. We all worked hard, had the time of our lives and raised $4000. Not much, but it got us the attention of the fund givers and within two years we had a building and qualified personnel doing their stuff with educables and ineducables in proper quarters and surroundings. The fair with modifications became an annual event. Freddie's Horse Show became a fixture on the national circuit, E-Town expanded its community facilities, and the funding agencies continued to deploy generosity in appreciation of a town which got off its butt and did something for itself.

* * *

The research programme of my division got under way after I had cleared up the problems associated with using humans as experimental subjects. Molnar was doing his thing with the mathematics of thermodynamics using a roomful of what in those days passed for a computer. Hadley and his group were doing some sophisticated work on the circulation of the kidney and its function under experimental conditions. Jasper was into the biochemistry of acclimatisation at the tissue level. Dooley was doing laboratory and field work in bacteriology. Joy was helping me and doing work on his own using human subjects exposed to cold under experimental and field conditions in the Arctic. Poe and Frohlich were into metabolic tissue changes due to acclimatisation, and so on.

These investigations moved along happily on their own motivation and momentum. My colleagues and assistants working on my projects became well versed in the objectives and procedures of our research programme. Once under way, it needed little attention from me personally which was just as well. Washington started to make heavy demands on my time for policy planning and for the solution of practical problems. Since this called on the pragmatic part of my make up, I was happy to respond.

* * *

Research in academic institutions is carried out under the banner of academic freedom and the importance of establishing basic truths. This is essentially the PhD trained researcher's approach and he defends it to the last. Medical research tends to bend more toward the solution of practical medical problems. Often these approaches clash and is one of the reasons PhDs and MDs often do not see eye to eye.

Research in military facilities often demands practical solutions to practical problems and the military does not care much for the search for the purity of truths. So there is usually a running battle between Washington and its financially supported research institutions to deliver the goods it thinks it is paying for. The research the military would like done is not often on the mind or the agenda of MDs or PhDs. Like others in similar positions, I saw myself caught between the devil and the deep blue sea. My research essentially involved establishing a truth, but it could easily be justified as militarily relevant. Nevertheless, I needed to respond to what I saw as the legitimate wishes of Washington.

On reviewing the capability of my senior staff to respond to these wishes, I could come up with only two or three young medicos who would remotely consider such propositions. The rest of the staff were into basic research, some of which was difficult to justify in practical military terms. So it was left to me and a couple of my medicos to respond to the demands and take the heat off those doing the more basic research. I had no difficulty myself in responding because the pragmatic part of me liked solving practical problems. Our burden was enlarged to accept these practical research projects.

* * *

One of the practical projects in which I became intimately involved concerned that important item to an infantry soldier, his footwear. This may sound like a subject not worthy of the attention of even the meanest of scientists. Even Napoleon thought the stomach was what soldiers marched on. Chaka, on the other hand, saw the problem as serious enough to ban the wearing of footwear by his warriors thereby forcing them to develop thickened skin on their feet capable of withstanding the most rugged of terrain and the biggest spikes of African thorns. I was brought up barefooted and prided myself in my ability to chase umoemoe (a tropical fish) over live coral into the seaweed and capture them using my bare feet.

Before my arrival at USAMRL, a group stationed there had collected information on the feet of 7000 soldiers at Fort Knox. From this data they were able to describe the physical characteristics of the foot of man in its every shape and convolution expressed in means, standard deviations, standard errors and graphic illustrations. This statistical treatment does more than simply describe a series of characteristics. It also gives the units of measurement within which the proportion of a characteristic of the foot can be accommodated.

Into one standard deviation 66 percent of the feet of soldiers can be fitted, while into two standard deviations, 98 percent of feet can be accommodated. This is a mathematical fact. Therefore, if the measurement value of a standard deviation is not outlandish, 98 percent of the variations within a characteristic can be made to fit within tolerable limits.

In the case of the foot of man, if all the variations of the different characteristics which make up the foot are not outlandish, the probability of coming up with footwear that fitted the majority of feet well and the rest tolerably well is high. There was no reason to believe that the feet of 7000 US soldiers did not represent the shape of feet of all Americans if not those of most humans.

Up to that time, as far as I know, footwear had been designed on the premise of what shoe-last makers and shoemakers thought was the shape of feet. No attempt had been made to measure and describe the actual foot of man. This was a very comprehensive first, but it lay in the dusty archives of USAMRL until some shoe-last makers at the Army facilities at Natick in Massachusetts unearthed it and made shoe-lasts out of the information and made shoes from them. They tried their products on themselves and others. For fit and comfort they were highly satisfactory, they thought, and they became dedicated to the quest of bringing better footwear to soldiers in particular and mankind in general.

Colonel Tim Timmerman, when made familiar with the product, was impressed enough to send the people involved to his practical research fall guy, me. I did not want to get involved with footwear and feet. For a product to break into an area already dominated by products which had already walked soldiers and their generals out of mud, fire and hell, had to be outstanding.

Encouraged by Colonel Timmerman, the bosses of the last makers talked to me of the virtues of their product including how they would do away with half sizes, thus easing the logistic problems of manufacture and supply. It sounded great, but I was not interested. My research was going fine. My involvement in the space programme was exciting and time consuming. My other duties of a more medical nature were occupying my time nicely. I did not need to add a task that involved convincing the conservative military world of the United States that it needed to jump out of its old boots to which they were emotionally adhered and slip into new ones. In the end I was overpowered by becoming impressed by trying out the footwear myself. I thought it needed a better chance than it had been given so far.

We used the footwear at the Army test facilities of Fort Lee on its artificially ruggedised trails. We put them on our subjects in the climatic chambers. As part of general military exercises, we put them on paratroopers and took them on parachute jumps and jungle manoeuvres in Panama. We marched soldiers in the heat until their feet blistered more in the old boots than in the new ones. My efforts to get this footwear on to every soldier, sailor, marine, paratrooper, general and admiral, became a joke on the home front and in headquarters in Washington the project was referred to as one 'nearest and dearest to Tom's heart.'

The infantry was the easiest to convince and they accepted the new product without much ado as did the Air Force and the Navy. The Marines and the Paratroopers were another story. Several visits to Paris Island and Fort Bragg were necessary to get the job done. The fact that the footwear of their choice were ill fitting to the extent that their feet were scarred and deformed, made little difference to their resistance to the new product. The footwear worn by these two services had achieved a unique status in each. They represented an important and distinctive part of their uniform. They shone with Kiwi polish to a brilliance unequalled in the other services and this, combined with their beautifully pressed and groomed uniforms, was a sight I never tired of beholding. in the end my dedication won the day. The Marines were the last bastion and we finally had to concede and provide them with a boot 2 inches shorter in height than the rest. In contrast commercial shoe manufacturers had already put the last into commission on a commercial basis.

* * *

Another of these practical projects which took a great deal of my time was the result of my own doing and concerned my personal interest in space. This interest still gnawed at me from those medical student days in my not so snow-proof digs designing a life support system to sustain man in space. In those medical school days, there were no vehicles capable of delivering my system into space. Now in 1955, there were potential vehicles in the form of ballistic missiles being tested one after the other at Cape Canaveral (now Cape Kennedy). Almost from the time of my arrival in Kentucky I had realised that next door in Huntsville, Alabama, was the Army's facility for building missiles under the guidance of Werner Von Braun.

At that time there was no National Aeronautic and Space Administration (NASA). The Army, the Air Force and the Navy had independently taken it upon themselves to develop their own nuclear warhead, rocket driven, ballistic delivery systems. Each developed their own approaches with their own failures and successes. But none seemed more successful than Von Braun's group at the Huntsville Army facility.

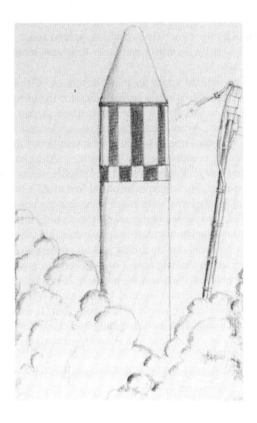

Washington thought that developing missiles by the three branches of the Armed Forces working independently on the same project was an expensive duplication of effort. In my opinion this is not generally true, at least for the developmental part of projects. It may be true for the expensive aspect, but I am not sure of that either. When several people or groups work independently on the same project, the chances of covering all the creative developmental possibilities are greater and the cross fertilisation that takes place increases the chances of rapid progress. This is not taking into consideration the driving power of competition. A single organisation tends to settle into the groove it has created for itself and has difficulties in getting out of it. Administratively this view is unpopular, but, within certain limits, it has merit.

Missiles from these three sources were being test flown with empty nose cones, planned to carry nuclear warheads. I made frequent requests to be given the opportunity to put biological specimens in these empty nose cones to test the effects of space on them. These requests were ignored. Then the break came. The antinuclear buffs seemed suddenly to realise that the activity at the Cape was a great deal more than the regular testing of rocket systems. They were seriously working on systems for delivering nuclear warheads. In effect the antinuclear group, by their vociferous protests, helped space agencies speed up a man in space effort by diverting emphasis to it and away from its nuclear warhead purposes.

Suddenly I was offered space in the nose cones of the Army's ballistic missiles and was made Chief of Bioastronautics for the army. This fitted very well into my wishes to further my interests in space, begun those many years before. At that time the Army's ballistic missile under test was the Jupiter. It had a failure rate less than one in twelve which was better than missiles being tested at that time. By comparison, the Air Force's Atlas had a failure rate of three in five and the Navy's Polaris, a solid fuel missile, was a little better. These failures were expensive, but very spectacular. Most missile tests seemed to take place at night and the failures were more spectacular than any big fireworks display. We never tired of watching take-offs accompanied by the tingling anticipation of a possible spectacularly explosive sequel.

No matter how far away our launching pad was from that of a missile taking off, the thundering, earth shaking power of a rocket was always awe-inspiring. The colour of the Navy's Polaris was the prettiest. It was heliotrope with shades of purple intermixed with that special orange/yellow hue associated with burning sodium. One night we saw it in full splendour. It took off on schedule, but at about two thousand feet the front end blew off and it slowed to a static position spewing its beautiful coloured flame from both ends like a large two ended Roman Candle.

The failures of the Atlas, being a large long-range missile, were always worth seeing. We always looked forward to its scheduled lift-offs. A Jupiter in which we had some black mice had a failure in one of its flight path controlling switches. It turned into a spectacular unguided missile cum Catherine Wheel at a relatively low altitude. Our personnel, watching from a normally safe distance, instinctively dived for cover.

* * *

The struggle for space superiority between the armed forces in the face of Washington's wish to implement its fight against duplication of effort, had given the Air Force the go ahead responsibility for long range rocketry while the Army and the Navy were limited to short range categories. The Jupiter was in the short range group, but it was reliable and would serve our purpose. Washington was never fully successful in its fight against duplication of effort.

Despite its enforced limitations on power and distance capability, Von Braun overcame them and eventually provided NASA with the only space vehicle with the power to launch the Apollo programme and keep the US in competition for the man in space race with the USSR. Von Braun did this by tieing 8 Jupiters together as the booster and hitching them to a Redstone to make up the Saturn which took the astronauts to the moon one after the other. This vehicle was ready and waiting to do this job in 1959. I saw it at the Huntsville facility standing several stories high sticking out through the roof which had to be modified to house it. It was not called upon to do its thing until ten years later. Dr Werner Von Braun was a remarkable man.

* * *

I got as many as were interested at the US Army Medical Research Laboratories to start putting together a co-ordinated effort to mount a meaningful bioastronautic programme. The area of space which most concerned everybody at that time was the possible deleterious effects of a variety of types of radiation in space. These were inhibited from reaching the earth by the atmosphere and other radiation deterring forces. So our early efforts were concerned with putting biological specimens into space which would be sensitive to the effects of radiation. We chose black mice to show the effects of cosmic particle radiation because a strike on the black fur would whiten it. We sent up grass seeds and sea urchin eggs which would show any significant effects of radiation by altering their maturation characteristics and finally we used monkeys to evaluate effects on physiological parameters during space flight. This series of experiments were carried out between 1956 and 1958 and all indicated that travel in space, protected only by the structural materials of the nose cone and the capsule in it, produced no discernible deleterious effects on biological systems.

* * *

In those early days of space research, in common with man faced with new horizons throughout history, we were plagued with fears of the unknown. We were also plagued with fears of equipment failure which would act strongly against support of our efforts. In those early days support funds rested on shaky grounds. Most considered us dreamers playing with something that was still decades, if not centuries, away. In my cover article for the *Atlantic Monthly,* published a month before Gargarin's flight, my opening sentence said that space travel for man was imminent. This caused much trouble with the editor, Ted Weeks, who firmly believed that this was not going to take place until well into the next century. I stuck to my guns and the sentence remained unchanged.[17] The editor's surprise at Gargarin's flight within a month or so after the article appeared in press has remained a mute subject between us.

* * *

Some of our complex bioastronautic experiments were seriously criticised from as high as the President. It was not until the time of President Kennedy that we could breathe more easily. We dispensed with some of the secrecy that many of our projects were cloaked in order to protect them from our own people. But we had our champions and, for the Army effort, the most prominent were General George Medaris and General Jumping Jim Gavin who were able to divert sufficient funds to keep us going.

The fight to mount some of our projects was at times so great that we lost sight of the gravity of the situation if we failed. It would not be until the last few hours of a 4 to 6 month count down that we would be suddenly struck with the enormity of what we were doing and what it meant, if the experiment or the hundreds of things that could go wrong went wrong. It would spell an expensive finis to months of long hours of co-ordinated work between engineers, PhDs, medical doctors, experimental psychologists, behaviouralists, biochemists and technicians and deter further support to our already fragile and unofficial status.

It was always with humble anticipation, silence, or hushed whispers and numerous cups of coffee and cigarettes that we waited with nail biting tension for each critical stage of the last hour, minutes and seconds of the count down to come up and pass into the sequential stages of ignition, lift off, programming down range, burn out, the glide and splash down. Our separate tensions released themselves in our own separate ways. Some of us would just sigh and smile, others would give a whoop and, if you were from the south, an awe inspiring rebel yell was the likely response. Others would just open their mouths and let whatever was inside come out as shattering sound.

When we got into the Manned Mercury Project, these tensions were heightened several fold and I do not think that I was the only one who never became inured to these tensions. The long daily hours of simulations at Langley Air Force Base and even more intense simulations on site at the various monitoring stations throughout the world must have helped, but when the day of the actual mission came around, we all seemed to be keyed up to fever pitch.

For me these tensions at the beginning were heightened by the fact that we were now flying human beings instead of monkeys, mice, sea urchin eggs or grass seeds and were using a vehicle, the Atlas, which had a history of high failure rates. The fact that President Eisenhower had proclaimed that those responsible for the high failure rates would have to be accountable for them was only marginally comforting. It was only time and the record of absence of failures that took this aspect of my personal fears out of the picture.

Around 1958, Von Braun met those of us in the Army interested in space and informed us that we now had the rocket power capability to put a small village into space and for a trip to the moon. He was, of course, referring to Saturn sitting on its lonesome, waiting patiently to do its stuff. No doubt as a result of this, twenty of us were unceremoniously removed from wherever we were and summonsed forthwith to the Walter Reid Army Hospital in Washington. I was giving a paper at Atlantic City when my presentation was interrupted and I was told to get on the next plane to Washington. They would inform my family, I was told. Others related similar experiences.

At Walter Reid we were given private rooms after which we were called together and told that we were to put together a programme to take man to the moon. Each of us was assigned a chapter to write. Mine was the environment required in the capsule for two to three men to live for the duration of the flight. My chapter was also to include the type of environment to be expected on the moon surface and the landing place where temperatures would be tolerable. We were given two weeks to complete our assignments and were not to communicate with anybody outside our group. Beyond Walter Reid was out of bounds and what we were about to do was Top Secret. Most of us knew one another, but our respective assignments kept us busy and apart. We were to use the Walter Reid library for our reference needs and runners were available to obtain what we needed from the Library of Congress. To make a long story short we came up with a document which became the Bible for the Apollo programme.

The late fifties and early sixties was a time of intense creative thinking for those involved in the space programme. The foundation for the Apollo Programme was laid and only modifications were made as it came to fruition over a period of ten years. Saturn, the rocket to achieve it, remained unchanged over this period. The shuttle concept was being put together and a portion of our time at the Mercury Project monitoring stations was spent on it. The drawings being sketched were little different from the eventual product. The piggy back test system concept was fully developed, but in the absence of a Boeing 747, the B 52 bomber was to be the carrier.

It was approximately 20 years after it was conceived that the first shuttle flight was made. The basic concept has stood the test of time. The unfortunate accident with Challenger should not detract from its value for delivering equipment into space, maintaining it, removing and replacing it as the need arises. No other system exists or is likely to in the foreseeable future to carry out these operations as efficiently. Systems which put satellites into space and forget about them after they cease operating, will end up in an untidy space.

* * *

It was only after NASA was formed with its first facilities at Langley Air Force Base in Virginia, that NASA drew heavily on my time for the Mercury Project series of space flights involving the first seven astronauts. NASA's existence did not have an effect on the Military efforts and it still depended on the existing rockets developed by the military for its program. It also depended heavily on the experience of personnel from the military establishments such as my own for support which we were happy to provide.

My site for medical responsibility for most of the NASA flights was at Guaymus, Mexico, except for the Cooper flight which was Zanzibar. Both of these were stations which had the final check of the capsule and the astronaut before procedures for re-entry were initiated. From Guaymus, splash down was in the Atlantic and from Zanzibar it was in the Pacific. At the Guaymus station, I was teamed up with, among others, Wally Shira for most of the missions and with Scott Carpenter and Deke Slayton for the others in which Wally was involved as an astronaut or was required for duties at base.

Work on site for the most part consisted of daily simulations carried out at the same hours as would occur during the mission. This meant that we were at it at all hours for about 3 weeks before the mission. With such close contact, Wally and I became close friends and shared most of our off-duty hours in each others company. All the astronauts were exceptional men and I shared Deke's disappointment in not being allowed to fly a mission because of a functional heart anomaly which, in my opinion, should not have disqualified him. I made strong personal attempts for a reversal of the decision, but over-caution in those early stages was the order of the day. It was with joy on his behalf that I received the news that Deke flew in one of the much later missions.

* * *

My research on acclimatisation in the climatic chambers with human subjects was going according to plan. The results were no different from those which had been observed on myself and my friends and on rats. They were just more definitive and more convincing to the unbelievers. Subjects not normally inured to cold, shed their shivering response gradually over a period of three weeks when exposed in a climatic chamber to a temperature of 40F (plus 5 Celsius) for six hours daily, dressed only in shorts. This was accompanied by a statistically significant decrease in the consumption of oxygen (about 40 to 50 percent) and an increase in subjective comfort levels in the cold.[19] During all of my testing of human subjects in the cold with reduced clothing, I never came across anyone suffering from the common cold as a result of it.

In the field (Greenland and Alaska) these adaptive changes occurred much more rapidly (within one week in Greenland) when subjects were exposed to outside temperatures and conditions for four to six hours daily, dressed in long johns and windproof clothing and exposed to temperatures varying between minus 20 degrees to minus 50 degrees F.20,43 again with a significant decrease in oxygen consumption indicating a substantial saving in fuel to overcome the same degree of cold. Subjects were always tested under the same conditions of plus 40 degrees F in shorts lying on an open mesh cot.

We were also able to demonstrate adaptive changes as a result of seasonal acclimatization of soldiers living in Fort Knox under normal circumstances.[18] More importantly we found that subjects could be acclimatized to heat and cold at one and the same time.[21] I have no doubt we could have added altitude acclimatization as well. This can take place because the physiologic mechanisms for each are different and they can coexist without ill effects to one another. Thus, if one cared to, one can, with little effort, produce a global soldier inured to perform in any climatic condition he might need to. Such a soldier would, besides being instantly efficient, be more resistant to the deleterious effects of these hostile environments.[22] Towards the end of this series of experiments, the subjects requested to be given the opportunity to expose themselves to lower and lower chamber temperatures to see what the limit of acclimatization might be. After the subjects had staged themselves at weekly intervals through 30 degrees F, 20 degrees F and 10 degrees F, dressed only in shorts, I stopped the experiment. They would have continued to lower temperatures if I had allowed them.

Our extensive experience with human subjects in the cold indicated a small percentage who were unable to adapt to cold. One in the Greenland experiment was physiologically incapable of acclimatizing to the cold over the six week period on the Greenland Ice Cap. I would place the existence of such individuals at less than one percent. We also came across one individual who was allergic to cold in the form of giant urticaria (an allergic response characterised by giant wheals on the skin) every time he was exposed to cold in the nude. We were unable to find any other agent which might have produced the response. Strangely he was a Tibetan who had never been at an altitude less than 11,000 feet. and generally lived at 14,000 to 17,000 feet. Our tests on him and his colleagues were performed at 13,000 ft. Normally he did not appear to be distressed by his condition.

* * *

Physiological adaptation to cold was a difficult concept for some to swallow. Some wanted to believe that what we were really demonstrating was psychological and/or behavioural adaptation. Why these should be easier to swallow always escaped me. Certainly the changes perceived and not perceived were dramatic, but no more dramatic than those occurring in acclimatization to altitude. Acclimatisation to heat was accepted, but only in its minor form of adjustments of pulse rate, blood pressure and one or two other parameters over a three day period. Longer term adjustments at the biochemical levels were not at that time seriously sought. The importance of these adjustments to athletes competing at the Olympics also seems to have escaped trainers and coaches.

It is not very remarkable that Kenyans do well in long distance events as they have trained at altitude and naturally built up a polycythemia (increase in red cells) that gives them an advantage as blood doping (transfusing blood into an athlete before an event) which is said to increase stamina. Nor is it remarkable that the boxing champion loses to a hometown favourite he is fighting at altitude. The experience at the Melbourne Olympics in the heat must have taught some lessons. The hot country boys took away the medals. Physical training itself is a physiologic and biochemical adaptive process, though it has psychological dimensions.

My biochemical background was insufficient to follow up the chemical adaptations which took place as a result of acclimatization. I felt convinced that muscle changed its role from one of producing heat by physical contractions in the unacclimatized state to one of producing heat by biochemical means in the acclimatized state. Since the revival of the chemical thermogenesis theory, others such as Cottle, Carlson, Depocas, Hart, Heroux, Jansky, Sellers and Weiss had indicated that the seat of chemical thermogenesis was outside the abdominal visceral organs. Muscle was strongly implicated.

In a dramatic experiment my technicians and I carried out in the dog, we isolated the circulation of the hindlimb by perfusing it with blood and measuring its oxygen uptake in the unacclimatized and acclimatized animal exposed to cold.[26] This confirmed once and for all that muscle was an important organ in chemical thermogenesis. Bone in the hindleg was the only other candidate, but this was ruled out as unlikely.

By 1958 we had convinced the majority of disbelievers. Chemical thermogenesis, or as I preferred to call it, non-shivering thermogenesis, had been revived and it looked like it was here to stay.

[16], [28] Alan Burton of Canada had been one of the first to accept the validity of our findings and our close personal friendship and student/master relationship remained until his death which to me was a personal loss. Our association, which had started in conflict, had grown to one of professional respect and finally personal friendship. Alan was much older than I and his guidance, advice, constructive criticism and encouragement played a major role in my quest. Otto Edholm visited our laboratory and witnessed a subject from the Greenland experiment exposed to cold in shorts lie comfortably on his mesh cot while his control counterpart bounced with uncontrollable shivering alongside him. He went back to England and, as Director of the Medical Research Council, redirected its environmental research programme to take into account his acceptance that chemical thermogenesis not only existed, but that it was the prime producer of heat in the cold in acclimatized people. Jim Hardy of Yale remained unconvinced to the last.

* * *

In Fort Knox, my personal quest for the Holy Grail had come to its conclusion. It was as much as I could do as a medical doctor and as a research physiologist. The problem now was a biochemical one for which I was not well equipped. But others were and any further role I might have in the elucidation of the question was to do for others what Stare, Mayer, Blair, Burton, Belding and others had done for me. Into this picture came the newer breed such as Hannon, Theriault, Vaughan, Masoro and a host of others.

For reasons of its own, the Army transferred Reece Blair. This was a blow to Floyd Odel and me. We had had a good working relationship. Reece by his understanding leadership had lifted the United States Army Medical Laboratories out of the doldrums it had lain in before he took command. It was a normal change of command, but his loss was deeply felt. He was replaced by a medical colonel and apart from some difficulties with an article on man in space I had been assigned by the *Atlantic Monthly* to write, we managed quite well.[17] At this time I was made a PL313, the highest rank which can be attained by a public servant in the United States.

Then, again, for reasons of its own, the Army transferred my operations to Natick, Massachusetts. This suited me, as I would be back with friends, but at the expense of leaving good friends in Kentucky. Except for some important members of my staff who were bound by family and fortune to the area, we moved holus bolus to the Natick Laboratories. It is difficult to put into words the loyalty of this staff. Some of them stayed with me for sixteen years. I often wish that I had acceded to the wish of some to come and face life back in the Cook Islands with me, but even I did not know what was in store for me in the strange world of politics in the Pacific.

CHAPTER ELEVEN

The Himalayas

Do not vainly lament, but realise that nothing is permanent and learn from it the emptiness of human life. Do not cherish the unworthy desire that the changeable might become unchanging. BUDDHIST TEACHING

Worship through work, worship through teaching, worship through meditation. HINDU TEACHING

If we say religion is opposed to science we either lack knowledge of true science or true religion, for both are founded upon the premises and conclusions of reason and both must bear its test. BAHA'I TEACHING

Moving from Kentucky to Massachusetts was reasonably easy with the help of the very efficient US moving companies that come, pack and load with no help from you and the family. I love them. I hate packing.

The United States government is less generous than other governments in financial assistance to public servants making moves of this nature. At that time travel on behalf of the government was often costly for the public servant. You were given a daily stipend from which accommodation, taxis, meals and incidentals had to be paid, and unless you found the cheapest hotels, motels and diners, you were out of luck. Rebates for chits and pieces of paper worked, but who cared to do that at every twist and turn of one's travel. Rebates were not always made without argument. What it cost was not deductible as an income tax expense. The many days in a year we travelled on behalf of NASA were particularly expensive for us. It was not NASA's fault as it was part of a uniform system throughout the Armed Services and the Public Service.

This move from Kentucky to Massachusetts was particularly expensive. While the cost of living went up, the stipend stayed put until long after there was need for an adjustment. More importantly owing to a depressed market, we made a substantial loss on the home we had built. We had to buy a house in Massachusetts on a temporary basis until we could find what we wanted and. when that occurred, we made another loss.

Although nothing much could be done about the exigencies of the housing market, I felt that it was time something was done about other costs incurred in moving and travel. So I totted up everything and made a case to our nearest tax office in Framingham. My plea was for costs incurred in such cases to be tax deductible. My PL 313 status must have had some effect, because in a very short time Washington passed the necessary legislation. However, the chief tax man in Framingham. on calling to inform me, seemed most happy to also inform me that the changes applied from the time of the legislation and mine did not qualify. He seemed discomfited when I told him I knew that from the beginning.

The PL 313 status was a prestigious one which seemed to carry a fair bit of authority. Whenever I went into government offices anywhere in the country and in US embassies overseas, I was aware of a sense of awe from the staff and my wishes were always attended to immediately. My habit of travelling to military sites where our experiments might be in progress, caused a furore of camp clean up. My visits were not usually popular. I was supposed to be safely ensconced in some ivory tower and not wandering around upsetting the activities of normal people. I had to be very careful what I said or proposed because they seemed always to be taken seriously.

I settled into my job to carry on research using human subjects. It seemed to be the wish of the Army high-ups in Washington that we were to turn these facilities into a kind of "Institute of Man" to carry out applied research on environmental problems which would use human subjects. The name of the facility was changed to The United States Army Institute of Environmental Medicine. It could be visualised that these would deal with problems associated with exposure of man to heat, cold, altitude and other hostile environments.

I had no objections to this concept, particularly as it was along the lines of my personal interest. With the right balance between fundamental and applied research this could be rewarding. But it would not be as easy a task as was being visualised. One does not just reach into the blue and come up with creative and meaningful research using little more than the availability of human subjects as the principle motive.

Similar concepts had been tried before with strange happenings and even stranger results. It is a characteristic of some administrators to hang the work of a research institution on biological specimens as experimental subjects rather than on research problems with the experimental species an incidental consideration. Such concepts may work very well for limited periods as has the Harvard Primate Centre, but sooner or later one runs out of meaningful research projects aimed specifically at the species selected.

The most celebrated of these were the experiments carried out by the Nazis on the inmates of death camps. Earlier I had been requested to examine the reports on these and analyse them for anything useful. I was unable to come up with anything worthwhile that these inhuman experiments brought to light other than the fact that humans in poor physical condition die in a short time when exposed to icy water and other uncomfortable conditions.

I am not for a moment suggesting that what might be visualised for us would in the remotest manner end up that way. However, I am making the point that availability of human subjects is not a reason to experiment on them. It is the wrong end from which to start.

The right end is that there is a good reason, based on sound fundamental evidence, for research using human subjects. Clinical evaluation of the efficacy of medicines is one of them, provided that toxicity and side effects have been fully evaluated first and that the clinical tests for efficacy are properly designed so that placebo and other effects can be accounted for and probability mathematics can be applied to determine that the results could not have occurred by chance alone. There is a mass of evidence that, in most cases, results of research on animals can be applied to man and confirmation of this is another valid reason for using human subjects.

* * *

Soon after my arrival at Natick, the Indian government requested the United States to assist it investigate the problems the Indian Ministry of Defence was having operating at altitude and in the cold. The Chinese who had invaded Tibet and some remote parts of India and were threatening India's remaining Himalayan borders. The Indian government had named me as a necessary member of any assistance that might be given.

The request came in November 1962 and by January 1963 we were on our way. The Commanding Officer decided to lead the team and, as a medical man, he put together a program directed towards gathering of blood elements and blood chemistry data. This was his idea of meeting the requirements of the Indian request. Much of this had already been done. I did not think that we were, by this means, going to add to the state of the art. But the enthusiastic activity to follow this line inhibited me from discouraging it.

The specific request that I be included in the team indicated to me that what was probably foremost in their minds was a desire for pragmatic answers to their immediate problems of how to inure their soldiers to the conditions of altitude and cold. I packed my equipment in the hopes that I was right and I would somehow be able to use it. Team size restrictions, I was told, would not allow me to take the technicians who were normally required for its operation. It seemed I was just to tag along without any real role.

* * *

The Indian Army we were sent amongst was deployed in the Ladakh area of the Himalayas which is a little nearer to the western end of this magnificent and awe inspiring range of mountains. It is where headwaters of the river Indus lies. Although there had not been much combat, there had been enough military activity and patrols for the Indian army to realise that its troops were utterly unable to operate in the conditions of altitude and cold.

The most feared condition was the pulmonary oedema of altitude. This was first described by Houston and is known as Houston's disease. We contacted Dr Houston and obtained from him the essential features of the disease. Its most characteristic aspect was its apparent association with physical exercise at altitude, resulting in outpouring of fluid into the lungs with possible drowning in one's own fluid. A number of cases had occurred. Some had died and some had been flown to low altitude. If done quickly it saved lives.

This association between pulmonary oedema, altitude and exercise had brought the Indian army to a physical standstill. Until some other solution was found, Headquarters decided that the only recourse was to suspend all activities involving physical exertion. So it had for some time lain inert and bundled up against the cold. To the Indian Army, it seemed that the Chinese forces were undeterred in carrying out their operations in these conditions. Therefore, they must have a formula which our little group was to discover.

If the Chinese had been serious about invading more of India, they could have done so without much resistance. They could not have missed the fact that the Indian Army was laid low. The nature of the terrain demanded a high dependence on foot slogging by infantry soldiers.

* * *

The soldiers of the Indian Army consisted of a rank and file from the communities which lived and farmed the plains surrounding the area near Delhi. They were known as Jats. Their religion was Hindu, but they were officered by Sikhs. As best as I could judge this arrangement seemed to work with no evidence of friction.

Without any prompting from me, I was assigned three Medical Officers, Captains Nayar, Sinha and Nishith and one biochemist, Dr Rai. The Ministry of Defence in New Delhi must have sensed my dilemma of no assistants and solved it this way. It proved to be a very good solution for we worked well together and became good friends. We convinced Headquarters that it would be to the advantage of our mission if we could have a group of Jats assigned to us to test for responses to cold before they went to altitude and while they were at altitude. New nations tend to be sticklers for the word of the book and the number of Jats assigned to us as subjects was minimal. Our demands took these soldiers from their normal duties and this upset routine.

We found a merchant who very kindly let us use his potato and onion cooler as a cold chamber. It was ideal as it was large and its temperature of 3 degrees C was perfect for our purposes. The only modification needed was to restack bags of potatoes and onions to make enough room in the chamber for testing our subjects. We set up our instruments in the ante room. For a make shift facility it worked very well. When our tests were done, there was nothing to keep us from the heights of the Himalayas and what lay in store for us in its valleys, on its peaks and through its snow-drifted high passes.

Because I was dressed in work khakis and my already dusky complexion had been further darkened by some golf in the Indian sun, I was inadvertently shunted along with my Indian colleagues and subjects into a military troop plane. I kept my mouth shut and enjoyed the flight. I was informed later that my travelling in this manner was highly irregular and I could have been shot as a spy. Our plane and that of my Natick colleagues arrived at the Leh airport, the main settlement in Ladakh, 11,000 feet up, at about the same time. Leh is about 34 degrees Latitude north.

During our wait we had only a brief sight of Leh which in 1963 was a small town consisting of two or three storey contiguous buildings built of what looked like brick or stone around a central square which was about one hundred yards by fifty or seventy yards. As I remember it, there were gates in two of its opposing sides and small doors entering the square from these buildings which in effect formed a solid wall on all sides.

At the level of the second floor there were balconies built out over the square. The ancient game of polo was still being played in the square annually. When they played the doors and windows were barricaded and the two gates formed the goals, the teams of players on their ponies played to their hearts' content in the confines of the square while the spectators watched from the safety of the balconies. Building a town around one's favourite sport seemed to be a novel approach to town planning. But I remembered that we were little different with our village greens, football stadiums and other sports facilities dominating much of the scenery even in our biggest cities. It struck me that this plan may have been for defence reasons.

Although there were not many roads, there were enough to meet the needs of the military and the populace. One of these was touted as the highest road in the world and ran up to about 22,000 feet. We had the opportunity to drive this road to its very top and for fun we stepped out 100 metres and three of us ran the hundred meters dash. I was proud of my third placing.

* * *

I had looked forward to this venture. The Himalayas had always fascinated me as it must most people. Earlier we met with Sir Edmund Hillary in Washington and had taken full notice of his descriptions as to what to expect at altitude. At last, to be here on the very edge of the top of the world was exciting.

During our wait at the Leh Airport, I watched the profusion of planes that came in, unloaded and took off. I was surprised to see that at least half of them were Soviet Union planes and the rest were a mixture of United States and Indian aircraft. It was only then that I realised that the Soviet Union was supplying arms and the implements of war to the Indian army as, of course, was the United States.

I had thought that the USSR was on the side of the Chinese invaders of Tibet. It was later explained to me by a Sikh General that Russia and China have distrusted each other for centuries and Russia protected itself from the Chinese threat by ensuring the integrity of its buffer states of which Tibet had until recently been one.

Tibet's fall to the Chinese was considered by the Soviet Union as a serious threat to its security. The other buffer states were Sinkiang and Inner and Outer Mongolia, all of which the Soviet Union made certain remained militarily capable of acting in their buffer capacity between itself and China. But I could not help wondering what China thought about the Soviet Union's obvious active support of India's attempts to prevent China from attaining its presumed objectives. I could only conclude that this was probably an age old game between them which did not amount to much on the diplomatic front.

* * *

We left Delhi, a few hundred feet above sea level, at 8 am. Twelve hours later we were at 13,500 feet. Apart from some shortness of breath on climbing even slight slopes, I felt fine. We all had a hearty meal and went to our respective quarters consisting of Genghis Khan type yurts unchanged over centuries. It worked for his army, why would it not work for this army?

I and my Indian colleagues were separated from our Natick colleagues and were expected to work separately. Certainly my proposal of a work programme was quite different from theirs and physical separation did not affect either of our programmes.

* * *

My yurt was off on its own on the side of a mountain looking across a valley to a magnificent rugged line of mountains. The whole magnificent scene was bathed in the cold light of a nearly full moon. Each morning for the next six weeks I had the greatest pleasure of saying good morning to these mountains. Inside and in the light of my altitude-dimmed candle I examined my yurt. It was round and about 10 feet in diameter with a liquid fuel stove near the centre post. The wall was constructed of wood lattice work supported by wood uprights meeting the conical roof of radiating wooden rafters rising in a 20 degree slope towards the centre where the smoke stack of the stove poked through. There was full headroom. All of this was covered with felt and the whole gave a nice sense of cosiness.

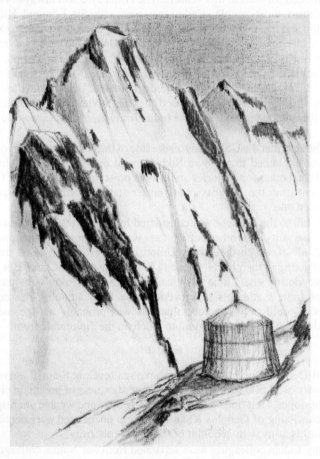

It was cold, but my arctic sleeping bag did its stuff and before I dozed off comfortably to sleep, I remembered thinking that my yurt was not very portable and would need at least one elephant or two camels or two yaks or three donkeys or six men to transport it. Then I slept like a baby.

At about 5 am, I sensed somebody moving quietly about and realised that someone was lighting the stove. I remembered sleepily thinking "how nice" and apparently fell off to sleep again until I was gently woken by a soft voice singing the strains of what I recognised as a Punjabi song. During our little time in New Delhi I had begun to familiarise myself with the music of India which was played nightly at the Ashoka Hotel where we stayed. The magnificent Indian orchestra did not often play the music of the Punjab, but after I had heard it for the first time, I had fallen in love with its lilting, rock and roll character. Now at 13,500 feet in the Himalayas of Ladakh, I was to be woken by it every morning at 6 am. All I needed was a jug of wine, a loaf of bread and thou to make my stay in these majestic surroundings complete.

My fire lighter turned out to be a Sikh assigned to be my batman in the British tradition. He spoke no English and I spoke no Punjabi or Hindi, but we became the closest of friends and needed no language to communicate with each other. His duties started at 5 every morning and consisted of lighting the stove, heating my bath water and, promptly at 6 am, he would softly sing me awake with those delightful, lilting, rolling rhythmic Punjabi songs. Often I would be awake when he entered, always very quietly. I always pretended to be asleep so that I would not disturb the quiet rhythm of his activities and eventually the rhythm of his waking up songs.

I would get up to a delightfully pre-heated atmosphere, acknowledge his presence with a friendly nod and smile, which he acknowledged in kind. Then I would make my way through the snow and ice to the latrine which was up the rise a little. On my way back, the hot water he had heated would be in a large basin waiting for me outside the yurt. I would strip and bathe in the nude in the open air, splashing soapy water over me in the cold chill of a bracing subzero Himalayan morning. After dressing, I would make my way to the mess hall and start the day with breakfast. He looked after me like a king. My clothes were always clean and well pressed and my boots shone with the spit shine he applied to them as often as they were not on my feet. When six weeks later we parted, we unabashedly cried on each other's shoulder.

* * *

I awaited the symptoms of altitude sickness characterised by headaches, nausea and vomiting, lack of appetite, a fast beating heart, breathlessness and loss of weight. Next day my companions were beginning to complain of these symptoms and most of them only toyed with breakfast. Apart from a little breathlessness on exertion, I felt fine and ate a hearty breakfast of buffalo steak, eggs, bread, butter, jam and coffee. As our mess was for Sikh officers, we had no worry about dietary restrictions. Dr Rai, our biochemist was a Brahman Hindu and subsisted on eggs and vegetables, the eggs being allowed under these special circumstances. I could not help being smug about not having altitude sickness symptoms, but refrained from making a point of it.

I spent the day with two young Sikh officers who I found timing each other running at full speed 100 or so yards up a steep hill behind the camp. I was impressed. These lads were not giving a darn about Houston's disease or the restrictions put on physical exercise by Headquarters. When we chatted they were of the opinion that the nabobs of the army were too conservative and that the way to overcome their problem at altitude was to face it and train in it.If they did this, their army would be as good as that of the Chinese whom they believed was doing just that.

This was exactly what I was looking for, so I discussed my investigative plans with them and enlisted their help. I told them that time was of the essence because I did not want the Jats I had brought with me to acclimatise both to cold and to altitude before testing them in the cold at altitude. They were enthusiastic at the opportunity of playing a part in getting their army into fighting form as they had done for themselves.

I brought my colleagues to meet them and plan our investigative programme, but their altitude sickness was making them green around the gills and not much more than a preliminary discussion was possible. We needed a tent which, with some judicious use of the available natural cold and some artificial heat, could be made into a test chamber at about the same conditions as our potato and onion cold chamber in New Delhi. We had done this in Greenland with success. We also wanted, besides our low altitude Jats, high altitude Jats who had been at altitude for at least six weeks for comparison.

We also needed a group of new Jat recruits straight from the plains for graduated increasing physical exercise for a period of three weeks or so to lay the ghost of Houston's disease to rest once and for all if that were possible. We believed that the disease appeared when troops new to altitude were put to a near full army physical work programme before they had acclimatised. When we disbanded at the end of that first session, I was elated. I felt that we had made a positive start and our new friends were going to be a great help.

That night I had a good dinner and played cards with our new colleagues. Then at about 11 pm, it hit me. I began to feel nauseated. I excused myself. If I did not look green, I certainly felt it. The approximate 20 degree climb to my yurt was a labour accompanied by a thumping headache, a wildly beating heart, extreme breathlessness, an uncontrollable wretched desire to vomit which culminated in the loss of my dinner and fearsome dry retching when there was nothing more to bring up. All I could think of was getting to my yurt and lying down.

Finally I made it, but things were worse lying down. I had stopped dry retching, but the nausea, the piercing headache and the fast pounding of my heart all seemed worse. I got up and walked around outside. The moon-washed valley and mountains which were so beautiful the night before was now a pain in the butt as thinking about it made my symptoms worse. If my batman had appeared singing his Punjabi songs, I would have thrown him bodily down that pallid valley. And as for that jug of wine, loaf of bread and thou crap, how could I?

At about three in the morning I forced myself to lie down and stoically put up with what was happening to me. At some time, I must have fallen asleep. The next thing I knew was listening to a Punjabi song and thinking how beautiful it was. All my symptoms were gone and it was six in the morning of our third day in the Himalayas.

It was not so good for Captain Nishith. His altitude sickness seemed implacable and he developed what was diagnosed as a heart attack with typical pains. He was flown out and we heard later that the diagnosis was confirmed. He recovered from his minor cardiac infarction without incident and after a period of convalescence was back to full duty at low altitude. We all had the pleasure of visiting him when we returned to find him in good health and full of needless apologies for letting the team down. Our commanding officer in charge of the other party never seemed to get over his altitude problems for the full time he was at altitude.

Altitude and the cold that goes with it obviously is not to be trifled with. Its effect varies greatly from individual to individual. Age may have a bearing. At the time we were approached, there had been some apprehension about my involvement because of my 45 years of age, yet in the final analysis the individual most seriously affected was Captain Nishith who, at 29, was the youngest member of the group.

* * *

Our tough minded officers, who were toughest on themselves, were true to their word. When they were free of their duties, they put together what we needed and helped set up our tent facilities and equipment. They also put together our high altitude test subjects and set up the test group for the graduated exercise and cold exposure programme for gradual acclimatisation to altitude and cold.

Under natural conditions, altitude is always accompanied by cold. In a programme of acclimatising to altitude and cold, one is faced with a situation where one is the antithesis of the other. Like acclimatisation to heat, acclimatisation to altitude is a physical performance requirement. It is a matter of increasing one's capability to do physical work in it. In the matter of cold acclimatisation it is a matter of increasing one's capability to produce heat in the absence of physical exercise.

To achieve these capabilities in our group, the cold adaptation programme was carried out in the morning over a four hour period of sitting around while exposed to natural cold in reduced clothing. The altitude adaptation programme was done in the afternoon with increasing physical activity demand over a period of four weeks. In the end we obtained soldiers who perhaps could not equal the physical capabilities at altitude of our highly motivated officers, but who could, we believed, produce a creditable performance good enough to give the Chinese a bad time if it ever came to open hostilities.

Our Sikh officers wanted to go one better. There were Tibetans in the area who had helped the Dalai Llama escape from Tibet when the Chinese invaded Tibet. Sadly they were now in limbo. They could not go back to Tibet without losing their heads and the Indian government would not allow them to come down into India proper. So they were left in this part of the Himalayas in a semi nomadic manner to fend for themselves as best they could. Our attempt to take them back to New Delhi for testing in our potato cooler at low altitude was firmly resisted by the authorities. These Tibetans, it was said, were capable of withstanding extremes of cold and physical ordeals at altitude. On this basis we considered them interesting to test.

The officers knew where some of them were camped and we visited them. I was amazed at the conditions under which they lived. This camp was at about 14,000 feet and consisted of no more than condemned army tents which did not keep out much cold. Neither could they have gained much of the heat produced by a small yak dung fire smouldering in one of them. This group had their families with them. The kids were running around without much clothing and some were walking in the snow with bare feet. This was not uncommon among the inhabitants of this region.

All of them exhibited the high blushing facial skin colour of polycythaemia (increased number of red blood cells) seen in people living at high altitude. There were not many of them, but we got six to undergo the same tests as the Jats. One of them was allergic to extreme cold in the form of giant urticaria (an allergic condition characterised by giant wheals in the skin) every time he was exposed directly to cold. His responses were atypical in that he shivered much more than the others and had a much higher oxygen consumption than his companions who typically exhibited the responses which we had come to associate with individuals acclimatised to cold. This allergic response to cold is rare, but not unknown. When dressed, he did not seem to be bothered by it.

In stark contrast to the tests carried out in New Delhi, the tests at altitude produced severe discomfort and inability to complete the one hour requirement of exposure to cold. Only 2 of the low altitude acclimatised subjects completed the required 60 minutes of the test under great discomfort, 3 of the 5 altitude acclimatised Jats completed the test. All of the Tibetans completed the test period without any show of discomfort. We excluded the allergic Tibetan from testing because of his atypical responses.

Failure to complete the tests was the result of unbearable pain in the feet, hyperventilation and general discomfort. Never in the numerous tests we had carried out at low altitude had we experienced such responses which required termination of testing. This was a strong indication that altitude seriously impaired the mechanisms responsible for tolerance to cold.

The Tibetans, who could be tested only at altitude, though exhibiting a low level of shivering, nevertheless shivered, further indicating that the impairment to cold tolerance at altitude was probably due to an impairment of the non-shivering mechanisms of thermogenesis. They, however, were dramatically more able to withstand the conditions of the test. Those Jats who had been at altitude for some time were better able to do so than the group we had brought with us, but compared with the Tibetans they still had a long way to go. We reported the applied results with our accompanying advice to the Ministry of Defence and reported its scientific aspects as separate reports.[23], [25]

We formulated for the Indian Ministry of Defence a programme to minimise further cases of pulmonary oedema, and to acclimatise troops to both altitude and cold to greatly improve their military performance at altitude. The Ministry sanctioned the graduated exercise and cold acclimatisation programmes. They later reported they were very happy with the results and were experiencing no further cases of Houston's disease at these altitudes in acclimatised troops. However, we could not guarantee that this would be the case at higher altitudes. Now that they were better prepared to face the Chinese threat, formal hostilities came to an end. India lost a sizable amount of territory in this forbidding area. It has maintained troops up to around 25,000 feet to this day and, at these heights, cases of pulmonary oedema still take place.

* * *

The beauty of the Himalayas is not exaggerated. My yurt, perched on the side of the mountain, overlooked a valley which stretched up into the distance high into the sky. A Ladakh village, surrounded by fruit trees, nestled in the valley which, as it rose into the heights, became a snow covered rift two or three miles wide, narrowing to a pass some miles further at the very top. In the clear crystal air of these mountains on fine days, it was difficult to judge distances.

I could not help wondering what a beautiful ski slope it made and tried to rustle up some downhill skis, but skis were not part of travelling equipment in these parts. The mountains on either side of the valley and high pass were magnificent, massive and majestic. They emanated the sense of the "rock of ages".

Amongst these mountains, was a perfect place to study the religions of the East, or religions of anywhere for that matter. It is from the Himalayas, in Lhasa, where Buddhism blossomed. It is here that the Holy Men have meditated and practised the essence of the teachings of Christ, Buddha, Lord Krishna and others to the ultimate of their meaning, mindless of the bitter winds or the penetrating cold of extreme altitudes. It is here that the stories of the supernatural are born and filter down to a world below, mostly unheeded, misunderstood or unbelieved.

I purposely took no reading matter with me other than that pertaining to the teachings of Muhammad, excerpts from the vast literature on Hinduism, Buddhism, Sikhism and some selected works on India. In the comfort of my yurt, but in candle light visibly dimmed by the low oxygen levels at these altitudes, I did not get through all of them. However, delving into them gave me a fresher outlook on religion and washed away misconceptions and any intolerance which I may have had towards other religions than the Christianity I was brought up in. I was not attracted to pursuing any of them in preference to Christianity, but this experience gave me a more holistic view of religion and put each one into a perspective which gave depth and equal weight in my considerations of them as a way to enrich my own life.

I found the fundamental teachings, though varied in approach, all reaching towards the same objectives of service, sacrifice and love for one another, the worthlessness of worldly goods and the right way to live our lives. Perhaps being a scientist, I tended to view what each had to offer as philosophies of how to live this life rather than as teachings of religion for a better after life. In this sense they differed little from the teachings and truths expressed by philosophers and seekers of truth, knowledge and a better way untinged by religious fervour.

Throughout life I had become conscious of the fact that the teachings of the great religious leaders had often been distorted to suit the wishes of their adherents. What was heavenly in them was often made earthly. What was pure was often contaminated. These distortions of man had made them acceptable to some, unacceptable to others and to be avoided at all costs by still others. The gamut of religions and schisms available to man perhaps reflects little else than the numerous manifestations of these distortions. One who cannot find God in one, is unlikely to find God in another. Finding that one of these distortions is more suitable to one's imagery of what is suitable, does not mean that one has found God. That is why I stick to my own brand of distortions. Any other is likely to be as distorted.

The parable equivalents of the Hindu teachings were profuse and many of them most delightful and meaningful. Buddhism, with which I was already familiar, continued to fascinate me, but the difficulty of ever achieving the potentially beautiful state of nirvana still frustrates me. Maybe I can at some quieter and mellower time in the future. Muhammad seemed a bit too strict and militant for me and dwelt too much on the self righteousness of the exclusive faithful. The propensity of its followers towards Jihad or holy wars as a means to an end does not endear it to me personally.

The religion of the Sikhs fathered by Govind Singh to oust the marauding hordes of the Mogul Empire, which had taken over India, was pretty straight forward. It was militant, but it was also tolerant, having developed out of Hinduism which is the most tolerant of all religions. Sikhism's basic require-ments of the long hair, the knife, the bangle and the underwear symbolising cleanliness, warriorship, bondship with one another and good health, did not repel me. I did not feel any untoward feelings when three of us were, at their wish, inducted into it in a simple ceremony in a simple temple at 13,500 feet. The religious schisms with "hallelujahs", "praise the Lords" and a great deal of shouting, proposing that a state of mental hysteria is a manifestation of the presence of the Holy Ghost do not attract me.

* * *

Since before our arrival, the normal level of snowfall had not taken place. The inhabitants were worried because the well-being of the crops when spring and summer came around depended on the snowfall during the winter and its melt in the spring.

The monks in their monasteries and the people in the villages whirled their prayer wheels, chanted their "Om mane padme um"(s) and rang their tinkling bells daily and with extra force whenever it looked like snowing. When there was some snow, these activities were doubly intensified. Although the village was well down from where we were, from my yurt I could hear the tinkling of the bells which I found comforting for they reminded me that I was not too isolated from normal human beings doing the normal things human beings do.

These bells, though sounding different, were akin to the wooden gongs (pate) which used to be struck in our villages back home calling us to early morning prayer. Eventually their efforts were rewarded with a healthy fall of snow in early February which put their world on track again. The joyous ringing of bells went on until the snow stopped falling. But some tinkled on sporadically, with increasing intervals between, as though unwilling to give up their expressions of gratitude.

* * *

Throughout Ladakh there were many monasteries perched on the steepest peaks. I pitied those who daily climbed to provide the monks with food and their daily needs. We visited one of the most celebrated. To get to it we went several miles by jeep until we came to the Indus river which here was more like a large creek. We crossed high above it by a rope swing bridge which was not without its frightening aspects. On the other side, we made a slow climb up to the monastery.

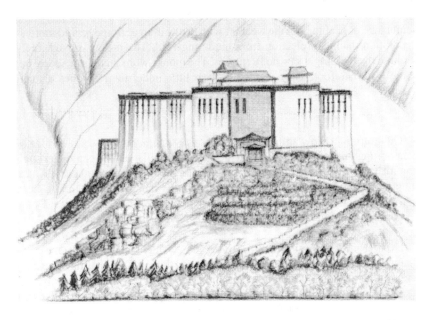

Although the way up was not as steep as some we had observed, it was and will ever be the most difficult and exhausting climb I have ever made. Some members of our party gave up and waited for our return. During the climb we were nearly always in sight of the monastery which, like them all, rose upwards like fairy towers springing from and rooted in the very rocks upon which they stood.

As soon as the monks saw us they came down to accompany us the rest of the way. Unlike us, they ran up and down the path with little effort. they were obviously frustrated by our wheezing and puffing slow pace, punctuated with frequent rests. By now we had been at altitude for about three to four weeks and I could not help thinking that any altitude acclimatisation we might have acquired could be nothing more than a fraction of the potential that could be attained. The monks were dressed in red robes and most of those who accompanied us on our tour of inspection were mere boys. They appeared to be not much more than twelve to fifteen years of age.

The climb was worth the effort, not only for the magnificent view, but also for the monastery. It was large with a large image of Buddha taking up two of its stories.

Surrounding this central figure was an extensive library with shelves reaching high and packed with books bound in wooden covers. I regretted that there was no time to examine them more closely.

The rest of the monastery, extending in directions away from this central part, was full of halls and rooms most of which were without furnishings or starkly furnished. I was struck with the open architecture. Some windows had some semblance of keeping out the weather with heavy drapes. Some served more as decoration than as protection from the biting cold. The breeze moved freely through the building. I saw no fireplaces. The monks wore sandals or shoes, but some were barefoot. They seemed to wear little under the red robes of their order.

* * *

On returning to low altitude, we spent some time in the New and Old Delhi area putting our report together, We became as familiar as one can under such circumstances with the Indian way of life. To me the most impressive single thing was the massive abundance of humanity that pervaded the scenery wherever one went. From morning to late at night one was beset on all sides by humans going about their own business or, by their vending endeavours, making one part of it.

Every form of earning a little living was evident all around. One man manufacturers of trinkets of all kinds. They plied their trade with little more than a few embers of charcoal, a blow pipe and pieces of wire. Side walk mechanics fixed vehicles of all kinds aided only by young boys and a few tools. Weavers of delicate cloth used simple looms. The ability of artisans to do so much with so little was impressive.

I watched them work and could not help thinking that, with the right kind of effort, these masses of people could be organised into a very potent and effective resource to increase their individual and national wealth. By this means they could reduce the poverty, overpopulation and disease, all problems besetting

India. There were also, holy men, beggars and the exhibition of the deformed for alms.

Poverty, over-population and high morbidity/mortality rates are inseparable symptoms of an elite economic system. It is characterised by 90 percent or more of the wealth and power in the hands of 10 percent or less of the population. It may be disguised in different forms, but this is its principle characteristic. In its particular form India was one of these.

Without changing the economic system, little change can be made to alleviate the problems that go with poverty. In 1954 while I was on the Staff of the Harvard School of Public Health, the Department of Epidemiology instituted a research programme under the leadership of Dr John Wyon who was a class mate of mine. The proposition was to examine the effect of providing contraceptive and educational aids to control the high birth rate in the Punjab.

To test the programme, they selected three villages, as like one another as they could be. One was to be a control village in which data was obtained but nothing done to it. Another was to have the contraceptive methods available but nothing else. The third was to be the experimental village. It had contraceptives available and staff to provide educational and other assistance to ensure that all women in the reproductive age received full information on the use of the contraceptives as well as the desirability of fewer births. The study was to continue for twenty years.

My experience in the Cook Islands in the forties and early fifties and my general interest in the problem had made me predict that no differences would be found between the villages. The forces which determine birthrate and over population are more complex and greater than could be overcome by the simple measures incorporated in the study plan.

At the end of 17 years, John thought that enough had been learned. I was then in Kentucky. Because of my former involvement in the study, I was invited to the unveiling of the results in Boston. The village which had nothing done to it had a slightly better result than the other two, but this difference was not statistically significant. In essence, all efforts to reduce the birth rate in the experimental village had no effect.

This study confirmed what some of us suspected: the economic reasons for having or not having children are far stronger than any force or good sense which might dictate otherwise. We can speculate that the high fertility rate could be due to the high mortality rate in children providing a feed back stimulus to overcompensate and produce more children. Perhaps the driving force is the subsistent life which may be best dealt with by having enough children to work. Children become low cost labour as well as insurance to care for parents in their old age. In a very risky environment, children are perhaps one's best investment. However, when it comes to dividing the land amongst them, their lot can only be worse.

The pattern of poverty and all that goes with it is also seen in urban areas where the stimuli to provide a work force is largely absent. However, the feed back stimuli of a high child mortality rate to compensate for deaths is present and may be more important than we think.

Whatever our speculations, poverty is always accompanied by high fertility and high mortality. The converse is just as true. Australia, earlier in this century, brought in the high fertility Europeans to boost its stagnant population. In one generation the immigrants had attained the standard of living enjoyed by other Australians, and began exhibiting the same fertility rates as them. I believe that the most effective way to reduce fertility is to improve standards of living. Although this is easier said than done, I believe it will produce the desired result. In Rarotonga, the population census found the average family was six, by 1985 it was four. During this period there was a phenomenal increase in the economy. A small sample may be, but not an indication to be passed without note. The unhealthy problems associated with loss of "living room" seen inn both animals and man as population densities increase needs to be faced now. Our attempts at simplistic solutions have not born fruit.

One would have thought that India would industrialise and lift itself economically and in other ways into the twentieth century. Instead it continued to bog itself down in an elite economic system with more interest in power fighting at the top than in dealing with the economic and social problems besetting its people. However, perhaps we should keep our judgement open because there may be a better way than the one Europe and America followed and Japan copied, with India at last showing signs of doing the same. I have no idea what that economic system might be, other than doing what we believe is a better way and doing it more perfectly than we have done to date.

* * *

The Taj Mahal is in Agra some one hundred and twenty miles south of New Delhi. I tend to scorn tourist attractions, preferring the unbeaten paths to satisfy my interest in new places. But I felt drawn to the Taj Mahal. I looked for ways to combine this with my usual method of discovering in new places.

Being a lover of motor cycles for their fresh air, free ranging and other attributes, I decided that this was the only way to go to Agra. Hiring a motor-cycle proved to be difficult. There were none to be found. Finally a Sikh taxi driver friend said he knew somebody who might hire his. A bargain was struck and the following Saturday morning was set for departure.

When my intentions became known, there was much consternation from friends and from staff of the US Embassy. John Kenneth Galbraith was the Ambassador, but he seemed never to have entered the picture. The arguments against my mode of travel were that the Dacoits, the robber bands of India, or the Thuggees, the assassins of India, would "get" me. They told me stories of bus and train loads of people being held up and robbed. My counter argument that this proved that travelling by motorcycle would ensure my safety, was not well received.

A reputed millionaire I had befriended offered to pay for a charter plane to take me to Agra, if I would give up this insane travel plan. I thanked him, but told him that seeing and feeling India from the air was not the idea I had in mind. Don Theriault, a member of our team from Natick, was my room mate at the Ashoka Hotel and he became enthused with the idea and expressed his wish to accompany me as pillion rider. This seemed to put arguments against the venture to rest. I supposed it was thought that there was safety in numbers. I, of course, welcomed Don's companionship.

On Saturday morning, the cycle was duly delivered. We donned the best motor cycle riding outfits we could contrive from what we had on hand. We obtained sandwiches from the hotel kitchen and, armed with a bottle of Johnnie Walker Black Label and minimum spare clothing in a rucksack, we were off to see the Taj Mahal.

It was a beautiful cool morning with a clear sky, made to order for motor-cyclists. We both shouted with the joy of the open air and the cool morning breeze on our faces. We did not even think of goggles. We had none. Nor did we have sunglasses. On this cool, clean, balmy, bright, sunny, yellow-tinged early morning, we needed nothing to hinder close contact with the sensual feel, sight, smell and sound of the environment. For an appreciable time, we both revelled in it and loudly acclaimed how great it all was.

Soon we were out of the elite part where the Ashoka Hotel was situated and into the morning traffic of the edge of New Delhi. The traffic was thick and our pace through it was slow. If you imagine this to be a traffic of motor vehicles as met with in the large cities of the Western World, you would be wrong. Mostly it was a traffic of people with loads of one kind or another on their heads or hung on the ends of poles on their shoulders. Interspersed liberally in this human pedestrian horde were bullock carts loaded to teetering heights, two wheeled carts with people and goods atop them, drawn by skinny ponies, one to a cart. There were camels, their heads topping everything else, striding majestically and gazing aloofly into the distance. Not to be out done, there were automobiles and trucks in all states of disrepair, depending on their horns rather than their motors and steering wheels to wend their way through it all. It seemed reasonable to look around for an elephant or two, but there were none.

Our motorcycle, with its narrow frontal area, did a little better than other wheeled vehicles, but it took us a considerable time to reach the less congested area of the country proper. I imagined that these were representative of the farmlands worked by the Jats who we used as subjects in our tests. The farmlands were well planted with lentils, mustard and other farm products I could not identify clearly. All gave a variegated green and orange hue to the flatlands stretching beyond the two lane highway broken only by some low hills, clumps of trees and shrubs.

Once clear of the heavy traffic, I wound the accelerator grip to get us moving, but found that 30 mph was the best we could get out of our cycle. We tried everything to overcome the problem, but to no avail. This fiddling and the slow pace through the traffic had taken time. We trundled along without any real idea how far we had come towards our destination. Our map did not help much because we had lost count of which village was which and found some of our own on the way. Darkness literally fell and, as it did, the rear wheel locked and we came to a shuddering stop. The engine was still running and still in gear.

From past experience I knew the chain had come off and had jammed between the rear wheel sprocket and the wheel. This had sheared the shear pin in the gear box (that is why it is called a shear pin) and now the power from the engine could not be transferred to the rear wheel even if the chain was restored to its rightful position.

Disaster. It was now pitch dark. Being a moon phase watcher, I knew that a near full moon would soon come over the horizon. We sat in the dark and cursed ourselves for not having checked the tension on the chain and for not having the foresight to bring a flashlight. We sat on the side of the road and waited.

In the starlight, we were conscious of people passing us. We accosted them in English, but failed to communicate. They were farm workers returning home with their implements over their shoulders. Finally a huge, near full moon popped over the horizon, showing that the people passing were not armed dacoits or thuggees. In the moonlight we managed to get the chain back in place which freed the rear wheel. We again resumed our sitting and waiting. Experience had taught me that when in trouble sitting and waiting was a sure way of getting help.

Eventually someone, without our prompting, detached himself from the passers-by and asked, "You being having any troubles?" In unison we both exploded in the affirmative. "You coming to my residence. I taking care of you." He instructed a boy we presumed was his son to wheel the bike while we walked empty handed with his father. In his broken English he informed us that he was a school teacher and that he would put us up in his cow byre, at least that is what we thought he said. I believed him because I had read travellers' stories of being put up for the night in rooms attached to cow byres in India.

After a fairly long walk we arrived at his residence. He turned to a building opposite and entered a room which was indeed next to the cows. We could hear them through the wall scuffling and snorting and their milky dungy odour permeated the room. He lit a kerosene lamp and we found ourselves in a low roofed and fairly spacious room with two iron beds and little else. We bathed with water from the well just outside the back door.

Our host brought some curried hot vegetables floating in what I took to be ghee. We were hungry and ate with relish. Our host came back with "loose clothing" and several people to meet us. One of them, in perfect English, informed us he was an advocate working in Delhi and the school teacher who rescued us was his younger brother. He was visiting for the weekend. The others with him were elders of the town who had expressed a wish to meet us.

We were soon lost in conversation with our new found friends. With the advocate translating, we talked about the war in the mountains and a number of topical and world events. They expressed strong anti-socialistic feelings. They did not think much of Nehru. They were admirers of Gandhi, and talked, I thought, very intelligently about the problems of India and the world in general. I had not expected this and, from their expressed thoughts about their political leaders, I do not think their leaders would have expected this either.

Half way through, I developed a thirst, but I was a little afraid of the water. When we used the well, I had evaluated it with a professional eye. It looked pretty good. It had a wall around it, as all wells should, to stop spillage and contamination going back into it. The water inside I hoped would be as good.

I thought that a shot of Johnny Walker Black Label would just be the thing to ensure that any stray bugs in the water would be put out of action. The efficacy of this theory I have never tested by the scientific method, so I cannot unreservedly recommend it. It did all right for me this time as it has done many times in the past. But I was concerned with the effects that taking alcohol might have on the sensibilities of our hosts who, as Hindus, would likely be teetotallers.

Anyway it was time for Don and I to overcome our, so far, admirable restraint from broaching the contents of our bottle. So in all seriousness I interrupted our discussions and, after paying homage to their teetotal leanings, I bluntly, but as sensitively as I could, expressed our desire for a glass of water each into which we were going to add some alcohol in the form of scotch. The advocate passed this message on and there was a bit of a discussion which made me believe that I had made the blunder that I so fervently wished to avoid. I waited with bated breath for some indication of this, but the advocate only urged us to wait. One of the company, the youngest, was sent out and we continued our discussions, as though nothing had happened. We held our glasses of scotch and water in front of us and waited while still participating in the discussion.

Finally the young man returned accompanied by a turbaned and dhoti clothed individual who sat opposite us holding out a shallow wooden bowl. The advocate explained that it was true that they were teetotallers and, to avoid any insult to us, their guests, they did not wish us to drink alone. To avoid this insult, the young man had fetched the village drunk so that he could join us on their behalf. Since he took only one drink to our two or three, he could not have been much of a village drunk. However, we appreciated the gesture and said so.

When we said goodnight, we had had a most interesting day with many plusses, generously sprinkled with the kindness and goodwill of our hosts, all of which made the disaster to our motorcycle a small matter. During the night, the cattle next door made snufflings and noisy bumps to the wall between us. Otherwise we slept very well until 4 am when the noise of their being hitched up for work in the fields woke us. It turned out they were not cows but huge brahman oxen, the kind that American cowboys ride at rodeos. I was later informed that crushed kidneys is a common complaint of handlers of these beasts.

Our hosts arranged a two wheeled horse cart to take us, motorcycle and all, to Mathura for repairs to the motor cycle. I was interested in having a look at Mathura as it was the birth place of Lord Krishna. It turned out to be a full morning trip. Here and there our little horse had to be given a little help. It was flat country with few rises and he bravely tripped along at a slow trot. In the early part of the morning, the scenery and the screaming parrakeets kept me interested. In Mathura, a side walk mechanic and his boy helpers fixed the motor cycle.

In the meantime we tried to have a look at Mathura, but with no great success. It was Sunday afternoon and I had to be back to do some tests on our Jats at the potato cooler next morning. So we returned to New Delhi. I felt no loss at not seeing the Taj Mahal. What we had done and what had happened to us met all my ideas of a good tour of a new place. Don seemed also not to be put out by our failure to reach our objective.

I returned the following weekend by more conventional means to have a look at the Taj Mahal. I was so enthralled by it I spent an extra day and sketched some of the designs on the arches in an attempt to understand them. The one that baffled me most was what an Indian gentleman, watching me sketching and puzzling over it, told me was the "diamond cutters" design. It was a puzzling motif because, as a whole, it was harmonious and met my criteria of an artistically interesting design. But in detail it was difficult to make out the very complicated pattern that made up the harmonious and delightful whole.

It would be foolish of me to attempt to describe the tremendous impact that the Taj Mahal made on me. You will have to see it for yourself.

* * *

I was sorry to leave India, but all good things must come to an end. Back at Natick I reviewed the results of my efforts to unravel the mysteries of my particular research interest and where it had lead me and what was needed for its future.

Our physiological research had helped to establish the existence of non-shivering thermogenesis. We had also determined that it was the primary mechanism for heat production in cold acclimatised, warm blooded animals including man. We established that skeletal muscle was the an important site for its production. This was quite independent of its heat production from voluntary or involuntary muscular contractions. The elucidation of the energy pathways by which chemical thermogenesis produced this heat was, I thought a biochemical problem. Accordingly I was amenable to providing them with facilities at Natick. I had identified three such biochemists who were willing to join us and proceed with the work, but there was a negative response to this plan that I was not able to overcome. I felt that to continue my physiological approach to the problem would be repetitious and unrewarding. The subject needed a new dimension which I was not able to give it on my own. So I resigned to seek new fields of endeavour.

CHAPTER TWELVE

Racing, Research and Consulting

Economic institutions change rather rapidly; large corporations and their relations with the community and state are especially in flux. And with such change comes new information, new insight. In consequence the rate of obsolescence in economic knowledge is high. JOHN KENNETH GALBRAITH

After resigning, I was at a loss as to know what to do next. We were not badly off financially, but could not go on too long without income. I raced my Alfa Romeo at Thompson race track and found the other Alfas fitted with ever more expensive accessories to achieve greater speeds. Previously prohibited, an increasing range of "production" ancillary speed equipment was now permitted. This equipment was expensive and my poor standard production Alfa had to do some extra hairy things to just keep the pack in sight, let alone to win. It was no longer competitive. I was prepared to go the extra expense, but my resignation put an end to that.

This saddened me because I loved motor racing and had had a go at most of the kinds available at that time. I enjoyed road racing best and enjoyed the fast acceleration and split second timing of drag racing enjoyable. I was never involved in the Indy 500 Classic except in fiction. This came about through a challenge by the Indianapolis Sports Car Club to race a team from our Kentucky Club in a time trials event during the Memorial Day weekend, the same Memorial day that Bettenhausen was killed in the Indy 500 Classic. I led the Kentucky team and we routed the opposition. Through some mix up, it was reported in the West Coast media that I had been killed in the same accident as Bettenhausen. I rather enjoyed replying to letters of condolence to Lydia in the vein that reports of my death were grossly exaggerated, a la Mark Twain.

I began amateur motor racing in 1956. Once I tried it, I was hooked. I loved racing cars more than any of the many sports in which I had participated. For the heck of it I had bought a second hand Triumph TR4 and joined the Kentucky Chapter of the Sports Car Club of America (SCCA). I drove in rallies with Lydia as navigator and found this enjoyable, very social, but, after a while, a little boring.

I unconsciously gravitated towards a few club members who occasionally turned up at our monthly club meetings. They seemed to be a breed apart. They were - they raced cars on the road racing circuits. I asked them how one went about getting into this so little advertised activity of the club. They told me to get a medical certificate, turn up with the car at the nearest race track and race six races as a novice. If you passed the judgement of a committee of race drivers, you qualified as a race car driver.

So I took off with son John, aged 13, as pit crew, to Lawrenceville in Southern Illinois where the next nearest race was being held. At that time, there was no minimum age limit for the pit crew. Our new found racing friends were there and helped John and me learn the ropes of becoming a race driver and a pit crew respectively. They showed us what was required to register, put the assigned number on the proper places on the car, go through technical inspection, find a pit space, get on the track for practice and get on the grid for racing. Some spectators from our Club were only too happy to join John as pit crew. John and I knew enough to bring a stop watch, a small blackboard for someone to write my lap times on, and our box of tools. It was not without some trepidation that I gave the car a final going over and tune up, put on my fireproof racing overalls, helmet and goggles and faced going out on the track for the mandatory two hours practice.

I got in the car, fastened my seat belt firmly, pulled my goggles down, started the engine and warmed her up. The bark of the open exhaust sounded right and I was ready to go. I felt nothing. No emotions. I sat staring at the way out of the pits on to the track. I had often felt like this before entering the boxing ring. Then I felt John's thump on my shoulder giving me the signal that the track was clear to go.

Many thoughts and feelings crowded into my consciousness. They seemed to be all about getting out there and finding out what it was all about. I shot on to the track and for the next half hour or so, I knew that up to the age of 38 years, I had, outside of sex, missed the best thing that I had ever experienced in my life. The elation was overwhelming. This was the sport of sports. This was the sport of Kings. This was for me.

Every driver seemed to be on the track a few seconds after my sortie on to it. I was having the time of my life with my foot on the accelerator, hard on the floor, weaving between the cars and being weaved through by the faster cars. At what I thought was the right time before the corner, I hit the brakes hard and the girling front brakes slowed the car straight and true. Why the lowly Triumph had Girling disk brakes was a mystery, but it gave that extra stopping power so necessary for full-out road racing. One could go deeper into corners than cars without them. Auto racing, besides other lesser things, is a play of hard on with the brakes when you are not flat down on the accelerator.

I was having the time of my life, but as the third lap came around, my car seemed to have lost power. It would not get up to speed on the straights. On the long back straight, I glanced at the speedometer and got a shock. We were doing over a hundred miles an hour and the tachometer was in the red. The Triumph was doing more than its recommended best. The illusion of doing much less was disappointing, but it was caused by my speeded up reflexes. A much faster car was needed if I was going to continue having fun.

Then I spotted the black flag being waved at me angrily. Humiliated, I shamefacedly pulled to the side of the track and stopped. The nearest safety official told me to proceed slowly and out of the way of the traffic to my pits and report to the starter.

The starter took no notice of me. I fretted at the time I was losing from my new found love of uninhibited speed on a track specially designed to test my driving skill under as many road conditions as could be contrived on a three mile lap race course: right angled corners, the esses, a hook, the chicanes, corners banked the wrong way to name a few and all of this with other drivers vieing for position and advantage, even in practice.

I could not help imagining this on the Nurburgring with its 14.7 miles lap of everything that road surface and corner combinations can challenge the driver and car. My lowly Triumph was practising in company with the high pitched whine of Ferraris, the unmistakable growling power of the Corvettes and the seemingly single banger grump of Porsche Carreras. They gave me a fright each time they roared noisily past. This was the reason for the black flag. I made my impatience obvious. This only made the starter's delaying tactics more prolonged, or so it seemed.

Finally the starter, who is the boss supreme of the event, gave me a liberal piece of his mind about my not keeping my eyes on the rear view mirror and not caring about what was happening behind me. I was in the way of the faster machinery and was not aware of it. I learnt my first lesson, caring for one's neighbour even on a race track.

I went back on the track for the rest of the day's practice and almost immediately learnt my second lesson. I went into a bend with too much exuberant speed and too little skill. I and my car went spinning down the track. One of the other lessons learnt that day was to keep a healthy distance from the hero drivers who drove with abandon and seldom finished a race. They usually did not last long in the game.

The spinning round and round down the track was a most extraordinary experience when encountered for the first time. To the novice that I was, it came without warning. The whizzing round and round seemed to be happening in slow motion and there was no control. Turning the wheel from full lock one way and then the other made no difference to the spins. Applying brakes or the accelerator made no difference either. I might as well have been on a sheet of ice. Later I recalled that throughout the spin, I was busily working out how I would be lined up when this thing came to an end and how I could quickly get back into the fray.

In reviewing the events of the day, I was happy. The illusion of slowness of the car, the slow motion during the spin-out and my working out while spinning as to how I could get back into the race quickly, told me that I was able to get my reflexes up to several times faster than usual and could react fast and logically to a situation that demanded it. This cheered me no end. Without this, one is vulnerable. This should not have been a surprise, I had been a boxing champion, a sprinter, a swimming champion, an A grade rugby player, a shooting champion and a runner-up for the New York Yacht Club Blue Water Cruising Medal. Why shouldn't my reflexes be good.

Finally my first novice race came up. There were about twenty of us from the several chapters of the SCCA in the nearby States. Since it was a novice race, there was a variety of machinery and a number of the cars were more powerfully engined than my Triumph. There were other Triumphs in the line-up, one driven by a redheaded youngster had drawn my attention during practice. The one Ace Bristol present bothered the hell out of me. Its 2000 cc engine had the same cubic capacity as the Triumph, but it cost three times as much as my second-hand Triumph. On the production line, it had received all the expensive "go goodies" which the Triumph had not.

I was given a position in the middle of the third row of the grid. Again, being a novice race, no one cared who was placed where on the grid. We all probably felt, as I did, "I'm lucky to be here at all." It was my first experience of a grid start or, for that matter, any start at all. Practice had given me some knowhow. At 38 years of age, I had my self confidence under some control. I had tried everything I could during those short hours of practice to learn. I tried to learn how to get the most out of the car and how to take advantage of the weaknesses and mistakes of the other drivers. I made many mistakes, but the trick is to pick these up. I hoped that I was better at picking up their mistakes than they were at picking up mine.

I was ready for my first race and so was the car. The Ace Bristol was in front of me and on the grid was giving me the heebie jeebies again. I was determined to beat it, even if I beat nobody else. I realised that this was my first novice race and first race ever on a race track. That is if we discount my racing to the home depot when I was a taxi driver as a student, a few hill climbs on my motorcycle, the Iron Duke, and some surreptitious flying quarter miles on back roads in New Zealand.

The Ace Bristol driver and others in the race were probably veterans compared to me. Most of them had some of the required six novice races under their belts. While these thoughts ran through my head, I saw the starter move to the front of the grid and say in a loud voice, "Gentlemen, start your engines!"

I was not ready for the thrill of a grid start. There was the roar of engines with open exhausts all revving up and down in unison and then in asynchrony with a beat note cacophony. Helmets could not keep the noise out. the smell of fuming castor oil permeated the air. Whether the castor oil concoction did any good or not, we paid a premium price for it, and its burning smell was beautiful. It became part of the nostalgia of the starting scene along with the barking, thundering noise of suddenly released power, the fast build up of adrenalin, the conscious keying of already speeded up reflexes, the nearness of other cars and competitors. They all gave the grid start a special thrill no matter how many times I experienced it.

It seemed no time at all from starting our engines to the drop of the starter's flag and we were off to a scrambling, noisy, smelly, no touch, pushing and shoving melee of cars trying for best position for the first turn, usually a right angle. There are other kinds of starts, the Le Mans, the Pace Car and others. In the following years we experienced them all, but for me, none can equal the "standing grid start" and the close scramble for the first turn.

In the noise and jostling melee of the start we were, in no time at all, at the first corner, a right hand right angle turn, with the brake lights of the cars ahead of me blinking on, I found myself standing hard on the brakes. In the mess of surrounding cars we made it around this corner, but a number did not. Some ran straight on. Some skidded off the track taking markers and hay bales with them and some went into half hearted spins. The low speed at this point did not allow them to get into real healthy, screaming spins. We, who were still on the track, by good fortune rather than good management, were having trouble avoiding each other in a seeming tangle of machinery. But we made it.

Once around and in the clear, with accelerator hard to the floor, I took stock of my rivals and found Ginger a little ahead of me but nothing of the Ace Bristol in front or behind. Ahead of Ginger were a couple of Austin Healeys, an XK120 Jaguar and a couple of other machines. I had not done too badly. Now it was a matter of settling down to watch the competition ahead, picking up their weaknesses, especially in the corners, and waiting my chance.

Once I had decided to participate in the sport, my mind created many imaginary situations of what could be done. In these day dreams I even made noises simulating the whine of engines to increase the realism. Some of these imaginings were Superman stuff and not remotely possible. Some were only marginally possible and even Stirling Moss, the wild man of road racing, would not have attempted them.

On the track, hardly any of the tactics of my grand imaginings were feasible. Like everything else in life, it was going to be decided by hard work and concentration. If there was a magic formula, it was eluding me. I was not even able to consciously pick up the mistakes of others.

On the second lap, I saw the Ace Bristol on the side of the track, its driver with helmet still on, his hands, still in his nice new driving gloves, gripping the steering wheel and staring into space.

Later I was told that his pit crew had to pry him from the wheel and lift him out. He had spun and frozen or, perhaps, frozen and spun. He wisely never raced again. In the meantime I was following Ginger, bumper to bumper, and by the fifth lap we had got by all the machinery except the Jaguar. I tried everything I knew, little as this was, to pass Ginger, but could not, and we finished in that order.

After several more practice sessions I managed to turn some of the tactics and strategies of my imaginings into realities and won the next two races from Ginger. Joy of joys, both Ginger and I were given our full racing licenses after only three novice races. It was the start of many years of road racing, a sport I enjoyed more than any other. I never had a serious accident. I won some, I lost some, but there was not one moment that I can look back on without a sense of enjoyment and satisfaction. So it was with a heavy heart that I hung up my helmet. I hoped it was temporary, but that was not to be. Racing had become too costly and my next job demanded a great deal of time, Now that I was near the sea again, I went back to my other love, boating. It proved just as costly.

* * *

I was now in the market place for a job for the first time since being appointed Medical Officer to the Cook Islands in 1945. Fred Stare typically made me a very generous offer to return to the Department of Nutrition of the Harvard School of Public Health. He also told me that Arthur D. Little Inc., over the other side of the Charles River in Cambridge, was interested in my medical and research background to provide clinical research qualifications to their Life Sciences Division headed by Dr Charles J. Kensler.

Fred advised me to take my time about making up my mind, but thought that Arthur D. Little Inc. (ADL) might suit me very well. He gave me a little background and I visited several times and was interviewed by several of the senior personnel. The way the company operated appealed to me and, after some serious thinking, I accepted the position of Research and Consulting Physician, newly created for my benefit.

* * *

Arthur D. Little Inc. is the oldest research and consulting Company of its kind in existence. It was founded by Arthur D. Little in 1886 along rather novel lines as to how its research staff was to operate. Being a registered commercial company, it had a Board with a Chairman, a President, and Vice Presidents of Divisions. Beyond that there were groups working under professionals from all scientific disciplines who formed them ad hoc to meet various research demands.

Within this minimum structure, obligated for the most part by requirements for registration of a company, there were groups forming and reforming to respond to the dynamics of demands in the major fields of scientific disciplines which formed the Divisions of the Company.

Basic to this concept was the rule that whoever came up with a project was in charge of it, regardless of status within the company. All projects at ADL were called cases and we boasted that there was no realistic research project that anyone could dream up that we could not investigate and answer.

This modus operandi of Arthur D. Little was not much different from that in universities and similar to that engendered by Fred Stare under which I had worked in the past. If one wants creativity, as one must in the creative business of research, one must follow something along these lines.

Often the low output of government research and other institutions is caused by the failure to recognise these considerations. However, there were some important differences at ADL which assisted the researcher. One was the superb support facilities available to researchers at ADL. It was generally recognised that ADL was the commercial and applied research arm of the basic research capabilities of the universities around Boston and the Massachusetts Institute of Technology (MIT).

The Accounting Department was very efficient. In other research situations, financial accounting was a broad brush affair in which one did not know, except after a long delay, and then only within uncertain limits, the status of one's financial support. It did not matter much in most situations as somebody else usually took the rap for overspending and it was your own fault if you underspent. But at ADL, within one to three hours of requesting it, you had a full statement on any or all of your cases up to the time of your request.

Another important area of support was the library services. A support staff of qualified librarians searched the literature and provided a written memo with comments on the value of the findings. Our ADL library was pretty good and other libraries, the most important of which were the Harvard Conant library and the Library of Congress in Washington, were also available to us.

These were important facilities because most of my work and much of that of others was evaluating the published literature and coming up with a review of what it said, what it meant, what credibility could be given it and its value as a basis for advice to the client. In general, our clients were more interested in a "state of the art" review than in original research. However, we did a great deal of fundamental research where information was lacking or confirmation was required.

Facilities such as laboratory space and equipment and changing these to suit the work at hand was never a problem. At one time I needed a swimming pool and measuring techniques devised by us to be built on the premises with facilities for all the needs of human subjects to be tested in the programme. These were installed with no hassle at all. The installation of monkey quarters and extensive behavioural equipment for testing psychoactive drugs on their behaviour, as with setting up facilities for other simple or complex and multi-disciplinary research programmes, never posed any problems. Facilities were adapted to the needs of the client.

ADL financed its operations for private clients on personal charge rates which differed in accordance to the qualifications of the personnel involved. It was the policy of ADL to limit research and consulting for government to less than one third of its work load. It believed that if government supported more than a third of the work, it might make demands which were not to be in the best interests of ADL or its staff. There was always enough private sector work to prevent this.

These features of ADL came out in my initial interviews with the upper echelon of the company and suited the free wheeling approach. Also my working life had been involved with government and academia and I felt that involvement with business was now important to me personally, as one day I would need these skills back home for the benefit of my own people living in a Third World country.

Not everyone found this structureless free wheeling approach to business their cup of tea. Thus the turnover of staff within two years of joining ADL was high. Those who stayed more than two years, usually stayed forever, because they were unlikely to find any other work situation as acceptable. The formula was expressed this way: if you join ADL, within two years you will leave it; if you stay for more than two years, you will be there for life; if, after two years, you leave ADL, you will be back in two years. It often was so.

Many left because they could not find the ladder of hierarchy up which they could climb - there wasn't one. One's survival in ADL was based on performance and not company intrigue and political infighting. Many individuals find an organisation without a structure they can manipulate is anathema and they do not last long in it.

Insistence on this free working system ensured that the company attracted creative researchers with performance as their main motive. They put ADL's reputation at the very top. The system was reflected in the fact that, of the 1600 staff, 800 were professionally qualified.

It was a policy of ADL not to compete with its clients, so the manufacture of products which ADL developed were passed on to manufacturers who were interested in making them.

* * *

In this milieu I found myself with a spacious, well appointed office and a secretary, but nothing else. It was the Harvard scene all over again. Everything was up to me, but how to get it started was the question. This time I realised that research and consulting was mostly about getting clients with problems which needed some of my particular skills to solve. This would pay my salary and expenses and the support services that ADL supplied for my use and the use of my staff.

ADL had never employed a doctor of medicine on its staff to actually do research and consulting. Normally it contracted MD consultants from the various teaching and research institutions attached to medical schools, medical institutions and teaching hospitals in Boston, New York, Washington, Baltimore and beyond. These were always available, but they had never before been involved in more than calls for consultation. Therefore, there was no past experience upon which I could draw. However, it did not take long for things to begin happening.

There was a need for my research oriented skills in the pharmaceutical and food industry. Each had problems within themselves and both the pharmaceutical and food industries had problems with the FDA and vice versa. The problems arose out of misconceptions due to decisions being based on opinion and lack of application of the scientific method. Over ninety percent of studies for efficacy of drugs, for example, was based on clinical judgement when properly designed and conducted studies could have produced results to which probability mathematics could have been applied to determine whether or not they were due to chance alone. This could have removed the need for guessing games and differences of opinion. In the relationship between FDA and the food industry much of the problem between them was based on unsubstantiated claims on both sides as to what was good and what was not.

The special skill I could bring to bear on their problems had to do with my training in research design and probability statistics that I had acquired both at the University of Sydney and at Harvard. I had used them to analyse and evaluate all my research results where they applied. I had become particularly impressed by the way that probability statistics could remove the "guess and by God" practises of evaluation that were in vogue in biological and medical research at that time. It was the root of the trouble the pharmaceutical companies were having in testing their drugs as it was the root of the trouble that the medical personnel of FDA were having in interpreting them.

This area of my interest was described by Charlie Kensler, our Life Sciences Vice President, as a "can of worms". He tried to convince me to leave it alone. Charlie defined many of my cases as "cans of worms", but I told him that my training and experience had given me a good handle on understanding the problems and solutions in this area. Because I knew I had some of the answers, it would be unethical not to try to do something about it. He mumbled something about letting it "be on my own head" etc. but he kept an eye on such cases.

Charlie, as a PhD, could not be blamed for seeing my medical research field as a strange unfamiliar area with approaches and techniques quite different from those normally encountered by non-medical researchers. It was an area where the scientific method met up with a profession which was likely not to know much about it, or, if it did, was unwilling to give up its artistically derived conclusions based on professional judgement, clinical experience and training. For the most part, this is perfectly valid in its place at the bedside of the sick.

Knowledge of the symptoms, signs and laboratory analysis results exhibited by the patient and how these come together to give a diagnosis is not based on any scientific method. Only professional judgement, clinical experience and training, together with the art to put it together properly can arrive at the correct conclusion. The artistry does not end there, for it is as much needed for the proper care of the patient as is the curative armamentarium available to the physician. A physician who does not have the artistry of the profession and who practises by numbers can never achieve a notable level of competence.

Having said that, we can see the problems when a physician turns his hand to clinical or other research. We can also see the difficulties Charlie and other PhDs were having looking from the outside at the resulting confusion. Physicians doing studies required for therapeutic drug applications tended to reject methodology which would test the veracity of their sacrosanct clinical judgements, made on the basis of their unscientific and uncontrolled studies. Because of this, the studies were not designed to take full or even moderate advantage of the methodology which would allow the application of statistical analyses. Clinicians took umbrage at any suggestion which might even faintly put their clinical judgement in the realm of suspect. However, research demands different approaches and skills from those required for healing the sick.

To overcome these shortcomings, the medical personnel of FDA were requesting a large number of studies on a large number of subjects. This resulted in a large number of applications for potentially therapeutic drugs which the MDs in the FDA were trying to evaluate with great difficulty, resulting in a large backlog of drug applications which were increasing at an alarming rate.

The large number of things being demanded and done was in the belief that numbers would provide a solution, but more of an unsatisfactory thing only produces more unsatisfactory things. The pharmaceutical companies were justifiably pressuring the FDA for a response to their applications. Tensions were high and had nowhere to go but up.

A short history of one of my cases might make these points clearer. Bill Holland of Cheeseborough Pond, just outside of New York City, called me. His company wanted to build a factory to process and manufacture proteolytic enzymes, touted to be THE thing for the treatment of bruises and injuries, particularly for sports, and as a general anti-inflammatory agent. A proteolytic enzyme is in the same family as a housewife's meat tenderiser. There are all sorts of proteolytic enzymes and all of them do much the same thing. In the previous five to ten years these enzymes had been promoted for the treatment of bruises and injuries on the speculation that, believe it or not, if one took it by mouth it would enter the blood stream and mop up the bruise.

One would think that any sensible person would question that a meat tenderiser taken by mouth as a pill or a capsule would, after it found its way into the bloodstream (if it did), make a beeline for that bruise and mop it up. Ten years of clinical studies had all said unanimously that, in the clinical judgement and opinion of the clinical investigators, that is exactly what it did.

We did a search of the literature in the hope that we could give Bill and his executives a considered good news answer. We found about 110 clinical investigations, of which only twelve were usable. Only seven of them had enough information to provide a basis for us to do a statistical analysis as to the efficacy of proteolytic enzymes not being the result of chance alone. Our analysis of the raw data provided by these seven studies showed that these agents were ineffective. Yet these and every other study of the 110 total stated that in the opinion of the investigators the proteolytic enzymes tested were efficacious. On that basis the FDA had passed the drug applications for their clinical use.

I presented my report to Bill and his colleagues which advised the company not to proceed with the manufacture of this agent. Unknown to me they had already spent over a half million dollars on the proposed production facilities. Their disappointment was sad to see. I had visions of losing the company as a client. I carefully went over the information upon which I based my advice so that they would have some understanding of it. In the end they were convinced and obligingly told me that they had requested my opinion and would abide by it. One year later Bill called to inform me that my advice had saved them millions of dollars because the drug had just been put off the market by FDA for lack of efficacy.

This case history can be repeated over and over again for a variety of therapeutic drugs being clinically tested for drug applications to the FDA. It became an obsession with me and I spent a great deal of my spare time working out ways and means to assist the Food and Drug Administration, the pharmaceutical companies and the clinical investigators to understand their dilemmas and overcome them. On the positive side, pharmaceutical companies on both sides of the Atlantic were using me more and more to plan and supervise their clinical studies for efficacy because FDA was accepting these with fewer hassles.

* * *

My obsession to assist FDA in overcoming the increasing load of drug applications seemed hopeless. At the beginning of my interest, the FDA was reputed to be about 3000 drug applications behind and FDA's insistence that enough studies be done on each of these, created a horrendous number of studies to be evaluated by the less than thirty MDs in FDA. I felt sorry for them because they had the highest of motives. They were doing what they thought best to protect the public from ineffective drugs. But the more they tried, the more difficult it became to achieve their goal.

The pharmaceutical companies were responding to the requests of FDA the best way they could. The problem was that clinical studies,based on nothing more than the clinical opinion of the investigators, could not be assessed. They were performed without using the scientific method and providing the information to provide a statistical probability that the drug was or was not efficacious. Clinical investigators who were untrained in the scientific method were doing their best in a mystical sort of way. Faith in professional opinion is the way they had been brought up.

However, things were sorting themselves out. The FDA and the pharmaceutical companies were coming along fine on controlled studies using blind procedures. This is nothing more than investigators making their evaluations on the patient without knowing whether the patient was receiving the drug under test, or a control drug, or a fake pill made to look like the real thing and called the placebo. Therefore, the investigator would be making his assessments blind. Placebo effects, where the patient feels better even though he is taking fake pills, can affect the results by as much as 30 percent and must be taken into account in the design and evaluation of clinical studies. Without going into technical details, suffice it to say that properly designed and executed clinical studies can take all the guess work out of determinations of the efficacy of therapeutic agents. Gradually both the FDA and the companies moved in this direction.

This was fine, but it did not solve the problem of the backlog of studies for drug applications up to that time. A great deal of effort, time and money had gone into these more than 3000 reputed drug applications with about 50 to 100 separate studies in each, making a large total of individual studies to be evaluated. Experienced medical statisticians know that only about five to seven percent of these can be salvaged. It may be easier and cheaper to throw the lot in the rubbish bin and start all over again, but a great deal of effort and money went into them. The problem was how to sort out the small amount of wheat from the large amount of chaff. I mulled over this problem for some time and came up with what I thought was a workable answer.

I did not have the ear of the FDA. Perhaps it was because I had unwittingly embarrassed it on some nutritional cases. Then out of the blue two ADLers from Business Management walked into my office. They had been doing business management work for FDA and had completed their assignment with about $2000 left over. While doing their stuff at FDA, they learnt about the horrendous backlog. They had also heard of my interest in dealing with this problem. Like good ADLers they wanted to help and asked me to prepare a report on how it may be resolved. The money did not mean a damn, I would have done it for nothing. What was important was that, through these fellows, I had a way into FDA with the information I thought they needed and get rid of an obsession to boot.

Since only about 5 percent of the individual studies had any worth, if we could sort these out we would have only a small total to worry about. It is relatively easy to sort out studies which have no value. They are the majority which supply no numerical data. No matter how long one stares at them, they will not produce one iota of factual information except to tell you in the summary

that in the professional opinion of the investigator the drug is or is not efficacious. He can't prove it and neither can you. So waste no time on them. Discard
them.

Then come those studies with numerical data which may be presented as
means only or means with ranges or means with standard deviations or standard
errors. The ones with ranges only can be thrown out unless the ranges do not
overlap. Although probabilities of efficacy cannot be mathematically ascertained, the fact that the ranges do not overlap is proof enough of efficacy.

Studies giving raw data are generally acceptable because the data can be
analysed. Studies which present analysed data are, of course, entirely acceptable, but they were a rarity in those days.

I suggested in my report that this separation could be done by employing
technicians and teaching them how to recognise useful studies which could be
handed to statisticians for computer analysis. The reports on these studies follow
a standard pattern of introduction, methods, results, comments and conclusions.
The only part of any value in the efficacy determination is in the results section,
the rest can be ignored provided that the methodology followed acceptable lines
to produce acceptable data. For clarity I added a chart showing the programming
steps and avenues to follow for the programming of statistical analyses in a
computer to give the degree of probability of efficacy.

On this basis I prepared the report for my friends from Business Management
to add to their other reports for the FDA. They were delighted and expressed
their certainty that FDA would also be delighted. I was not so sure, I had had
too many bad experiences with this kind of innovation, but felt reassured and
happy that I had at last reached FDA in this matter and it was off my list of
obsessions.

A few days later, the physicians of FDA went public and I found myself being
castigated coast to coast in the media for even suggesting such an approach and
expecting technicians and non-medics to make decisions that only professionals
could possibly make and a whole lot more of other words that tore my medical
character to little shreds. *The Washington Post*, the *Boston Globe*, the *Chicago
Tribune* and the West Coast papers carried the story. I was devastated. So much
for wanting to help.

The Chairman and the Board of ADL were equally devastated and convened
a meeting at which I was asked to attend. They got my story and indicated that
they were fully behind what I had proposed, but what were we to do to counter
the public attack? Everybody put on his thinking cap. Everybody except me. I
just was not capable of any coherent thought. I sat there like a dummy.

Then Charlie Kensler asked me if we had any reputable medical consultants
who were also consultants to FDA. If so I should send them the Boston Globe
release and my paper and ask them to give a critique on my proposal. All agreed
this was a good idea. I was in no fit state of mind to think whether it was good
or bad, but I did what was agreed and the response was a happy one in that the
consultants in effect said that the ideas expressed in my report were what FDA
needed and that FDA should follow my suggestions. I breathed a sigh of relief,

but Charlie again warned me against my tendency to get involved in cases that were "cans of worms".

If all interested parties, the clinicians doing the studies, the clinicians evaluating the studies and the pharmaceutical companies, were rejecting the very means by which their problem could be solved, their dilemma was simply going to become worse and proportional to the number of studies and subjects being demanded. From the time of my first involvement with the problem I had approached it with the caution of a cat stalking a highly suspicious mouse, but even that did not prevent me getting into trouble.

Preliminary efforts I had made in the very beginning to orient my potential clients to the concepts of research design and the application of probability mathematics to replace professional opinion, produced so much alarm that I had to back off fast, but not fast enough to avoid the wrath of the FDA MDs. However, the cost to pharmaceutical companies was so great and the light down the tunnel so dim that they were willing to consider anything I suggested. So I went to work. It was the only hope I had of cracking this so unnecessary dilemma which was costing everybody a mint and leaving large numbers of suffering patients without even a potential means for relief.

* * *

This was a time when new breakthroughs, especially in drugs for the treatment of a variety of mental conditions, were being made. The possible new compound formulations and permutations of the promising basic chemical structures needed to be pursued with vigour and rapid evaluation. This could not be done as long as clinicians doing the test studies and those evaluating them were having difficulties in accepting methodology which verified their professional opinions. It would also bring to an end the continuous confrontations between the pharmaceutical companies and the FDA. It was often said that if aspirin was a new drug, it would never get past the FDA and on to the market.

I concentrated on the pharmaceutical companies because, next to the patients, their need was the greatest. They needed to perform their studies properly. I patiently went through with them the design concepts that must be incorporated in each study and explained how the statistical probability mathematics could verify the efficacy of their new drugs.

They saw the good sense in this, but showed some concern because such methods could also show their drugs to be ineffective. I pointed out that this would be a better result if it could be shown rapidly and save them pursuing something which would be proved ineffective anyway. An ineffective drug even after receiving the approval of the FDA, will eventually in from three to five years fall by the wayside. This can take place through nothing more than the integration of the experience of clinicians using them.

They were impressed by the cost argument but were faced with the dilemma that sales for three to five years are mighty good returns. In their experience, poor evaluation techniques had often allowed drugs to escape on to the market and had earned good money before being removed. Some had come to accept this as normal and not of great moral consequence! However, I managed to convince them that verifying efficacy was the better way to go. They indicated some concern that the clinicians who did the studies for them would balk at having to do the studies in the manner I had described. I agreed, but asked them to let me try.

Slowly we began to put some of the available scientific methodology into the system which resulted in better scientific evaluations of efficacy. This was reflected by the ready acceptance of the studies by the FDA. It made the problems of putting together the enormous amount of material required by the FDA into a more organised and purposeful manner. It was my hope that the FDA would perceive their request for a large number of subjects and a large number of studies as being unnecessary. It made the evaluations by the medical personnel at FDA easier and their requirements less demanding. It provided the public and the medical profession with therapeutic products in which they could have confidence. All these benefits could be obtained at considerably less cost in both money and effort.

CHAPTER THIRTEEN

Food And Poisons

Our studies at Harvard among residents suggest that the average physician knows a little more about nutrition than the average secretary - unless the secretary has a weight problem, and then she probably knows more than the average physician. JEAN MAYER

Although my research and consulting work for pharmaceutical companies on both sides of the Atlantic concerned studies and evaluations of the efficacy of therapeutic agents, some of it was concerned with litigation over the ownership of interesting compounds and formulations with potential or actual therapeutic effects. In these I provided the expert medical input.

These were interesting, especially in the aspect of working closely with lawyers. What seemed to me logical, they found illogical and vice versa. One of these cases was with three lawyers from a famous firm in New York. The litigation concerned a potentially therapeutic compound in the psychoneurosis area. Two of the largest companies were claiming to be the first to find it. With everybody working furiously at new formulations and chemical permutations to form a variety of interesting chemical analogs in this area, it was possible for two companies to hit on the same compound to which each was now claiming exclusive rights. This may not have been the case in this instance.

The case was dealt with by deposition. This meant that our team met with their legal team and presented the arguments for both sides. All were taken down verbatim with coughs, laughs, ums, ahs, ers and pauses included for someone to adjudicate at some later date. This also meant that we met at a variety of places dictated by where the material under dispute was lodged or the principal witnesses were working or living. Each meeting lasted a week or so after which we would go back to our home bases and go about our normal activities until we received word as to when and where the next session was to take place.

Our three lawyers consisted of the senior partner of the firm, ably assisted by two young lawyers. The senior partner's experience was matched only by his strange ability to work with illogical conclusions which his younger colleagues accepted without a whimper. In the beginning, these conclusions disturbed me and I asked questions hoping to obtain a better understanding of why certain stands were being made. The answers sounded good, but at the end of it I was no wiser. Eventually I accepted the inevitable that I was there to give medical advice and to keep my nose out of what they did with it.

* * *

The junior lawyers were the greatest gourmets I ever met. One was tall, big and a little softly overweight. The other was medium sized, but by the way his clothes hung on him, I diagnosed he had been overweight. Regardless of where we met in the length and breadth of New Jersey, Pennsylvania and sometimes in other nearby states, the junior partners knew exactly where the best restaurants were, not just one or two, but seemingly all of them. They would drive us unerringly to a different one each evening.

The big junior partner was a five star gourmet. He carried his own ingredients for salad dressing: a bottle of olive oil, Coleman's English mustard and a neat sized pepper grinder which contained a most aromatic pepper. At each restaurant, he would produce these from his side pockets and alarm the waiter by ordering raw materials for a salad, a salad bowl, and proceed to make a salad for the four of us. Some waiters were disturbed by these performances and showed it. The gourmet took not the slightest notice. The smaller junior partner informed me that his method of dieting was to order a full meal and eat only half of it, which he proceeded to do. I also obtained the impression that he had gained the weight that he had now lost by at one time following in the gourmet footsteps of his friend. I thoroughly enjoyed these dinners and also gained weight in the process. I experimented with eating only half of what I ordered, but failed to carry it through. A gourmet restaurant is not the best place to experiment with diets.

* * *

At these meetings under the whip hand of the senior partner we worked very hard. We would start early, working over the material we had produced the day before and any other material we were given. We would continue our discussing the case over breakfast and, at nine o'clock we went to the rooms which served as a deposition court and proceed with a full day of fresh depositions from witnesses. These would usually end around five. We would rest a little, shower, dress and drive to our next gourmet restaurant. When we returned, the typed copies of the day's proceedings would be waiting for us in our rooms. Individually we went over these unless the senior partner called for a group discussion.

Our stenographer was a Kelly Girl and the same one attended all our meetings on this case. I could never work out how she managed to stenotype the day's proceedings, type them accurately with laughs, coughs, ums, ahs, ers and pauses included, make copies, have them in our rooms at nine in the evening, and next day look as fresh as a daisy and do it all over again. My praises go to her and others like her. This went on for some months until I was informed by the client it was all over, but that it would take time for the results of the hearing to be adjudicated. I never heard who won, if this is how to describe the result of our efforts.

* * *

Involvements of this nature took some getting used to. Being intermittent, routines were constantly interrupted at a moment's notice. Although ADLers worked in groups on a variety of widely unrelated subjects, there was a great deal of intercourse between the professional personnel. It became standard for me to be involved with a meeting of professionals at least once and sometimes three or four times a week. Since the Life Sciences Division was on Memorial

Drive next to MIT, it meant a drive of about four miles through traffic to attend these meetings at Acorn Park. This was the main facilities of ADL and was situated at the Concord end of Cambridge.

At one kind of meeting, there were usually 15 to 20 present, but up to 30 was not unusual. They were composed of some very senior down to some fairly junior professionals. The subjects discussed varied greatly. Sometimes they dealt with problems concerned with someone's current case. More often than not it was about some facet of a professional discipline with which we were having problems. Many times it was about an area which we considered worthwhile for ADL to explore. At times we met for no special reason, but we never failed to come up with an interesting topic for discussion. The membership of this group varied little from meeting to meeting. It was said that the group had much to do with the vitality of ADL and the policies it followed.

The other kind of group with which I became frequently involved was oriented to actual or proposed cases. These varied from business management to engineering, physics, equity, electronics and others. I welcomed the involvement with business management and economics because my past had been destitute of this kind of exposure. I also became involved with the Equity Group which dealt with patents. Among other responsibilities it offered inventors an avenue to develop their ideas, complete the development of their inventions, patent their efforts and market them.

The Equity group had grown out of inventions in which ADL personnel had been involved. The most important of these was synthetic penicillin in which personnel from ADL and MIT co-operated. This brought in a healthy income from royalties. The horizons of the group expanded to include inventions by inventors from outside ADL.

My role was to assist in evaluating inventions of all kinds commensurate with my background. Much of it was with inventions in medical electronics, therapeutic agents and medical devices. In completed inventions our job was to find a company which might be interested in purchasing or in some other rewarding way put the invention on the market. In uncompleted inventions we looked for companies which, by virtue of their interests, would be likely to take over an invention and develop it. If a company agreed, we would negotiate a goodwill price and royalties for the inventor.

Our reward was a share of the royalties commensurate with the degree of our involvement. Sometimes ADL would consider developing the invention itself. To me it was an interesting sideline activity. In terms of success rate, it was a low yield activity, though returns were generous when it was successful. Although the Equity group were not involved, ADL did fall flat on its face when it rejected the offer to participate in the development of the Xerox process!

* * *

ADL's workload fluctuated, but not badly during my time. We never had to take salary cuts, but in the fifties the staff took salary cuts and found difficulty in keeping gainfully employed. So some of them got together and explored ways they could amuse themselves and perhaps make a buck in the process. Arthur

D. Little's son, Royal, came up with an idea based on the old adage, "You can't make a silk purse out of a sow's ear." Through the magic of chemistry, they made a silk purse out of a sow's ear which for all practical purposes was indistinguishable from the real article. The result now sits in the Smithsonian Institute as does the first cryogenic apparatus for achieving ultra low temperatures which ADL developed. This allowed research into superconductivity and other low temperature phenomena to take place. I was proud to find the monkey experiment that I had been in charge of, among the space exhibits.

* * *

Sam Battista, who had the office next to mine, was a very organised person. He appeared to have on file every scientific trivia and non-trivia. This I found very convenient close at hand. The connecting door between our offices was usually open as Sam and I had many things going on together. Whenever Sam or his secretary heard me discussing a particularly complex assignment with a client on the phone, he or his secretary would place before me the right kinds of published reports to help me out. Thus on the phone I often gave clients the impression that I was a bottomless pit of knowledge. Sam, of course, used this repository of trivia to achieve the same effect.

Sam, Charlie and I often worked together. Some of our work involved testing the biological effects of cigarette smoke which is fundamentally composed of two phases: the particulate phase and the gaseous phase. The particulate phase is the part that you see as smoke. The invisible gaseous phase contains numerous products of which carbon monoxide, acrolein (tear gas) and formaldehyde (an irritating substance) are some of the more important ones affecting lung function and its tissues.

Although the unburnt part of tobacco in a cigarette and cellulose filters remove a proportion of smoke particles and tar, they have little effect on the components of the gaseous phase which pass through them into the lungs and to the delicate tissues and membranes of the alveolae (tiny thin walled sacs) of the lung designed by nature to allow ready transfer of oxygen into the blood stream and carbon dioxide out of it. We all know that inhaled carbon monoxide also readily passes into the blood stream and, because it sticks to haemoglobin better than oxygen, it deprives haemoglobin of its oxygen carrying capacity.

All smokers go through life with a portion of their haemoglobin out of action. We all know the irritating effect that acrolein (as tear gas) and formaldehyde has on biological tissues and, in the guinea pig, even very low concentrations of these cause severe gagging and airway constriction, reflecting the effects these substances have on lung tissue and lung function in man.

Sam developed a system of determining the lung effects of cigarette smoke inhaled by a guinea pig using bronchial constriction and increased airway pressure as a measure of the degree of this constriction. With this experimental system we were able to test the effects of cigarette smoke and its components on lung function. We could also test the effect of different filters on mitigating these effects. Out of it, the activated charcoal filter was evolved. It is the only filter which will absorb these harmful gases and to a significant degree protect the lungs from their effects. The charcoal filter was incorporated into the Lark cigarette produced by Ligget Meyers who supported some of our research on this subject. [24], [27]

The link between cigarette smoking and lung cancer and emphysema is now well established. Charcoal filter or not, smoking is a serious health hazard. The fact that smoking also affects the health of those nearby who are non smokers, there is every reason for legislation against smoking to be a reasonable proposition.

The populace of the third world are either ignorant of the deleterious effects of smoking or they do not care, for the proportion of smokers in it are higher than those of developed countries. In the Cook Islands, although it has clambered out of the third world status to a large degree, has a higher proportion of smokers than New Zealand or Australia. Education, however, is having a significant effect in that the proportion of non smokers in Rarotonga is far greater than those in the outer Islands. As yet legislation against smoking is virtually absent. Many legislators are smokers.

Marijuana is particularly destructive to the lungs in the causation of emphysema because of the way it is smoked. It is more often than not smoked by taking a big drag, inhaling it and holding the smoke in the lungs for as long as possible. This ensures that the drug passes into the blood stream, but it also ensures that the destructive effects of the irritants is playing havoc with the tissues of the lungs.

* * *

My consulting and research work took me back into the field of nutrition. It involved me with products of the major manufacturing companies and foundations of certain areas of the food industry. It was natural that I leaned on my former colleagues in the Department of Nutrition at Harvard for assistance. At that time, few MDs had training in nutrition. Rife amongst them were beliefs about nutrition which caused problems for the food companies. This led medical personnel in the FDA to wage campaigns against food companies which perhaps should have been taken with a greater degree of restraint.

I became involved in these confrontations between FDA and the food industry. One of these involved an attack on the makers of cereals on the basis that cereals had little or no nutritional value. The Food and Drug Administration set out on a programme to promote the idea that legislation should be instituted to prevent the advertising of cereals as a breakfast food, which was aimed primarily at children on the Saturday morning TV children's programmes. The Cereal Institute contacted me to see what I could do to counter these attacks.

Cereals may not be the greatest food, no food by itself is, but they fill a void which is important in our average daily nutritional needs. The nutritional value of cereals is in direct relationship with the nutrient value of its cereal base and the amount of processing it has undergone. Cereals from oats will have a higher proportion of protein than most. Maize contains a protein of low biological quality.

Companies may add vitamins and minerals in an attempt to increase the overall nutrient content. The overall price may have a variable proportion of cost included in packaging and advertising. This supplementation of a basic food and the glorifying of it in advertising and packaging may be questionable practices. However, to attack it on the basis of low nutritional value is hardly a sensible recommendation. The nutritional value of cereals and the long chain carbohydrates it contains is the basis of the development of man in Europe from a hunter and food gatherer to an organised and settled society. The addition of sufficient protein in adequate proportions to the cereal base of man's diet is a recent innovation in most societies. Although this added a whole new dimension to the potential of physical and mental development of man, it should in no way denigrate cereal as an important component of man's diet.

In a balanced diet we consume our main nutrients in a proportion of about two of carbohydrate, one of protein and one of fat. On top of this we need all the other nutrients of vitamins, minerals and trace elements. Also of importance are the foods providing bulk and fibre which play a role in the proper operation of our alimentary system. If we consume foods in the variety which provide the main source of our nutrients in these proportions, much of the vitamins, minerals, trace elements and fibre and bulk would be made available to our bodies. Unfortunately we do not seem to consume all the foods of the right kinds or in the right proportions to give us the full potential of a healthy body and mind.

Being high in carbohydrates, cereals are an important provider of this nutrient and supply our energy needs which is the main function of carbohydrates. Eating cereals for breakfast makes a great deal of sense because, overnight, one's stores of fuel have been depleted and blood glucose is at its lowest level. A cereal is a good way to face the day's energy requirements with a proper load of fuel. Adding milk and fruit does no harm.

It did not need nutritionists to tell the peoples of most of the world this fact. Cereals provide some of the vitamin B needs and, of course, much of one's bulk and fibre needs. It is devoid of cholesterol and, if low cholesterol in the diet lowers the incidence of heart disease, what better food should one entertain than cereals. On this basis I produced a document which successfully defended the cereal industry from the efforts of FDA to discourage Americans of their traditional breakfast of cereals.

* * *

The next nutritional mission of FDA was to rid the market of supplementary vitamins and minerals. Not just one or two, but the lot. Again this was initiated by the strongly held opinion of the medical profession at large that advertising and providing these preparations to the public was a misrepresentation. The American diet, they argued, provided more than enough vitamins and minerals. Particularly under attack were the producers of preparations which provided the minimum daily needs of vitamins and minerals as set out by the FDA.

Miles Laboratories a client of mine in other matters, depended on their One-A-Day preparation as a vital part of their existence. They wanted me to determine whether or not they had a case to fight the FDA on this issue. Miles Laboratories needed an answer quickly because the case was coming up for a hearing in six weeks. I mentally reviewed the extensive literature with which I was already familiar.

I remembered this literature as having arrived at the general conclusion that most Americans did not eat a diet which supplied even the recommended daily requirements as set out by FDA. I had always considered these minimal and on this basis I accepted the case. A phone call to my friend, Professor Stan Gershoff, at my old department at the Harvard School of Public Health obtained his agreement to participate in the research required to support Miles' position. In addition Miles made Dr Dean Gamble from its staff available to help us.

In addition to Stan and Dean, I organised the ADL library staff to obtain the published reports we would review to give Miles the relevant information. Only a partial review of the literature revealed that Americans were ingesting diets which were deficient in the majority of vitamins and minerals. Therefore, In considerably less than six weeks we had the required short answer and presented our findings to the company with enough evidence to demonstrate that they had a strong case to fight the FDA in court and win.

We had worked hard to obtain this advice in the short time allowed only to find that the court hearings had been delayed and there was no time set for when it would be held. The indications were that it would not be for about three to four months. So Miles asked us to continue working on the case to obtain as complete a report as possible on the information needed to substantiate their case. We prepared a report which at any time could be presented as evidence in court and at the same time could be updated as new information was gathered, reviewed and fitted in.

The court hearings were continually delayed due to depositions being taken by FDA's lawyers from scientists and medical doctors from all over the United States and Europe. In effect these testified that there was no nutritional need for vitamin and mineral supplements and that their sale should be banned; the use of vitamins and minerals, they said, should be restricted to those prescribed by physicians for patients with conditions requiring their therapeutic use.

There were, I was told, 86 such witnesses. I was not able to ascertain whether any of them were reputable nutritionists as I was not privy to who they were unless I attended the hearings. This was economically and for other reasons out of the question. After many months with no call to a hearing, we felt that we had obtained all we could from the literature and we published the results in the *Journal of Nutrition Education*, as a supplement. Added to this were comments from the leading nutritionists of the time. Miles Laboratories submitted reprints of the article to the court as their deposition in the case.[29]

Very soon after, I was summoned to one of the courts in Washington to present Miles Laboratories' side of the argument supported by their lawyers. When I arrived, Stan Gershoff and Jean Mayer were there to give me moral support and help if I needed it. I really appreciated this genuine concern for my welfare.

When I entered the court, the FDA counsel took me to an adjoining room and I noticed that he held a copy of our published report in his hand. Holding it up before me, he said without rancour, "This has stifled all the arguments on which FDA has spent so much money, time and effort to put vitamins and mineral supplements off the market. We have absolutely no case to counter it, but," he said, still without rancour, "I am going to try to confuse you every way I can in court."

When he took me aside, our lawyers looked highly concerned, but could not prevent it. When I returned, our counsel agitatedly inquired what had transpired. All I had time to say before entering the witness box was, "They admit defeat, but are going to try and confuse me." On the stand, their counsel kept his promise.

The Judge sustained all our counsel's objections and apart from answering the standard questions of who and what I was, what my qualifications were and my involvement in the preparation of the report, I said nothing. My time on the stand before the case was dismissed could not have been more than five or ten minutes. This whim of the medical profession and those who believed in their unsubstantiated claims and the insistence of FDA in pursuing them had cost Miles and the government a large sum of money, time and effort not to mention embarrassment to more than a few.

There were other similar cases involving products of different kinds but most of these did not reach these proportions of expenditure of money and human effort and sometimes I sit in my Pacific Island home and wonder whether similar dramas are still taking place and if someone is taking care of potential victims.

* * *

In the free market system of the United States in which competition aims to be the guarantee of quality and a fair price, developing new products and new ways of doing things occupies a fair portion of the effort of those providing goods and services. As part of this, the protection of existing goods and services also becomes an important and time consuming effort.

A new product has only a limited time within which to make returns for a company before someone else has something equally good or better competing against it. We already saw this in the case of the two pharmaceutical companies litigating about who developed a potential product first and companies protecting their products from the FDA in pursuit of its watch dog responsibilities.

These depredations can be substantial in the field of food and weight consciousness where new products can replace old ones very rapidly or take over a substantial share of the market. This change, more often than not, has little or no basis in fact. I have friends, and so do you, who do not take sugar in the belief that sugar is fattening which of course it is. I have medical doctor friends who do not take sugar in tea or coffee because this allows them to have cocktails later instead. A teaspoon of sugar is sixteen calories whereas a cocktail is about one hundred. This type of thinking makes losing weight and ways of doing it open to all sorts of abuse and misunderstandings.

Much of it is due to the public wanting a magic formula to solve their problem of overweight rather than facing the reality that a particular diet, unless there is a restriction of calories, will not solve one's problem any easier than eating a good diet, but eating less of it. Diets being foisted on the public, especially in women's magazines, advise what one should or should not eat to lose weight. What we were told not to eat several months ago is now on the menu and something else has fallen into disrepute as a weight reducer.

Some "unbalanced" diets can make one lose weight, but they need to be used with the supervision of a doctor who knows their dangers and understands the biochemistry that takes place in the body as a result of following them. Since few physicians are trained in nutrition and the biochemistry of it, not many can give qualified advice. One of the most common unbalanced diets is the ketogenic diet in which one can eat as much protein and fat as one likes, but no carbohydrates.

The literature that has been floating around the Cook Islands in recent years, and no doubt elsewhere also, is interpreted by unsupervised dieters as meaning they can eat as much protein and fat as they wish, but absolutely no carbohydrate. This results in a severe negative fuel balance with symptoms of severe lassitude and weakness. The literature, inadvertently perhaps, emphasises that eating fat does not affect the weight loss, so nearly all on this diet eat more fat than before. This puts a strain on fat metabolising mechanisms and the dieter can smell of acetone because the unnecessary fat they consume is being imperfectly metabolised as a result of the abnormally low carbohydrate intake.

Proper supervision would have advised a low intake of fat and allowed the right amount of carbohydrate to allow it to be metabolised. One married couple proudly told me that the diet permitted them a breakfast of eggs and delicious fat bacon every morning. When I asked them to consider having a slice of bread and a glass of fruit juice or some fruit with this breakfast, I was given a look of pity for my ignorance. Fresh fruit for breakfast, a slice of whole meal bread or a glass of sugar free fruit juice would have helped prevent the severe symptoms they and others later developed due to following the imperfect and unsupervised advice of this information. All sooner or later exhibited lassitude and lack of energy. One swore that she was at death's door. She probably was.

* * *

In this world of weight consciousness, sugar has been given a bad name. So low or non-caloric preparations have been put on the market one after another to substitute for the 16 odd calories that a teaspoon of sugar provides. Hardly worth it one would think. One of these was cyclamate. Its manufacturers claimed that after it provided the sweet taste in the mouth, it passed through the alimentary tract, unabsorbed, and excreted in the faeces unchanged. On this basis its manufacturers were given a license by FDA to produce and market it and for some years any of us who were conscious of being overweight used one pill of cyclamate as a substitute for one teaspoon of sugar. This seriously reduced the market sales of sugar.

Then in 1966, reports started indicating that all was not as claimed by the manufacturers and that cyclamate was being absorbed and metabolised in the body. We were asked by the International Sugar Research Foundation Inc. to confirm the truth of these reports. We drew up a research plan using human subjects. One group of subjects would consume three grams of cyclamate a day in three divided doses before each of the three meals and another group would consume one gram in one dose before lunch each day. This regimen, we thought, should go on for three weeks.

For a week before the experiment, subjects were to give up soft drinks, diet foods and other foods which contained or might contain cyclamate. At the end of this period they were to be tested to insure that no cyclamate was present in their faeces or urine. I lined up those who had the necessary equipment. Norman Adler of ADL, because he had a gas-liquid chromatograph and other analytical equipment, was in the study right from the start.

Now that we had a case and a research plan, what about human subjects, I was asked. I was already working on it. Through the years I had become good friends with the Manager of the Sheraton Plaza Hotel. Dr Jeannette Opsahl was the physician in residence for the staff and guests of the hotel as well as a physician in attendance at the Peter Bent Brigham Hospital. As soon as the case was confirmed, I titillated Dan, the Manager, and Jeannette about the case. Jeannette, who had always wanted to be a researcher, showed her enthusiasm and with high pitched pleas of, "Let's do it, Dan. Let's do it. Please, Dan, let's do it." Who could refuse a full-bodied, mature, Scandinavian blond. Not Dan. Nor I for that matter. He gave us the OK to use the staff of the hotel as subjects, if we could get them on a voluntary basis. Jeannette volunteered to recruit them and, after a couple of martinis, I left them to it.

Jeannette recruited enough subjects and was briefed fully on her role. She was to feed the two groups the required doses of cyclamate and teach the subjects how to collect their faeces in two litre ice cream buckets and their urine in milk shake containers, both of which were to be closed with the lids that come with them. The lot driven over to the Life Sciences Division at 30 Memorial Drive each day.

Phil Schepis, one of my most capable technicians, volunteered to take charge of the processing of samples on their arrival at ADL. Phil had commandeered part of the basement for the purpose and had set up scales, blenders and an exhaust ventilating fan to do this job. He was ably assisted in this irksome and unsavoury task by technicians from Norman's laboratory at Acorn Park.

Although there was little evidence of any distaste on their part of doing this part of the project, I felt their noble sacrifice deeply enough to visit them in their premises, chat with them awhile and silently cheer them on at least once a day. I must admit I was not unhappy to escape from their processing plant. Up the back stairs, I was sure I detected a faint aroma, but no one of the staff not involved in the project ever mentioned it and I put this down to their long sufferance of things scientists did in their search for knowledge.

All through the studies, Jeannette's subjects were most co-operative and never failed to provide us with samples in the manner required. The Hotel manager was also co-operative to the end although he said that what we were looking for could not be worth fooling around with all that shit and piss. Because it was all for the sake of 16 calories, I heartily agreed with him, but perhaps not as much as Phil and his gang would have if Dan had said it to them. The study proved conclusively that cyclamate does not provide just sweetening and pass through the alimentary tract unchanged. It is absorbed into the blood stream and metabolised into cyclohexamine and possibly other metabolites and excreted in the faeces and the urine, the maximum of which is reached in about 2 weeks. Cyclohexamine is a recognised and listed toxin. Cyclamate was put off the market by FDA. For good and perhaps just reasons the sugar industry was able to retrieve its share of the sweetening market, at least from this competitor.[30]

* * *

The Food and Drug Administration is a watch dog organisation necessary for ensuring that the food and therapeutic drugs and agents manufacturers wish to place on the market do indeed perform in the manner claimed and without toxic and side effects. In order to ensure the therapeutic standards for drugs, it must demand that tests are performed to establish their safety as well as their therapeutic efficacy when used for medical conditions indicated by the manufacturer.

Apart from the clinical studies for efficacy, we were also well equipped to carry out the studies required for testing the toxicity of therapeutic and other agents. Sam Battista did the studies to determine dosage curves and basic toxic effects using mice and rabbits or guinea pigs. From there, my staff and I picked it up for undue effects on dogs and or monkeys and eventually, if these tests showed reasonably low toxicity and side effects, on human subjects using outside clinical medical investigators.

We were very careful that our animals were not in any way harmed by this toxicity testing. Permanent damage was particularly avoided. We used beagle dogs as our mainstay and squirrel and rhesus monkeys in cases where we needed some definition of effects on primates as being closest to man. These animals received the best of care. The dogs in particular knew what was expected of them and seemed to enjoy cooperating with the procedures required of them. The Squirrel monkeys, because of their sometimes lengthy behavioural training were particularly cared for against harm and habituation effects. The writings of my political enemies that I was cruel to them and caused their deaths were utterly untrue. Even if we did not need to protect them from harm for the purposes of the tests, they were expensive animals. The loss of one was to lose what amounted to a coworker which could not be replaced without the expense and effort of training a replacement.

* * *

Statistical methods for determining the probability that the data obtained in tests are not the result of chance alone have been available for the past 60 years or more. Medical and biological scientists in general downgraded their value and shunned their use. They preferred to rely on their personal judgements which are subject to bias and influence. This is a normal and unavoidable part of our human make-up. The scientific method has means of overcoming our proneness to want results to come out the way we want them to.

Because of reluctance to use the scientific method, only five to seven percent of studies done on the efficacy of drugs were usable as measures of the efficacy of therapeutic agents. The medical field was one of the last to grudgingly accept test methods to allow the application of statistical probability techniques to ensure that the results were not due to chance alone.

It was in the interest of the objectives of the FDA that its medical personnel accept and insist that these methods and techniques be applied to the testing of therapeutic drugs for both safety and efficacy. It was no less in the interest of pharmaceutical companies to do the same for economic reasons if for no other. It turns the altruistic motives of both away from the chaos of guessing games and gives their products lasting value and benefit to those needing them.

CHAPTER FOURTEEN

Destination Rarotonga

Home is the sailor, home from sea. ROBERT LOUIS STEVENSON

Sadly in August 1967, Lydia and I came to the parting of the ways for reasons probably no different from those of many others who do the same thing. From that time on, I lived on my thirty seven foot lobster boat which I soon exchanged for the Bob Tom, a forty two foot six inch cutter rigged motorsailer which I renamed the Torea after one of my grandfather's schooners. It was appropriate as the Torea is the migratory golden plover, a bird which spends from about August to April in the Cook Islands and other South Pacific islands and then flies non-stop to the Arctic to breed. I made my living quarters on the Torea berthed at the marina in Winthrop. My work with ADL went on unhindered. My youngest son, Robert Teremoana, and I eventually sailed her to Rarotonga in 1972.

In the summer I sailed with friends and we often had some good fishing off her. Mainly we cruised around the nearby waters and made trips in her to watch most of the America's Cup challenges of that time which mostly involved unsuccessful challenges by Australia with Gretel II making the best showing. In the winter, the Torea was iced in and I was grateful for my Shipmate wood and coal stove. It could always be relied on to warm things up to comfortable levels even at below 0 degrees F (32 degrees F below freezing or -18 degrees C) outside temperatures.

When the fire in the stove was allowed to die out, as was the case when I was away at work, I resorted to all sorts of ruses to protect things from the effects of freezing. Water was kept from freezing by putting a 150 watt lamp under the tank and turning it on whenever I left the boat for the day. I also kept a heater going in the main cabin, but this kept the cabin only just above freezing. It was a cold welcome when I came home from work at night. During the night I had to add coal once or twice, if I wanted to get up to a reasonably warm cabin.

The first thing I did when I came home in the evening was to fire up the Shipmate and stay bundled up until the cabin warmed. The Torea had a canvas cover which fitted over the spacious cockpit. This made the deckhouse and the cockpit one large enclosed area. I put it up in the fall and left it up until spring. When the Shipmate was going strong, I could open the double doors to the main cabin and the shelter would be quite comfortable to use when I had a number of guests or when I just wanted to luxuriate in more living space. The Shipmate could produce any kind of cooked meal I fancied. With my cats for company, a TV, a stereo, a telephone and visits from friends, it was a pleasant way to live. There was an ADLer living nearby on his boat in the same marina under similar circumstances. We saw a great deal of each other and swapped tricks on ways to live on a boat in all seasons.

When the thaw came I had a problem. The cats had come aboard in the beginning of the freeze and grown up playing on the ice. When the thaw came they thought water was ice and leaped over board for their usual play. One wetting was all they needed to learn the difference.

* * *

Over the years since 1968 I received audio cassettes of the voices of my relatives and friends back home saying that the political scene there was not good. Typically there were no details, only some weeping and pleas to come home and do something about it. These pleas were becoming more insistent and were coming from individuals I could not ignore through both rank and friendship. The most important was Makea Nui Teremoana Ariki, my cousin and Paramount Chief of the district of Te Au o Tonga in Rarotonga.

Also of importance was my friend and former mentor, Vainerere Tangatapoto, from the island of Atiu. He and I had worked on a number of community projects in the past. He was a Member of Parliament and had been so for a long time in all the forms that our legislative process had taken in the past. Albert Henry was now the Premier. His methods were not appreciated in many quarters. There was an opposition in accordance with the Westminster type of government and Albert was, I was told, using harsh methods and victimising those who did not support him.

* * *

Quite consciously, I had prepared myself over the years in the knowledge that one day my country would call on me to assist in its development. I must admit that this was also nurtured by personal ambition. It was always my belief that the secret of our success, if this was ever going to occur, would be in economic development. Spurred on by the requests from home, my attention consciously turned to the field of economics and finance so that, if that day ever came, I would not be found wanting.

The experience with Arthur D. Little Inc. had given me the opportunity to examine economics in operation first hand and my deep personal interest in it made my observations bear fruit as to how the system operated in the United States. My attention also turned to the economies of other countries as much as it did to that of the United States and, after a time, I was able to discriminate between them as to the relative value of one over another and what driving forces operated within them and which aspects of which might suit us better than another.

Watching how the large and small businesses worked and attempting to discern the thinking of the managements who steered them became a pastime. Attempts were made to understand the thinking of governments towards the dynamics of the economic mechanisms working in the private sector. Tax structures and the major areas from which revenue derived was delved into.

The dynamics of international trading and their relative value to a country were examined. The thinking behind the value of subsidies and antitrust laws was looked at. These and more seeped into my consciousness in a more or less jumbled manner for sorting out at some future date. Neither immediately nor for some time could I make good sense of what was being absorbed. The idea was to put everything into storage.

Some books on economics helped, some did not. It did not worry me and I did not try very hard to put things in order in my mind as they have appeared in these chapters. When the time came to put what was being absorbed to use, the right trivia, it was hoped, would pop up at the right time, in the right place and for the right reasons. It had done so for me before in other matters.

My self-imposed interest in economics, desultory as this might have been, had led me to the conclusion that it was a young subject still trying to get to grips with itself as a discipline. This is not surprising perhaps since there was no apparent need for it until the industrial revolution of Europe in the eighteenth century. However, this is hardly a sufficient reason. The biological and physical sciences did not make any advances of note until about the same time. These were able to form themselves into fairly organised disciplines with the development of the scientific method to test the validities of their propositions and theories.

Nevertheless, a fair proportion of this book is devoted to the slowness with which medicine and the biological sciences accepted the scientific method and probability mathematics to take the guess out of tests used to validate theories and propositions. When one comes right down to it, all the sciences are relatively new inventions or perhaps better termed as new revolutions. Some of them are slightly ahead of others but, if at some time in the future we can look back, historically speaking, it all happened at the same time. We will probably give this "Scientific Revolution" a name all to itself.

Economics should be no less scientific than the biological and physical sciences. It is just as important. In fact in terms of human social and political progress and as a force in the development of world harmony it may be more important. I am not speaking of it only as a monetary discipline, but also as a social and political force distinct from its lesser application as a solution to our interminable economic difficulties. In this sense, it has not so far proved its value in a reliable manner.

In my life as a scientist, I often said, "If a unit of measurement can be applied to a problem, its solution is a foregone conclusion." The science of economics has such a unit, the dollar. Any other currency and their equivalents can be used. This opens a whole vista of economic processes with which to study and understand the economic, social and political future of the world, provided we accept the interdependence and interactions of the triad of economic, social and political factors and stop dealing with them as unrelated entities.

* * *

Throughout my working life I had dealt with budgets. The first was as Medical Officer to the Cook Islands and I found working on budgets and making them balance both enjoyable and easy. It became second nature to sense spending in accordance with the demands of the budgets I had set up. I found this equally true of research budgets at Harvard, in the Armed Forces and at

Arthur D. Little Inc. It was rare for my departments and projects to overspend cost estimates and, although it may not have been a big thing for others, I took private and personal pleasure in the performance of tasks in accordance with their planned budget objectives. Later, as Minister of Finance and Economic Development, I took just as much pleasure and pride in doing the same.

Early in my years of financial responsibility, I developed a method of looking at individual financial areas in two dimensional or even three dimensional pieces, the sizes of which represented the sums of money involved, their relationship to work to be achieved and to the total budget. These could be recalled at will and translated into dollar values when needed, allowing the state of my budgets to be determined at any time. I don't know how common this conceptual way of keeping budgets up to date in one's mind is, but it was within the bounds of acceptable numerical accuracy to be of great assistance in dealing with my financial responsibilities.

* * *

On several occasions in the United States I had been involved in the problems of poverty and hunger. I developed some fairly firm, though perhaps impractical, ideas about the question and had given written testimony before McGovern's committee. The United States was not immune to the problems of poverty within its own boundaries. However, the proportion and severity in the population was much less than that of its neighbours south of the border. Although poverty exists in direct relationship to economic freedom, some of the US efforts to overcome its problems in this area, I thought, highlighted America's inexperience in dealing with social problems. It did not mean that anybody else's was much better. The US tended to believe in large injections of money rather than judiciously considered correction of social faults in the system.

* * *

Apart from existing contracts which required my personal attention, there was nothing to stop me from returning home to respond to the requests of my people, but I was not so sure that the problems were in such serious proportions as they appeared to those who contacted me. I needed to look for myself.

The United States had been good to me in every way and I did not really want to leave what I had. On the other hand, I had often felt guilty and remiss that I had for many years now assisted the United States in achieving many of its national and other goals, while my own country languished in the Third World with all the social, political and economic ills that always go with it. These guilts and thoughts were real, but there were also rationalisations.

The letters and audio tapes from home had disturbed me. They were from a place where I had been brought up with compassion, love and a lot of spoiling. In effect the opportunity to return to the womb was not unattractive.

By now a pattern of changing my life and employment every seven or eight years had emerged. The reasons for this I believe were related to my personality make-up that made these decisions of change attractive, and staying on unattractive. The work on each objective as time went by soon became repetitive or the objective had been achieved. Perhaps the work had become just plain boring. I was never able to empathise with those who could stay in one job all their lives. Neither was I ever able to appreciate the promise of a pension as a determinant to what I did with my life.

The pattern of my life indicated that at the end of each seven year period, I had made a significant change in the application of my professional and other skills. For the most part I was not concerned with what the next seven or so years had in store for me. In several of these changes I lost pensions without caring a hoot. In some I gave up substantial salaries as well as pensions. In some I went to remunerations below the poverty line until what I was to do for the ensuing years made itself clear in its own time. This does not mean that I did not have an objective in mind. It just took time for it to line itself up. If the changes had an altruistic content, I was pleased and worked hard to keep it so. During each era I worked hard and no doubt made others work hard also. Some appreciated this, others did not.

* * *

The care that my upbringing had nurtured in me for responsibility towards the society of my birth would often, without the slightest warning, reach up from the depths of me and make emotional if not rational demands. Since joining ADL my work had changed from doing things for the national good to doing things for the survival and financial betterment of companies in the private sector and myself. Since a fair proportion of what I did for them was indirectly for the national good, it was no big thing. However, my continued failure to respond to the needs of my own people had become increasingly demanding of my conscious attention. It also promised a new life and new fields to conquer with pretty attractive rewards of another kind.

Moreover, if I were going to respond and that meant entering politics, I would have to make up my mind soon. The Cook Islands general elections were due in 1972 and there were such things as residential qualifications and more to be complied with. So without further ado, I pulled my finger out, booked the necessary flights, took some leave and, in July 1971, was on my way. Just to have a look.

The booking of the flights necessary to get me to Rarotonga showed me that, since 1965 when the Cook Islands became self governing, nothing had changed with respect to the number of flights into Rarotonga. It was once a fortnight in 1945, it was once a fortnight in 1965, and it was still once a fortnight in 1971. I marvelled at this ability for a country and its leaders to stagnate. It was little wonder that many of our people of all ages were doing everything they could to escape to greener fields. This picture was repeated in country after country in the Pacific. After Western Samoa, we had been the first to become self governing and, like her, we had had time to do something. Neither of us had done so. I was beginning to doubt the virtue of the dreams I had and the time spent in accumulating the type of knowledge and experience that I fondly thought might be applied to give our people a better life, but I reserved my judgement. After all, stagnating is what most small and some large places did everywhere in the world.

* * *

The flight from Boston took me to Los Angeles for an overnight stop, across the north-east Pacific Ocean to Honolulu for another overnight stop, then to Nadi, Fiji, for two nights to await the Air New Zealand "Coral Route" flight. On that occasion we went via Pago Pago, American Samoa, for a short stop before the last leg to Rarotonga. It was a long haul and it brought back to mind the immense size of the Pacific and the United States. Little wonder that I had not come home for nearly 20 years. It was just too far away.

It was during the one hour stop-over in Pago Pago, that it hit me that I was going home. I became increasingly excited at this prospect after nearly twenty years. I found it hard to grasp that within a couple of hours or so, I would really be home. All my life I had never thought of any other place as home. All other places had been temporary abodes. I had been away from the Cook Islands more than I had been in it. From the age of twelve, I was away for sixteen years except for that month my sister, Mary. and I returned for a holiday in 1933. Then more schooling and medical school had kept me away until 1945 when I came back to take up my medical duties.

Now, after another seemingly interminable period, I was on the last leg of this return journey to see if it was really necessary for me to leave the United States, try to enter the entirely unfamiliar arena of politics, which had never interested me as a career, and eventually do what I could for my country. In reviewing my interest in politics, it hit me that, while resident for all those years in New Zealand, I had voted only once and that was for the purpose of voting for the referendum to have the pubs open after 6 pm. In the United States I had also voted once and that was for the express purpose of helping JFK into office. I had no illusions about the difficulties I would have to go through if my decision was to respond to the wishes of my relations and friends.

Now that I was close to home, I remembered that Polynesian custom demanded I do what was being requested. There was really no escape unless I could come up with a good argument which nobody would take any notice of anyway. Up to now, my sojourn in foreign countries had made me forget this custom. I realised I was caught and eventually I would have to give in even if things were not as bad as they said. I realised I had not come to make a decision. The decision had already been made for me by custom. My life as a Cook Islander would be in many ways finished if I did not do what they asked.

* * *

At last there was Rarotonga, its high peaks rising jagged to the usual cloud formation that hung above them. For a moment I overcame my emotions and remembered the times I had gazed on Rarotonga from afar and thought how this so little island encompassed all the problems and emotions usually ascribed to inhabitants of much larger places. I had in the past put this down to those steep and rugged mountain ridges and soaring peaks reflecting themselves in the character of the people. I had also put this down to the fact that Rarotonga was one of the 'Avaiki (variants: Hawai'i, Havaiki, Hawaiki, Savai'i, Havai'i) of the three in South Eastern Polynesia. The others being Ra'iatea, the central one and Nuku Hiva in the Marquesas, the one to the north-east. These were the centres of culture in the area and their people tended to be traditionally sure of themselves and proud of the code they lived by. They also tended to be the setters of cultural and social mores in their respective spheres of influence.

For the first time since leaving Boston, I wondered how I would be received after twenty years of absence. I had kept some kind of touch over the years and after all I had been asked to return and set to rights whatever might be wrong in a nation which received its independence only six years previously in 1965.

The requests had come from people who were close to me and whom I loved and respected. They were also loved and respected by a substantial proportion of the population, so it was likely that I need not worry on that score. The plane landed and it was as of old with crowds to meet me with mountains of eis (leis). And the old familiar faces were there.

* * *

I spent two weeks having a good look, redundant as this may have been for my fate was already sealed. The two weeks was not needed, but, if I had wanted to leave, I could not because there was only one plane every two weeks. My examination of the situation indicated that things were not as they should be. The Westminster style of politics had been taken to its literal extent and the existing two parties had polarised the Cook Islands into two factions with an ill feeling between them equivalent to the intensity of feelings seen in civil strife elsewhere.

The ruling party had nearly seventy five percent of support at the last elections and they had been making good use of this majority to the detriment of the opposition and those who did not support them. A recent by-election had indicated that they had lost some ground. The reports that those known to support the ruling party received most of the goodies that political favour can bestow was not exaggerated. The important public service posts were held by important Party members, some of whom obviously did not qualify for the posts they held. Nepotism was present and the ruling party managed to make the fear of reprisals tangibly real.

Despite the welcome at the airport, it was easy to see that many of my old friends preferred not to be seen associating with me. There were too many cases of people avoiding me in public not to realise that the old convivial, jovial and friendly way of life was no longer present. The fabric of the society that I knew and loved was in tatters. Community was against community, family against family, parents divided against their children and so on to the extent that there were cases of children leaving home for political reasons.

These antipathies, arisen over a period of six short years, were now deep seated. They created a society which spent the major portion of its energies in political wrangling without the slightest regard for the harm it was doing to the well being of the country. Politics was more important per se than what it was supposed to be doing for the country.

From what I could gather, the economy had suffered and was continuing to suffer, but no one knew what to do about it or what was causing it, least of all the politicians. They were doing their thing the only way they knew how and that was to ape their metropolitan brother politicians. However, what they were aping best were the superficial trappings which did nobody much good. I did not have all the answers, but it would have been criminal not to heed the cry for help and come back home to do my best to overcome some of the problems that beset my little country. Soberly I thought to myself, if I did nothing else, I would do all I could to return the smiling friendliness of my people.

* * *

This wish to return to a people who had given me special treatment while growing up had worked its will on me and returned me amongst them as a doctor of medicine. It was now working its will on me again, albeit abetted by the lure of becoming the leader of my country and the opportunity to apply what I had learnt and gleaned as to the best way to tackle its problems. It was not a new ambition. Neither was the wish to return to the womb where I had been nurtured, loved and spoilt a new emotion. It had welled up in me many times while in the United States.

As soberly, I also thought to myself that many of the politicians in opposition, who were supporting the bid for my return, with some notable exceptions, would probably be no different if they were in government. I had held some sessions with their party and I got the feeling that perhaps some of them deserved no better than to be in opposition. Their policies lacked depth, humanity and purpose and dealt with mundane things that had little to do with getting a country on to its feet as a nation. it had little to do with the business of building a country and achieving a better standard of living for its people. The policies of the government in power were no better and no worse.

Albert Henry met with me several times to ask me to join him and not those "fools" as he put it. When he did not come himself, he sent others in his party whom he knew had been close to me in the past. I enjoyed these visits with old friends, but my conversations with them and especially with Albert brought out their strong adherence to the socialistic line as practised to a degree in New Zealand. Albert himself was closely associated with leaders of the New Zealand Communist Party which had little possibility, even if it were more realistic, of doing any good for the country. It was based on a socialism which was to be paid by somebody else who, they said, owed it to us anyway.

The metropolitan countries that surround the Pacific Basin and especially those which had been "colonial masters" in the area were the ones who were going to pay the bill. It was many years later at the second Lome Convention that I heard the same arguments from the leaders of the African states. There was little or nothing in their thinking about people using their independence to independently work out something which they themselves could do to better their own situation.

It also became apparent that there was absolutely no understanding of economics or business. The sum total amounted to the belief that anybody in business was automatically a millionaire and a thief. It was not surprising that I learnt that the private sector received little assistance or sympathy from government. The opposition side which had a few business men in it, at least understood these things better. I decided to stay with those who first requested my return, even though it was a much longer way to travel to get where we could do something positive.

In any event the die was cast. I returned to Boston to wind up my affairs and get back to Rarotonga and start another new life with an assignment that proved to be tougher than any I had ever tackled before.

* * *

When I got back to Boston I informed Charlie Kensler of my decision and the reasons for it. He probably did not comprehend the Polynesian part which made escape from this fate nigh impossible. No doubt he also privately thought that I was again into another "can of worms", but he did not say it aloud. If he only knew it, for probably the first time, he would have been dead right.

On the flights back to Boston I had given much thought to how I would distribute my cases to other ADlers and how my clients would feel about this. Three of them especially bothered me that I would not be able to be there to help complete them. One was a human engineering case with the Coast Guard. Another was a comprehensive one on chemical pollution of water in the United States and its possible toxic, carcinogenic, teratogenic and mutagenic effects on man for the Department of the Interior and the third was my consulting work with the Pharmaceutical arm of Phillips, whose main plant was situated near Amsterdam.

The case with the U.S. Coast Guard had caused me some problems with the Engineering Division of ADL because of the policy that the case leader should preferentially be the individual who obtained the contract. The engineers considered the problem as a purely engineering one. Whether it was or not, my bid had been the successful one against, as I learned later, some very tough competition. We also had differences of opinion on the matter of the rationale behind the research design.

The case was based on the Coast Guard's need for basic information on the buoyancy (floating) and stability (resistance to capsizing) characteristics of the human body to assist them in the design and evaluation of life jackets. Current life jackets were said to be unsatisfactory in cases where individuals were unconscious in the water, as happens when accumulated petrol fumes in the bilge explode, or during collisions at sea. Existing life jackets would not reliably turn an unconscious victim, who was face down, to the preferred face up position. The large and rapidly growing area of boating recreation had brought this problem into sharp focus.

When I saw the Request for Proposal in a publication put out for publicising such requests, I jumped at it for several reasons. The important ones were based on my biological statistical background, my avocation in naval architecture which I indulged in as a hobby and the fact that there was absolutely no information on the buoyancy and stability characteristics of the human body. I was interested in knowing about it.

The panorama of how the human body could be measured for buoyancy and stability like that of a boat, how the density and displacement characteristics of different parts of the body contributing to the overall buoyancy and stability characteristics of the human body could be obtained, the kind of experiments needed to measure its stability characteristics, and how the data could be statistically analysed to give a true picture of what was needed to do what was proposed, flashed excitingly through my mind.

I immediately wrote the proposal and presented it to the Coast Guard. I called in the engineers to assist me in its preparation. The engineering input was based on a research design using a mathematical model. The trouble with mathematical models is that they are as good as the information you put into them. There was no information in existence on the buoyancy and stability characteristics of the human body and how they varied from person to person within the sexes, between the sexes and with age.

I happened to have obtained enough clues from my contact with the Coast Guard to know that this was not what they were looking for. They had already been down that obvious and facile road. Nevertheless, I included the engineers' approach in the proposals with comments on its fallibility and presented the bioengineering statistical approach I thought would best meet the objectives of the Coast Guard.

This approach was to measure the parameters which allowed definition of the characteristics in question by involving volunteer families (these turned out to consist mainly of families of ADLers who proved to be very co-operative and enjoyable to work with as human subjects). Enough families would give a statistically valid sampling of these characteristics by sex and age.

A swimming pool, twelve feet in diameter and about ten feet deep, comfortable waiting rooms, change rooms and showers were built. Adjoining this, the devices we had evolved for measuring the vertical distribution of body density were constructed. This consisted of a complex system which weighed the body, section by section, in air and in water in accordance with Archimedes principle. These requirements necessitated two floor levels built in a part of a high ceilinged workshop at Acorn Park which, when completed, painted and furnished, formed a very impressive complex. It was visited by many local and distant dignitaries, curious and interested in our, to them, novel goings on.

The case proceeded well in partnership with Dick Stone and his staff of the Physics Department who provided the physics and engineering input. Much of the work was done before I left, but I was sorry that I was not there for the final days. The differences in stability and buoyancy characteristics were most marked between the sexes. Males had the major part of their buoyancy in the upper part of the body while females had theirs in the lower part. This made the females characteristically less stable in the water than males.

This basic difference was present regardless of individual differences in breast size or body fat and density distribution and must ultimately have an effect on the design and performance of life jackets. Dick and I were starting to get into the theoretical possibilities this may have on the design of personal life jackets when I left.

* * *

The case on Chemical Pollution of Water was also well on the way towards completion and I had no problem in leaving the completion of it to young Dr Alan Burg who with the library staff under the leadership of Bella Wadler, who spoke something like ten languages, were both well into the work required. I regretted not being available for the final report because of the medical input and its implications.

The case was interesting in that the Europeans and other countries had done much more work in this area than the United States. Therefore, what could be happening in the United States had to be largely extrapolated from the European and Russian data and it was one of the areas which I felt needed my medical attention.

* * *

I flew to Europe to wind up my cases there, the chief one of which was with Phillips Pharmaceuticals. I particularly regretted having to cut short my consultancy with this company. Their pharmaceutical company near Amsterdam was relatively small compared to those of Hoffman La Roche, Upjohn, and others which were my pharmaceutical clients in the US.

The staff of Phillips in all areas had a particularly good grasp of what was needed for a chemical development programme in search of interesting compounds and their medical doctors were very receptive to better clinical research designs and data analysis techniques for defining the efficacy of their new products. This was not the case for many of the other pharmaceutical firms in Europe, probably because there was no real equivalent of an FDA to make the necessary demands or which had the knowledge to know what to demand in order that the products which end up on the market do what they claim. Phillips, on the other hand, even without stringent regulatory requirements, did everything possible to produce therapeutic agents that met their own high standards and much of my work with them was to assist in doing just that.

When I told the president of the parent company that our association would have to come to an end, he was genuinely sorry. When I pointed out the location of Rarotonga on the huge map of the world on the wall behind his desk, he expostulated, "That fly speck!" and stared at me in amazement. But when I explained as best I could why it was necessary, he was solicitous and wished me all the best.

Back at ADL, I worked like fury to put as much of myself as I could into the cases before I was forced to abandon them to those who were to take them over. Finally it was time to go. As always it was hard to part with friends.

ADL gave me a farewell which Dick Stone, my partner in the Coast Guard case, said was most interesting because of the people who were present. He said there were people there who never came to functions of this nature and he thought their presence was their way of paying me tribute. One of them quietly informed me that he was sorry I was leaving because I was one of the few who could put multidisciplinary research programmes together and make them work. On the other hand, he said he was pleased because an ADLer was getting the opportunity to play a direct role in the welfare and development of a Third World state, a subject in which they were most interested. I was flattered and humbled to say the least.

But he was not talking idly. ADL had been for some years involved in a substantial case with the Nigerian government for the economic development of that country. It involved ADLers in Nigeria with a back-up team in Cambridge. I had often made inputs to the work of the home team, as also to the development of Brasilia. Sandy Walcott, now Sandy Clark, who had worked effectively with me on several of my medically oriented cases, was put full time on various aspects of the development of the health programme for Brasilia. And there were others in which I was not directly involved. Therefore, this member of the Board was not just making conversation, but I did not enlighten him that, because the Cook Islands was a poor country as were the other Pacific Island states, it was unlikely that the expertise of ADL would ever be called upon.

* * *

On 1 October 1971, Teremoana and I, with a young man and his girl friend who said they wanted a ride to anywhere we were going, cast off the lines of the Torea from the marina at Winthrop after saying farewell to friends, some of whom shed tears.

Up to that time, Teremoana, my youngest son, was known by his first name, Bobby, for Robert. Teremoana, meaning "Ocean Voyage" was his second name, given to commemorate the voyage of the Miru. This Polynesian custom can be very confusing because a person can have a number of names, each of which can be used according to occasion or by different groups of people. Court records and electoral rolls might use any of the names and it is an important duty of supporters of a candidate for election to peruse the electoral rolls for evidence of a person having registered himself more than once using his many names.

These names can be given at the christening or any time in his or her life by those giving it and announcing it. These extra names are to commemorate important occasions in the family. Common occasions are when someone goes overseas to school, Tereapii, meaning "Voyage to school", and Terepa'i, "Voyage by boat". Other names commemorate deaths of relatives and are literally called death names. Marriage or a twenty first birthday are also occasions for changing or adding names, and there are many other reasons.

Names have special relevance to Polynesians. Everything is named. All botanical specimens are named. In many, their different stages of maturity require different names for the whole plant as is also the case with species of fish. Canoes were given personal names as were their outriggers and sometimes their sails and other parts. They were thus truly personalised, and their qualities given a human dimension. The language is full of these fine distinctions.

So when we set off from the marina in Winthrop, it was fitting that Bobby should now use the name appropriate to this occasion and the future. So Teremoana is what he has been called from that day to now. This has been shortened to Tere. In Polynesian languages, all vowels are sounded and the vowel sounds are always pure, therefore, the ees in Tere are both sounded as the e in ten, bet, get, etc.

We sailed out of Winthrop, past the Boston Lighthouse with the Boston Lightship well out to sea and headed south in the gentle breeze of a hazy October morning. On our way we wanted a last look at New York so, after transiting Cape Cod Canal and passing Block Island, we slipped into Long Island sound, leaving Long Island to port and, in due time, passed Manhattan's majestic skyscrapers to starboard, whisking past them in a strong outgoing tide of the East River, dodging tugs and their barge tows, and exchanging waving greetings with the tugmen. We all enjoyed this fast last look at New York with its skyscrapers. From our vantage point, it was dominated by the United Nations building all sparkling in the sunshine of a clear blue sky. We passed the Statue of Liberty, albeit demurely, and then sailed past Sandy Hook and out to sea. Off Delaware Bay we ran into onshore gale winds which forced us to heave to for about twenty four hours with steep seas which the Torea handled very nicely.

Time was getting short and, before we left, I knew that I would probably have to leave the boat under the care of Teremoana in order to fly to Rarotonga to meet my residential and other qualifications. The elections, the timing of which is at the whim of the Premier, had been called for March, 1972. I hoped we would have time to get back for me to meet the various requirements, but this was not to be. So I left the Torea in the tender hands of Teremoana at Fort Lauderdale, Florida, and flew back to Rarotonga.

* * *

During this break in the voyage, I won a seat in Parliament and became Leader of the Queen's Opposition. Its demands made it impossible for me to join Tere until August 1972.

* * *

On 28 August Tere and I sailed out of Fort Lauderdale to continue our voyage, we sailed through the Bahamas whose chain of islands and waters were familiar to us from previous cruises. We sailed through Paso de los Vientos running between Cuba and Haiti, to Kingston in Jamaica, to Colon and through the Panama Canal to Balboa. It was a nice sail, but with only two of us, the watches took their toll. Tere did not seem to be as affected as I was by this.

We stayed in Colon a few days at the Marina and did our final victualling. We were berthed among many yachts who were surprised when we said good bye to them because we were off to Tahiti. They asked how we could come in for a few days and set off across the Pacific. They had been berthed there for some time, some for as long as five years, getting ready for that long 5000 mile leap. We found it difficult to answer apart from saying that we were going home and did not want to waste time getting there. We transited the Canal on 17 September, found a young man in Balboa who wished to go to Tahiti, thereby solving our fatiguing watch-keeping problem considerably.

We had a relatively quick passage to the Galapagos of 6 days 4 hours and 30 minutes averaging around 150 miles a day which was a fast run for this leg normally plagued by calms and squalls resulting in slow passages. Almost every day there were spectacular cloud formations and beautiful displays of rainbows. It was the first and last time that I experienced a full circle double rainbow, going from under the boat on one side across the sky, each in a perfect circle, to pass under the boat again.

Because of the strange conditions, we took some readings of sea and air temperatures. Normally the water here is cold from the effects of the Humboldt Current. They were the reverse of what we expected with disparate readings as much as 74 degrees F (23.33 degrees C) for air and 78 degrees F (25.56 degrees C) for water. This was in contrast to the water temperatures encountered in this region on the voyage of the Miru, twenty years before, when they were decidedly colder in the mid sixties degrees F (15.56 degrees C).

The weather was blustery, but the wind kept to the starboard beam most of the time varying in velocity from about 15 to 25 knots with intermittent rain, wind squalls and calms. We did not know it at the time, but this was the El Nino year of 1972 and no doubt was the cause of the unusual conditions we were experiencing. It gave us a quicker than normal passage for this leg.

The Torea was proving to be a fine sea boat with speed better than expected in a cruising double ender of traditional Swedish design from Batvary where she was built in 1938. Her large cockpit with a hatch in the middle of it gave me some concern, but from Boston to Rarotonga the alternative open grilled cover which we had used to close it in Boston was never changed to the solid cover. The only sea that entered below was a small dollop of water that slopped over the quarter when we were rolling along at hull speed between Tahiti and Rarotonga.

* * *

El Nino is a recently discovered climatic phenomenon which affects the weather of the Pacific, the west coast of North and South America, New Zealand and Australia as well as the Indian Ocean and the Far East. It is suspected that it may have an influence even beyond these regions. Being a relatively newly discovered phenomenon, its characteristics and reasons for its development are ill-understood.

It is essentially a phenomenon brought about by a larger than normal upset of the swings of the barometric pressures found in the area of Indonesia and the

Eastern Pacific Ocean referred to as the Southern Oscillation. Normally these barometric pressures are characterised by a large "low" centred over Indonesia and a large "high" centred over Easter Island. It accounts for the general flow from east to west of the prevailing winds and ocean currents.

At around Christmas until March each year, the low pressure over Indonesia rises somewhat and the high pressure over Easter Island lowers somewhat. The pressure difference between the two systems lessens or may even reverse. This, it is supposed, causes a lessening of the winds that blow from east to west which piles up ocean water in the Western Pacific. When this east to west wind system (trade winds) lessens in intensity, which it does normally from December to March, the normal east to west current flow stops or may even reverse. This causes flows from west to east and warms up the waters off Peru.

The phenomenon, because it occurs around Christmas time, is called El Nino, the Christ Child, by the Peruvians. This is the normal picture. When the swing is deeper than normal and starts earlier than December, and does not end in March, we have what people outside of Peru call an El Nino year or years as it often affects two years in succession. What causes this deep swing is unknown.

An El Nino year is characterised by an increased frequency of cyclones in areas where normally cyclones occur, cyclones in areas not normally cyclone prone, floods and/or droughts. The most recent El Nino years of 1982-83 were characterised by a severe cyclone in Hawaii and cyclones in French Polynesia where cyclones are infrequent, a high frequency of cyclones in Fiji and the Melanesian area of the Western Pacific, droughts in New Zealand and Australia, and floods in California. The average frequency of a significant El Nino appears to be about once every eight years, but the variation is from five to eleven years.

※ ※ ※

After we passed the Galapagos Islands, we headed for the Marquesas, running west just south of the Equator. There were several days when we ran into poor winds, calms and strong winds from the south which pushed us north of the equator. It took us a day or so to cross back over it. When the winds were good and everything pointed to our doing our normal seven knots, the position sights showed we were doing less than a hundred miles a day. After three days of this, we decided that we might be in the counter equatorial current that normally runs west to east a few degrees north of the Equator. We should have been south of it. It must have shifted. On this tenuous premise, we fought our way to the south-west and found better day's runs, but still with unexpected weather conditions. When later we found that this was an El Nino year, it explained these anomalous conditions.

During this reach to the south-west the Torea excelled herself. She logged over 200 miles per day on six days, three of them consecutive. Her best day's run was 216 miles. During this time, I remember being on the ten to midnight helm watch. It was a moonlight night with dark clouds frequently interrupting the light of the moon, but the wind stayed steady on the beam which the Torea likes. Because of the strength of the wind, she was reaching under double reefed main and the small spitfire jib. She was storming along prancing like I imagined a springbok might with a sideways step and an extra lift upwards now and then. I was enthralled at the way she seemed to be enjoying herself romping and skipping along in this manner with me enjoying it with her. Her speed and behaviour so captivated me that I stayed on watch until 4 am when fatigue finally overcame me.

We met many humpback whales and were given a fine display of aquatic acrobatics by a huge, shining, black sperm whale, not more than two hundred yards away. Otherwise we just sailed on in variable winds and just when we were right in the middle of the Tuamotus, after running between Marutea and Tekokota in strong easterly winds, rain squalls started to form, the skies darkened, and the wind backed to the south and started to strengthen.

We kept bowling along with the wind on the port beam and increasing in strength. Visibility was negligible with the rain now becoming continuous. The currents around the Tuamotus are strong and unpredictable. So we set a course well to the south of Mototunga with little hope of seeing it in the rain and poor visibility. We must have been pushed to the north by a strong current and the wind, for, just before dark, the rain cleared momentarily and we saw we were heading straight for the reef of Mototunga. Tere threw the helm over and we came about, fortunately with enough room to clear the reef. We could not help talking all at the same time how lucky we were that the rain squalls had cleared just at that moment, for only a few seconds and just before dark. If it were not for this, we would have been on the reef of a Tuamotu island as many boats have before us. It was another of those times I let slip one of those prayers of thanks. It is not for nothing that these many atolls are also known as the Dangerous Archipelago.

Escaping this reef was not the end of our problems. We were now heading in the opposite direction with Haraiki, the nearest, Tekokota, Hiku'eru, Reitoru and other atolls across our bows further to the east. Worse still, to leeward of us were a host of atolls to the north with Makemo and its 50 odd miles of reefs broad across our lee. Except for the atoll Anaa we were clear to the south straight into the storm. We were what is classically referred to as "embayed". I was scared. We were all scared. I could not help recalling Shakespeare's scholarly description of the wreck in the "Tempest" and hoped Ariel and her ilk would deal with us better.

We triple reefed the mainsail and put on our storm jib. We were going to sail across the storm one way for three hours to free ourselves of Mototunga, come about and sail back for two hours, go about again for two hours and do it all over again and again until the storm abated and we could see what was happening to us. By this means it was hoped that we would keep clear of Haraiki to the east and Mototunga to the west. In addition we hoped that the Torea would be weatherly enough to keep from going to leeward and ending up on one of the many reefs to the north in our lee. That night we estimated the winds at 50 to 60 knots. Not a lot to write home about, but with reefs to the lee and in either direction across the wind, it was enough to worry about. It was, we agreed later, the worst night at sea that any of us has ever had or will ever likely have. Again I had to say to another brave ship of mine, "Old Girl, It's up to you."

We could not tell if we were losing to leeward or making good to windward or holding our own. We were not even sure that our two hours one way and two hours the other would keep us clear of Haraiki at one end and Motutunga at the other. Horizontal sheets of stinging rain took care of our visibility problems. These uncertainties and the expectation of hitting a reef at any moment during our two hour tacks, made these dark, windswept hours of biting rain interminable and full of anxiety. Later we found that Fiji was being hit hard by a devastating cyclone at the same time we were dodging reefs in the Tuamotus in our own lesser storm.

We went through the night without any sign of the storm letting up, but it was not getting worse. Painfully daylight struggled through, the storm fleeing with the night and the abating wind swinging to the south-east. We were able to see for quite a distance so we headed west expecting Anaa to be our next sight of land. We obtained a sight at 1300 hours which placed us well south of the reefs and atolls. Early on 25 October we sighted the forbidding surf-pounded small high island of Mehetia to the north of us. The Torea had sailed us out of the hole we were in and made good to windward better than anybody had any right to expect. We have never been able to reconcile how the Torea moved us so far into the teeth of the storm and away from danger.

A review of the log revealed several entries of my praises for this brave and able little ship. Here is an entry in the log made on 25 September, the day we sighted the Galapagos and before she made those consecutive runs of over 200 miles per day:

"The Torea is proving her worth despite her 34 years. At times we have driven her hard against head seas especially coming down Exuma Sound. This caused a loss of some caulking in the section of a seam two planks up from the keel, starboard of the mast. We caulked this from the inside at Clarence Harbour, Long Island, Bahamas and have had no trouble since. Later, in Jamaica, I put in a couple of fastenings."

Here are more entries made at different times on 23 October the day after our harrowing experience among the reefs of the Tuamotus:

"0300: Winds now 50+ knots...ship now in a highly vulnerable situation with atolls and reefs to leeward, strong northward current...attested to by coming up to Motutunga on a 17-20 degrees drift (to leeward)...this means that we have about 6-10 hours before being close by the reefs to leeward."

"1300: Obtained sights of pale sun which showed that the Torea had, during tacks, made considerably to windward and we were actually west and south of Motutunga at 17 degrees 10' S, 144 degrees 15' W. Behaviour of Torea in keeping us off reefs with no power was outstanding. Only damage was some caulking shaken out. Recaulked next morning from inside. All O.K. Bilges dry again."

"1600: Altogether we have sailed from Boston and weathered two 50+ knot storms with the lazerette (area below cockpit and stern decking) covered with the open grating (only). I have great confidence in this ship."

In the fresh south-easterly with everything up and drawing we headed for Tahiti which came into sight at the expected time. At the entrance to Papeete harbour we were in the usual calm of the lee that lies off the harbour of Papeete. Just an hour ago we had been foaming along the north-west shore in a strong 25 to 30 knot wind. The pilot came out and said, "Iaorana, Tomu." He remembered me and we chatted back and forth in my now rusty Tahitian which shook Tere to the core because he had not known that I could speak anything other than English.

We stayed a week or so in Tahiti spending time with old friends, new friends and relatives. While in Tahiti we were met with the news that one of my best friends and strongest political supporters, the former Chief of Police, Tangata Nekeare, had died. The death, it was said, was under suspicious circumstances, but he was buried quickly without a post mortem and nothing ever came to light which could confirm these suspicions.

We dragged ourselves from Tahiti and made another good passage to Rarotonga in 3 days, 23 hours for the more than 700 nautical miles. I eventually sold the Torea to David Brown, but not before one of my enemies, political and otherwise, bored holes in her and sank her at her moorings.

On behalf of David, Tere sailed her to New Zealand on two occasions where she, for the most part, operated out of Whangarei. In 1987 during Hurricane Sally, while on shore and in her cradle, she was damaged beyond repair. It was a sad day for those of us who knew her, but most especially for David Brown, Teremoana and me.

PART THREE

Home-Brew Politics

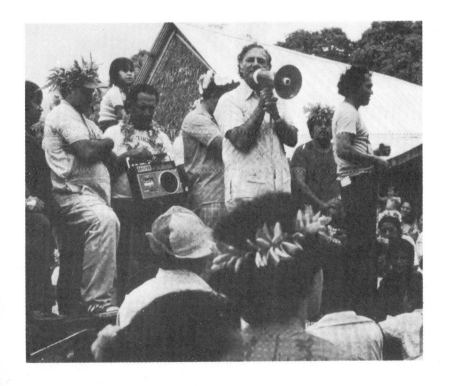

CHAPTER FIFTEEN

Home-brew Politics

We should not go to political philosophers as mentors in the practical art of government. DAVID THOMSON

I had never been interested in a political career. Even knowing for some time that some day I might have to use it as a means to an end, had not prompted me to do anything about learning about it. It was probably very remiss of me. The little I read about it did not particularly appeal as a way to make a living. The fact that corruption is always associated with it and the cautioning old adage that 'power corrupts and absolute power corrupts absolutely' did not make it attractive. So, perhaps unconsciously, I had avoided learning about it because of a sense of repugnance. My friends and colleagues seemed no better versed in politics than I was. This pretty much ensured that whatever politics we came up with would be a home-brew concoction. Perhaps this was not bad. We might come up with something better through ignorance and by accident.

Therefore, when the day came to face politics and use it, my knowledge of it was little more than that of a babe in arms. What I did know about politics and how I saw people practising it, often indicated to me that there was probably a better way of going about things. This was confirmed by an examination of some of the great leaders of history and how they went about fixing things. They hardly did things the way most politicians did or said they would. Anyway it was clear to me that my knowledge of politics was nothing to boast about and that must have been pretty obvious to everybody else too.

* * *

I got back to Rarotonga in late November 1971 with the elections set for March 1972. There was little time to whip something together, but it had to be done. Albert Henry made more overtures for me to join his party; at least he thought I knew enough politics to constitute a threat to him. For the reasons already expressed, his blandishments fell on barren ground.

We got to work immediately on my arrival in Rarotonga, starting with my decision to join the party in Opposition from where all the requests had come for me to return. It was not in very good shape. If I managed to obtain a seat, I would probably have to sit in Opposition for a few years. This did not seem a bad idea for there was much for me to learn about everything as it might affect the Cook Islands in my new role.

Albert Henry had a strong hold on the country and it was not going to be easy to shake him loose. Many years before, in 1946, we had together planned the future freedom of the Cook Islands to determine its own destiny. We had no delusions about each other. We both knew we were rivals. We differed in both philosophy and method, if not in objectives.

Albert had been greatly influenced by the New Zealand Communist Party and extreme left wing elements in the New Zealand Waterside Workers Union. In my opinion this philosophy was unacceptable for the development of our country in particular and underdeveloped countries in general. It lowered the productive capacity and personal integrity of the individual. This has to be the last thing a struggling Third World country needs. I felt we needed quite the opposite, to encourage and reward the creative productivity of every man, woman and child. This could only be achieved by everybody having the right to enter the market place and do his or her thing.

At that time I felt this more instinctively than consciously. As time went by and I learnt more about what makes a country economically viable, I became certain of the rightness of this simple philosophy. My future economic policies were based on this fundamental concept. Albert, on the other hand, believed in a politically controlled socialistic hand-out policy. No developing country can afford such a policy unless it has large hand-out budgets from developed countries which are prepared to hand out excess finances. I thought this was a most unreliable base for an economic policy. It also diverts the energy of a developing nation away from the self reliance it so badly needs to engender.

In following this line, my problems were doubled because we were closely associated with New Zealand. She is a country then committed to the philosophy of a welfare state. Cook Islanders tended to follow what they mistakenly thought were New Zealand ways. While the government of New Zealand provided an extensive range of services, the New Zealand economy was based on individual farmers, private industry and commerce. Banking, marketing, insurance, and commerce were private, but with government as a competitor. But government operated the monopolies such as railways, power and communications. Few Cook Islanders understood this and Albert Henry in particular was associated with a minority in New Zealand who favoured total socialisation, a policy which was never adopted.

Cook Islanders' experience of New Zealand was almost exclusively with its welfare state aspects such as education, medical services, postal services and family benefits. The only commercial ship owned by the New Zealand government ran to the Cook Islands because it was an uneconomic route. Cook Islanders had almost no contact with the side that paid for the welfare services, and did not understand the connection. When I became Prime Minister, this formed a serious communication barrier in putting my policies into place. There was no common ground or point of reference from which we could all work with understanding.

* * *

The time for the general elections moved inexorably closer. My cousin Emily and her husband Frank and Emily's sister, Nane, took care of me to the best of their ability and that was the best anybody could wish for. My half sister Tepaeru threw her weight into the secretarial work with help from others. Frank built us an office and made the furniture from scratch. I still use the table he built. We formed working committees and had planning meetings and all the things one usually associates with putting a political campaign and headquarters together. These were very much Cook Islands style.

It was all new to me and to most of us. Some had been through this with Albert Henry when they supported him and later on with the Opposition after they had changed allegiance. Up to this time all we were really doing was putting together the trappings of a political party. We were, Cook Islands' style, having too many meetings and talking too much. We had not turned our attention to what the party stood for and what its policies should be.

I also obtained the distinct feeling that what some wanted was revenge for real or imagined personal slights that Albert or the Cook Islands Party had perpetrated and I was to be the medium by which this could be achieved. The thought passed through my mind that I was building a political party based in a significant part on dissenters and defectors from Albert's Party. Such individuals generally expect much more in return for their support and vote than can reasonably be met. They could easily become my dissenters and defectors. Perhaps this is how political parties are normally built, and destroyed.

* * *

In reviewing the policy literature of both parties from former campaigns, I was not impressed. They dealt with little things that pertained to doing them or not doing them as they thought the voters wanted them. Much of it was on a personal basis and there was disregard for the percentages one way or the other. Initiative and leadership to lead us into something more worthy was not evident. Anything dealing with the economic and social welfare of the country was singularly absent. Pork Barrel politics was probably the best way to describe it.

They were all internal policies presented to attract votes. Most of them would not have attracted my vote. It was also obvious we were working from a position of great weakness. The previous election had gained the Opposition party only 26 percent of the total votes. A recent by-election had gained an encouraging 46 percent of votes, but it was not something to get excited about.

The worst feature against us was the tremendous polarisation of the voters with the resulting entrenched inimical feelings which would be difficult to sway one way or the other. By far the greater proportion of the polarised population fell to the Cook Islands Party of Albert Henry.

It appeared we had little chance of gaining votes, let alone new seats unless we could hit on some middle road with a new approach altogether. The voters needed something to look at for which they had no entrenched and intense feelings one way or another. To achieve this we needed a new party with a new image. This was agreed to and, for the want of a better name, we called it the Democratic party. Not very original.

Having settled that, we needed a new image. This would have to come out of a policy statement which would deal with broad issues, what they were and how we were going to deal with them. I put myself away for several of the remaining weeks to write a document with as much depth and sincerity as I could to give the voting public a picture of what the party stood for. It contained concepts which I knew would be difficult for our people to grasp. To simplify these, I believed, would make the document lack sincerity and force.

I did not share the opinion of some that we were dealing with a simple people. My seven years as a doctor of medicine amongst them had taught me otherwise. However, I felt that even if few could understand all of it, there were probably parts all could understand and like. This might make them believe in the parts they could not understand. A bit Irish, but it was the best I could come up with. It was also my hope that there were enough voters around who could understand what I was driving at and they would confirm that it was all good stuff.

All through this, except for close associates of whom Tangata Nekeare, the Chief of Police, was one, no one took the least notice of what we were up to. We seemed to have few supporters outside of ourselves. I just plugged away with the document I hoped would turn the trick.

At last it was completed, beautifully typed by Joanna, the then reigning Cook Islands Beauty Queen and beautifully translated by her father Taira Rere. It was printed and, at what we thought was the most propitious time, it was put to the public. Joy of joys! It caused a reaction and we started to have people declaring themselves open supporters despite full awareness of the danger that such a declaration might cost them their jobs or benefits. We had campaign rallies around Rarotonga. These were well attended and it began to look as though we might pull something off. We visited the outer islands and did our stuff there. At the elections, we polled 47.8 percent of the votes, but added only one seat, my own, bringing the total in Opposition to seven against government's fifteen.

* * *

Campaigns were torrid, rollicking affairs with much abuse, mud slinging, character assassinations and personal attacks thrown about with abandon. Meetings, held in strategic areas, consisted of the introduction of candidates and speakers on behalf of the party accompanied by music and singing. Our people are prolific song and lyric writers and we were not short of campaign songs, some of which are still around and have become part of the popular music fare.

These public meetings were attended liberally by our supporters with a fair sprinkling of the opposing party's supporters to add zest with tricky questions aimed to catch candidates off guard or intended to disclose something that the party or a candidate did not want aired. Heckling to disrupt meetings was not a feature at Cook Islands political gatherings. The campaigns usually stepped up in intensity and ferocity as election day drew closer with the last public meeting for the party out of office being held two days before election day and the incumbent party having their go the day before election day. The use of radio is essential in a country of tiny scattered islands and the radio was government owned. They kept the crucial last night for themselves. The duration of campaigning time was set by the incumbent party after discussion with the leaders of the other party. This was more or less the pattern in the 1972, 1974 and 1978 elections.

At the constituency level, frequent get-togethers were the usual mode of campaigning and these revolved around keeping as accurate a count of supporters and non-supporters as could be obtained and visiting those who might be wavering. Usually a candidate visited as many households as he could. In a large multiple candidate constituency this was a large order and some discretion had to be used as to the value of visiting some as opposed to others in the time available.

I had learnt that the chief electioneering characteristic of the Cook Islands was denigration of one's opponents. There was no pulling of punches in these attacks. In the vernacular it was known as akakino. The campaigning for the elections of March 1972 was no different. It was the prime political weapon. There was little offering of platforms, policies or issues, principally because very little of these were in the minds of the candidates or their supporters. It was all comedy entertainment and what better comedy entertainment than someone else's discomfiture.

Albert Henry was a past master at the entertainment of akakino. Attempts by his opponents to counter in like manner almost always failed because they lacked Albert's finesse. Traditionally Polynesians are great entertainers, but few could match Albert. Much to my amazement he dealt with me kindly. Whether this was in response to my personal policy not to use the method on anybody including him, I could not be sure. This led me to examine the technique more closely.

At public campaign meetings, the people loved akakino, at least on the surface, and would scream their delight. But I noticed that there were those who did not appreciate it immediately. There were even more who did not on cooler reflection later like it. It was perhaps because the person receiving the akakino was a relative or a friend. In a small community like ours a surprising proportion of people were one's relatives, in-laws or friends. Albert seemed to be aware of this and was very careful, I noted, who received his akakino and who did not. My long absence did not allow me to make that kind of discrimination and my policy of avoiding akakino altogether and especially with Albert was working points for me.

My Party despaired of my inability and lack of wish to be like Albert. It was the successful method and I was supposed to be able to parrot it. I became tired of listening to those who said, "Why don't you do it the way Albert does." I knew I never could. Moreover, I strongly believed that I would gain nothing by promoting someone else's image. I had my own to promote.

I resolved to avoid akakino and stick to issues. I had no choice. I was no entertainer. There were, as may be imagined, many issues. At first I allowed my colleagues to give as much akakino as they received as was the apparent custom, but, after closer examination, I came to the conclusion that, if our candidates would avoid akakino altogether, we could all win points. Accordingly, towards the close of the campaign I asked my candidates to avoid akakino altogether especially during the live radio broadcasts. This was particularly important because whoever one denigrated, there were relatives and friends listening. We needed their sympathy and if possible their votes, not their antagonism.

This seemed to be working to our advantage and we fired up the crowd by other means and we had enough good old Polynesian humour and humorists to do this without akakino. In response, the presentations of Albert and his party toned down with some confusion as how to take this new approach. My own group found this restriction very hard to accept. I pointed out that the screams of applause were coming from our supporters only and that we were not impressing the unbelievers. I tried to make them understand that the applause which was gladdening our hearts was turning away those we needed to swell our ranks with the substance of our policies.

The new campaign approach seemed to be working to our benefit and it became the rule, but each time, I had to remind everybody not to akakino, for the desire to do so was constantly present. Who, after all, does not want to hear the roar of the crowd when one is on stage.

Then came the fateful night, the last of three allowed live broadcasts just before election day. I again requested no akakino, but in vain. Tangata Nekeare and one other, our lady candidate, Mrs Poko Ingram, chose to break protocol and gave the supporters their fill of akakino. The supporters rose in their seats, screaming their pleasure, and apparently could not get enough of this kind of campaign fare. It was great entertainment.

I glanced around the hall and saw the sour faces sprinkled throughout the hall. My thoughts sprang to those listening in and I was sure that whatever chances we had of winning votes from the fence sitters were now gone. But our candidates were ecstatic. They thumped me after the meeting and said, "Listen to them. This is what they came for." As calmly as I could, I said, "We have just lost the election and the two of you will not win seats." I gained a seat and it was the only extra seat we gained. Perhaps that is all we would have gained no matter what we did. Tangata had been touted by all to win a seat for us, but he did not. In future campaigns, we stuck to issues more closely and the method of akakino, though now much out of favour, still bursts forth occasionally as I suppose it must.

* * *

On election day candidates put as many vehicles as they could on the road to transport electors to the polling booths. These were supposed to pick up voters in a non-partisan manner. Mostly a party's fleet of vehicles picked up their own supporters to make sure that all voted. Hopefully, those they were not sure of would vote for the party to which the vehicle belonged.

Some candidates offered large quantities of food at their homes or at a suitable not so blatant venue for all to come and have a feed and then be transported to the polling booths. Most, however, were more in line with the electoral act and took them to the food source after voting and before they were transported home. The former and blatant technique was the most common cause for post-election petitions under the guise of bribery and undue inducement. These petitions were not often successful because the defence plea was based on the custom of Polynesian hospitality. This is difficult to argue against.

All candidates were by law banned from being near the site of voting except for casting their vote. There were police to enforce this and scrutineers of candidates assigned to booth areas to make sure that the police did their job in this and other respects and generally see that no hanky panky took place. The population voting rate was usually high, at the 95 to 99 percent level.

The results were usually out well before midnight on the same day and were cause for great jubilation and taunting on the one hand and downhearted silence on the other. Radio and press interviews of the leaders were held and by next day or within a very short time the winning party government was in full swing especially if the same party won government again, which to us in Opposition was too frequent an occurrence.

* * *

No doubt you are asking how we could have polled 47.8 percent of the votes with a gain of only one seat. At that time the Cook Islands voting system was not based on the one vote, one candidate method. There were three constituencies in Rarotonga. The largest one had 4 seats, the next largest had 3 and the smallest had 2, making a total of 9 seats for Rarotonga. Aitutaki was considered as one constituency with 3 seats to represent it. This was also true for other islands with more than one seat.

In the largest constituency for Rarotonga where there were four candidates, a voter put the mark of his choice on only four of the candidates on the list. If he put his mark against more than four, the ballot was invalid. One could poll at any of the many booths within the electorate. All the votes for the constituency were counted for each candidate and the four who received the highest number of total votes were the ones elected to parliament. Within this electorate of four seats, there are four distinct areas and the candidates were, through natural and traditional circumstances, chosen to represent each of these. However, these areas were not equal in population and two of the largest were heavily for Albert's party.

Therefore, a candidate who had a high vote from his own area could be swamped out by votes not for him from another more populated area. Accordingly the party which received the highest number of overall votes in a more populated area swamped out anybody who may have received the highest vote from a more sparsely populated area. Thus the party which received the highest number of votes from the more populated areas went into parliament with an inordinate majority. This negated any representational aspects the Westminster system may have had and ensured an absolute majority for the Cook Islands Party.

Absolute majority was likely to produce a number of abuses. The government was likely to make changes in the constitution which might not be in the best interests of the country. A constitutional change required a two thirds majority for its passage. Just by having the numbers, government could believe that it had a mandate to do things which it otherwise would not. Often these were no more than abuse and disregard for consultative discussions with the Opposition. Often legislation was bulldozed through without regard for the views of the Opposition or the public. Guillotine motions were used if there was any resistance.

Between 1972 and 1978 while I was Leader of the Opposition, we had no offices or support services of any kind and for most of these years my salary was that of an ordinary member at $300 per annum. The adage that power corrupts is not just an idle saying. It happened to Albert's Party and it happened to mine in its due time.

* * *

There was not much that could be done in Opposition but wait and exercise patience. I watched the economy crumble. It had been bad enough during the days of New Zealand administration, probably no worse than it would have been under any other colonial administration, but now without the input of even minimal economic measures and with the antagonistic attitude of government towards the private sector, it was deteriorating at the rate, it was said, of 70 percent over the past eight years.

The per capita Gross Domestic Product was little better than that of Western Samoa which was the poorest of the Pacific Island States, but that was mainly because we received more New Zealand aid per capita, some of which was recycled in our domestic economy. Where we were better than other Pacific states, it was not saying much.

There was no understanding of inflation rates and their effect on purchasing power, earnings, budgets and the economy as a whole. When I introduced the subject in my policy statement, it confused nearly everybody. The concept and its effects were alien to almost all in positions of responsibility.

I spent several sessions trying to convince Albert that a policy which would stimulate business activity would start to lift the country on to its economic feet. It was impossible for him to see this in any other way than by government getting into business which, he said, it could not afford at that time. I explained that if the business sector did these things itself it would cost the government nothing. It was a hopeless task which I abandoned with reluctance.

He had not always been so anti-business. Albert had himself tried on several occasions in his career to become a private businessman, but had failed miserably. However, when he organised cooperatives using other peoples resources, he did not too badly, even though the cooperatives went bankrupt. The concept of self motivated enterprise had no point of reference from which he could start thinking about it. It was completely alien. Unfortunately it was alien to almost everybody else too. This included those in the business sector itself. They did not see that they were contributing to their own dilemma of stagnation by helping government strictly control business activity so that new businesses had little chance of starting up. Legislation already in place ensured that this stagnant state of affairs would continue.

I had no idea how far the economy had to deteriorate before I was given an opportunity to do something about it. I was going to sit it out no matter how long it took. Some of the ministers of government knew that I had ideas how to solve this problem and wanted the formula, but I had had enough experience of second hand knowledge making a mess of good ideas. Besides I did not know myself how exactly I was going to implement whatever formula I had. It could only be done with sensitivity at each step of the way. It would have to be done without alarming a population already entrenched in a system averse to the kind of measures that I had in mind. It was frustrating. There was little I could do about it until I was in a position to do it myself. That still seemed a long way off.

* * *

The debates in Parliament, at that time called The House of Assembly, were little more than sessions of one side of the house denigrating the other. The sessions were in English and Cook Islands Polynesian and were transmitted over the radio. It was entertaining, but in time that kind of entertainment begins to pall. At least it did for me. At every opportunity, I was attacked as a 'foreigner', as a 'Yankee' and along with this was added what they thought of Americans and my speaking 'through my nose'. There was always a variety of unsavoury epithets in both languages.

After one of my colleagues in Opposition recited my local lineage and family connections, one of the government side who was related to me denied I had any connections with his family. After the session I was pleased that his family gave him a bad time and forced him to take this back at the next sitting. Members of the clan also apologised profusely on his behalf when we met casually on the street.

Albert on the other hand was always pleased to point out our family connections, distant as they might be by European standards. To Polynesians, as alluded to elsewhere, family connections are as important as anything can be and to deny a relationship is serious. My education was attacked on the basis that it was useless theory in the practical world of hard knocks. I was able to hold up my end by ignoring these attacks as though they had never been made and confined my speaking time to the business at hand. My colleagues, however, made full use of these attacks to make their own points in rebuttal and it was not necessary for me to defend myself, even if I thought it prudent to do so.

We worked hard in Opposition and gave it all we could and became known as an effective Opposition. We discussed together all the bills that came before the House and many of them seemed of little consequence. Perhaps some were there to fill the order paper. Regardless, we gave them our full attention and caused some to be withdrawn. There were a number of constitutional changes which had little substantive effect, but with government having a two thirds majority our arguments were academic and made for political effect on listeners.

* * *

After the general elections of 1972 in which we had polled nearly 48 percent of the votes, our supporters were highly disappointed. A number of public servants and wage workers were fired on the basis that they were our supporters. Some were not. This caused so much consternation and fear this would spread that, between March 1972 and September 1974, 4040 people of all ages emigrated from the Cook Islands - over 20 percent of our total population. Albert kept tabs on this, as I did also. The exodus consisted mainly of Democratic Party supporters and their families. These were also the hard working artisans and skilled workers from our society. It was not going to be good for the Democratic Party's prospects at the next general elections. It was going to be worse for the country to lose this calibre of people in such numbers.

The great exodus which took place at this time was facilitated from 1972 on by the operational opening of the Rarotonga International Airport and easier access to New Zealand. Until this time there was only one small plane every two weeks and a small cargo ship once a month. Most places were taken by officials, medical cases or students going on courses. Ordinary citizens had to wait up to several months to get a passage.

By virtue of the fact that Cook Islanders are New Zealand citizens, they have free access to New Zealand and, since 1903, New Zealanders have had free access to Australia. This privilege was later extended to us. Thus there are now nearly three times as many Cook Islanders living in New Zealand and Australia as in the Cook Islands. This exodus caused problems for employers and in-house training programs. Young Cook Islanders took jobs at home for as long as it took them to obtain the money for a one way plane ticket.

This worked to the benefit of New Zealand during the good economic times when New Zealand needed a greater labour force than it could supply itself. It was also perhaps of benefit to the Cook Islands in relieving it of a potential over-population problem and poor prospects for employment. There were definite benefits to relatives from money remitted back home. Therefore, since the 1940s, Cook Islanders have used New Zealand as a safety valve for any potential over-population problem and when times have been economically difficult back home. However, if economic circumstances at home ever improved, this exodus could pose problems.

This migration is a one way affair because only a small proportion ever return to live in the Cook Islands. Cook Islanders are hard workers and, therefore, are the favourite Pacific Islanders for jobs in New Zealand and now in Australia. Many factories and work places in New Zealand employed Cook Islanders by preference.

The independence that the Cook Islands received in 1965 maintained this relationship of Cook Islanders retaining their New Zealand citizenship. In addition the relationship included New Zealand being responsible for the external affairs and defence of the Cook Islands subject to consultation between the Prime Ministers of the two countries. Since 1965 the Cook Islands has developed its own external affairs capability with New Zealand Foreign Affairs assisting in cases where our own facilities are not adequate.

The Cook Islands needed to develop its own foreign affairs capability for the development of its own economy. Although New Zealand is still nominally responsible for the defence of the Cook Islands, it is, with its past and present defence system, unable to do this for itself let alone for the Cook Islands. If it should face a moderate scale military operation against it and the Cook Islands, it would not be unreasonable to assume that it would sacrifice the Cook Islands in its own defence. It is, therefore, important for the Cook islands to develop and maintain good relations with its friends, large and small, near and far, as well as involve itself in universal efforts towards world peace as its best means of defence. It has no other. This in my view made the ANZUS Pact important not only to the Cook Islands, but also to other Pacific Islands States. Few of them openly admit that they relied on this protection.

* * *

At any rate both Albert and I were keeping tabs on this exodus to New Zealand. I saw our political prospects for the future fading into oblivion. We were severely damaged by it. Albert was in high glee and informed me he was wiping me and the Democratic Party off the face of the earth. I secretly could not but agree with him. In reality we had the numbers but they were emigrating. In the latter part of 1974, to make his threat a reality, Albert called a snap election for December, only two years into his four year term.

* * *

In this 1974 elections, the Democratic Party introduced the "flying voters" from New Zealand. We did this to recoup some of the supporters we had lost to New Zealand. The Electoral Act provided for overseas residents who had been away for not more than a year to vote, but they must return to the Cook Islands to do so. This virtually excluded all qualified overseas voters, as they could not afford the regular fare or be easily freed from their job commitments.

We chartered an Air Nauru 727 to fly those voters who paid in advance to vote at the Rarotonga Airport where special booths were set up. 95 voters flew in, but only 75 were eligible to vote. After voting, they flew out again. In setting up these "flying voters" we made absolutely certain that the flights were available to all voters regardless of their party affiliation and that they paid their own fares. The fact that the charter was known as "Demo" flights more or less ensured that few voters from Albert's Cook Islands Party would use them. One or two did avail themselves of the opportunity. This ploy must have helped, but our deficit was much greater than could be offset by this means.

I was just as surprised as Albert when we gained just over 48 percent of the total votes and added another seat. This broke his two thirds majority in Parliament. Albert was very upset and I don't think he ever really got over it. For us to have done this meant that we had taken a very healthy proportion of his support from him. Our winning only one more seat meant that our small majority of total voters had not been enough to overcome the disproportion of votes caused by the unbalanced distribution of voters in the multiple candidate constituencies.

* * *

In the Cook Islands Party 1974-1978 term, Albert's hold was beginning to visibly weaken. The country was not advancing in anything, it was still going backwards. We did not need experts to tell us this. The Airport had been opened by Queen Elizabeth II who at the same time, at the instigation of the New Zealand Government, knighted Albert, Sir Albert Henry KBE. The Rarotongan Hotel, owned jointly by the Cook Islands government, Air New Zealand and the New Zealand government, one third each, was opened. It was to be run by the New Zealand Tourist Hotel Corporation (THC), a New Zealand ad hoc government corporation, which pretty much ensured that it would never make a profit. In the ever eternal springing of hope that it might make a profit, permits were refused to our own people who had already built or were in the process of building tourist accommodation units. The restriction was imposed on the grounds that permits would be issued only after the Rarotongan Hotel had started to make a profit. Instead, its losses increased yearly and our people went ahead anyway and built their units.

It was plain that tourism was going to be important to the economy of the Cook Islands, but progress to make it happen was slow. There was fear of this relatively new thing. There had been tourists in small numbers, but not enough to have made an impact. Academics in the area were doing their bit to turn this fear into a panic which our people and our traditional leaders took to heart. "We don't want to be like Hawaii," many said. Others said, "Tourism will spoil our culture." Still others said, "Our country will be invaded by foreigners who will take what we have." The churches got in the act and said, "They will not respect our Sundays. They will go down the street in bathing suits and bikinis. In Tahiti they are sun-bathing without tops. These will all be bad examples for our mapu (youth)." The economic minded said, "You will not benefit from tourism. Only the investors in the hotels will benefit and we will all become nothing more than waiters, waitresses and housemaids." The real problem was that even our most educated and intelligent citizens could rarely see that economic gains in any sector benefited more than just the sector directly involved.

And so the anti tourism arguments went on, but it was inevitable that tourism would come about and that, if we did it right, everybody could benefit. Our natural resources were virtually non-existent. To me our own people going ahead and building accommodation units one or two at a time and adding units as time went on was most impressive. What they were doing imprinted itself on me as a way to keep benefits of tourism within our own hands. It looked even better for the farmers and fisherman if they could supply all the vegetables and some of the meat products and all of the fish requirements for the visitor trade. In the matter of farm products it should surpass exporting, with all the problems associated with that.

* * *

With the seemingly favourable events taking place in an election year, things should have been good for Albert. But they were not. Four of his Members of Parliament, two of them Ministers of the Crown, resigned for a number of reasons. Ineffective leadership, nepotism, administrative irregularities, persecution, partisanship, dictatorial tendencies, lack of development and a poor national image were some mentioned by Dr Joseph Williams in writing about his reasons for resigning.[59] The others would probably have given a similar list of grievances. But even prior to this and before my return from the United States, ministers had resigned, perhaps again for similar reasons. Albert's political sins were beginning to catch up with him and most were now coming home to roost.

At his request, we met many times regarding my joining him and taking over the Prime Ministership from him at some later date. I continued to resist these requests. Towards the end of his term, he publicly made his final request to me, walking the main street from his office to my surgery and announcing his intention to all as he went.

Despite our openness with each other and our liking for each other, I was probably his prime subject for persecution over the years. His political training would not allow him to do otherwise. Our openness with each other included discussions on the most intimate matters of a political nature affecting us and at no time did either of us breach these confidences.

Towards the end of his 1974-1978 term, a seat held by one of his members became vacant. In the by-election he lost the seat to our member, Iaveta Short. This was to presage what was to take place in the general elections of 1978.

* * *

From the beginning, I was having difficulties of my own. I had problems with the language after being away for so long. I was all right in normal conversation, but not in the specialised fine tuning of oratory and public debate. The fact of being away for so long was a problem in itself. I was out of touch, and many who knew me well were no longer with the living or had migrated. I had great difficulty in making economic and social concepts understood. These were not necessarily common place elsewhere, but they were central to my own philosophy. Often the difficulty was not as much a matter of language as of concepts which were new and strange to this part of the world. In either language, points of reference that I could appeal to were missing.

I agonised over these difficulties in an attempt to simplify their presentation, but with only partial success. This agonising stilted my presentations. It probably would have been better if I had sung some cowboy and old time Cook Islands' songs with my ukulele instead, or, as one late member of the legislative body once said, "Give them ice cream." It was, however, apparently sufficient for most to believe that the concepts had some validity because I polled next to Albert at the 1972 and 1974 elections and subsequently out-polled him. I depended heavily on sincerity. There was no way that I could compete with Albert in oratory. He was a master orator and none in the Pacific, a region traditionally famous in the art of oratory, could equal him.

* * *

From the beginning, I also had leadership problems. Even as early as 1972, the big thing going for me was my ability to pull in votes, but as soon as we came through an election, there were those who wanted to take over the leadership. It was also plain that there were those waiting on the sidelines with no willingness to involve themselves openly in the affairs of the party until it had gained enough strength. When this occurred they set themselves up as candidates and entered the craving for leadership group.

Between elections it was difficult keeping these ambitious adherents in some semblance of order, but at election times, they all lined up like good boys for the most part and for the short time necessary to get the elections over with. The attempts to take over leadership were abortive, but the hopes of the ambitious never waned. They seemed to be at it constantly and I came to accept their activities as part of the normal scene, realising that at some time in the future their efforts would be successful. It strengthened my own admonition on quiet occasions to candidates that to expect more than a fifty fifty chance of winning at the polls would someday cause disappointment.

Of all the challengers, Vincent Ingram, the first of a line of pretenders, was only one who followed the Party's constitutional requirement that the party leadership should be changed only at a Party Annual Conference by a vote of members present. When he failed in this attempt, his persistence was not in any way dampened. His political tactic seemed to be one in which, if he was not going to obtain the leadership he was going to spoil it for everyone else and in particular for me. I secretly referred to him as the Spoiler.

His next try was through a vote of no confidence in 1986, by which time I had been PM for eight years. It was to be supported by Geoffrey Henry, who was at this time my Deputy Prime Minister in the first coalition (he had been leader of the Opposition up to that time). Which of the two of them was to be the Prime Minister was never clear. The vote was ushered in with flags flying, reporters and a television crew replete with commentator flown in from New Zealand. The attempt was abortive.

I continued to ignore these constant threats of a vote of no confidence and the ambiguities within the constitution in the interest of getting on with the job, but knowing full well that some day one of these would be successful. All of the pretenders were anxious to get me out of the way on the premise that, once this was achieved, all their troubles would be solved. It never entered their heads that all of them could not be Prime Ministers and their troubles might just be starting once they got me out of the way.

* * *

The significant success of the Democratic Party was its worst enemy. Observations of political parties in general indicate that this may be true everywhere. Too much success brings out the worst in its members of parliament, particularly its ministers. Everybody wants to be the Prime Minister and the cohesive force of the adage "United we stand, divided we fall", which carries political parties to success, is pushed to the background and a series of divisive attempts by ambitious individuals to share the glory at the very top becomes evident. It happened to Albert and it was happening to me. In the Pacific Island States it seems to happen everywhere. Leaders are constantly being threatened with it or suffering from it. The simple arithmetic that spells disaster to these divisive internal conspiracies is ignored and the march of folly must stolidly tramp its way to an inevitable and predictable conclusion.

In the Cook islands the favoured way of taking over leadership was through a parliamentary vote of no confidence. This seems to be the favoured way in some other countries of the Pacific region also, especially Western Samoa, Solomon Islands and Papua New Guinea. This neatly avoids having to depend on the democratic process of overcoming any mandate the leader may have in carrying the success of the party at the polls. All one has to do is build up dissatisfactions of members in government into a large enough dissent and act on it. All one needs to complete the process is a head of state (usually a Governor General in the Pacific Commonwealth or, in our case, a Queen's Representative) to accede to it.

Votes of no confidence have become a political pastime in some Pacific Island States. It is either a predilection in the character of Pacific Islanders or a weakness in our constitutions, written so that it can too freely take place.

Albert Henry had successfully promoted the idea of a four year term and the constitution was changed to accommodate it. In his last term he promoted the idea of a five year term, but for one reason or another had not carried it through, presumably because of some resistance within his Party. When we came into office we pursued this successfully, although with some strong resistance from certain quarters of the public, mostly the New Zealand expatriate sector.

The argument for the four year term is sound. The three year term, as practised in New Zealand and Australia, appears to be too short for the government in power to put its policies into effect and stabilise them after a change of government.

Since we introduced the five year term, I have noted that during the fourth year, government members start to become increasingly more demanding of greater privileges and involvement in downright corrupt practices which I found very difficult to contain. An impending election at about this time I believe would have done a better job of containment. I am not saying that a five year term does not work for others, but for us, who may not be fully aware of what constitutes corruption, a four year term is enough. There is no more sobering prospect to a parliamentarian than an impending election before he has become tempted into bad habits.

CHAPTER SIXTEEN

Cancer and Charlatans

But ye are forgers of lies, ye are all physicians of no value.   JOB 13:4

During my term as Leader of the Opposition, I came in contact with a number of strange circumstances. We are so used to these that one often hears the comment "It couldn't happen anywhere but in the Cook Islands." Some of these affected me personally.

I have mentioned the purposeful sinking of the Torea, which I am happy to say was not done by indigenous Cook Islanders. A great deal of personal spite led to this episode by Chris Vaile who wanted to own the Torea on his own terms. He initiated the idea, Joe Cowan planned it and Paul Fry bored the holes. The episode may have been political in that they were all apparent supporters of Albert, but what they did, though perhaps abetted by political feelings, was motivated by personal antagonism. It may have been precipitated by a rumour that I was going to sail it to the Northern atolls to campaign and the sinking was to prevent me from doing so. Tere and I since 1972 had successfully used the Torea in reactivating the pearl shell trade. It was profitable, but very hard physical work and necessitated frequent trips to Penrhyn, 750 nautical miles to the north.

In the true style of Albert's politics, which was one of eliminating one's opponents by any means possible, I, as Leader of the Opposition, was a prime target.

* * *

Parliamentary sittings did not follow any predictable pattern. This would have required a co-ordinated effort between the Ministers as the lawmakers, legal advisers, draftsmen, printers and the parliamentary staff. This co-ordination never took place in a manner which might allow organised parliamentary sessions. Instead, they were at the whim of government depending on the readiness of bills pending and other factors. We generally accepted these circumstances except when bills were suddenly put before us with little and often no time to give them proper attention before they came to debate. In my own time as Prime Minister I was not able to overcome these shortcomings to any significant degree. Tomorrow is another day had much to do with it.

Between sessions and sittings, opposition members and ordinary government members had little to do. Moreover, the remuneration of ordinary members of the governing party and the opposition was only $300 per annum, later increased to $500 during our days in opposition. Therefore, most such members did other things to eke out a living. Since a Member of Parliament could not be employed by the Public Service, all work was in the private sector. Some worked for companies which indulged their absence during sittings, but most reverted to their respective callings. Lawyers practised law, storekeepers sold goods, growers planted. However, doctors in parliament did not practice medicine since all medical services were provided free by government doctors since 1901. Hospital care and medications were also free.

Except for Fred Story's father many years before and probably before there was an adequate government medical service, no doctor had ever thought of going into private medical practice. It was generally believed that, because of the comprehensive free medical service available, private medical practice would not be economic. But it seemed that there were people willing to pay for medical services if they could be assured of them being better than those available from government doctors.

On close examination, I felt certain that I could provide that service. It had been a long time since I had practised medicine seriously as most of my work in the United States had been in research, though I had never denied anybody who required my services, as had been the case in Alaska and elsewhere. I had kept up with the mainstream of developments through my medical research, clinical and pharmaceutical interests.

In any event I rented space and with the help of Frank, Emily's carpenter husband, we put up partitions and ended up with a fine surgery consisting of a waiting room with receptionist area, an examination cum treatment room and a consulting office. Very soon I had more patients than I had bargained for and after I became Prime Minister, these premises have since served two medical practitioners and are still doing sterling duty to this day.

In setting up in practice, Albert and the doctor in government who was also the Minister of Health, created as many barriers as they could to prevent me from practising. They even claimed that I was not properly qualified. Some government doctors regarded my practice as a slur on their competence and were not averse to aiding and abetting attempts to frustrate my efforts.

Having failed in this, they turned their attention to persecuting my patients. They were discriminated against by a charge of plus 30 percent above a liberal interpretation of cost on medications obtained on prescriptions signed by me and obtained from the government pharmacy, the only pharmacy at that time. A notice to this effect for the edification of my patients was prominently placed outside the pharmacy. This did not deter my patients. They paid for what they should have received free, and continued to be my patients.

Charges were also attempted for laboratory and other hospital services, but these came to nothing. I was banned from visiting patients I deemed in need of hospital care. In general I took no heed of this and visited them whenever I felt this was in their best interests and consulted with the doctors and nurses in charge of them as though we were in a normal patient/doctor, doctor/doctor and doctor/nurse relationship existing in more objective communities.

My returning to full time medical practice was greatly aided by the medical journals I subscribed to and particularly to a publication serving the New Zealand medical community called New Ethicals. Each monthly publication dealt with a few medical subjects contributed to by specialists in each field. Only a few, as few as three, were dealt with at a time, but these were presented in depth from the practical point of view as they affected the practising physician.

In very short order a practising physician can be updated in a variety of medical conditions that physicians face in the normal course of their practise. I found it and its companion publication, New Ethicals Catalogue, of infinite service in providing my patients with the most up to date treatment that the profession could provide.

* * *

Into this milieu entered Vlastimil Brych, usually referred to as Milan Brych. He had a charming personality and a plausible medical knowledge gained through being a medical orderly attached to a prison doctor for seven years while serving a prison sentence for robbery in Brno, Czechoslovakia. His criminal record were not known in New Zealand at that time. He claimed to be a qualified physician with special training in oncology (tumours).

Just how Vlastimil Brych came to apply for admission to New Zealand is not clear, but in 1968 New Zealand admitted a number of refugees from Czechoslovakia. He arrived by air in Auckland in November 1968 and was given a job as a technician at Auckland Hospital's central laboratory.

Through a series of events and fabricated information, Milan Brych was given a license to practise medicine in New Zealand. He was interviewed by a number of the most prominent luminaries of the profession. It is to his credit that he was able to con them into believing that he was qualified and had not only attended medical school in Brno in Czechoslovakia, but had attended institutions which gave him extra qualifications. He practised in Auckland, New Zealand, where he became famous as a cancer therapist. For a time there was overwhelming enthusiasm at Auckland Hospital and in the Health Department for what seemed to be a breakthrough in the treatment of cancer. His claims, however, could not be sustained by the results of his treatment in the longer term and by his unprofessional attitudes which became apparent as time went by.

He shrouded his treatments with secrecy on the plea that he had to protect his methods from pharmaceutical companies who would steal them. Although he promised to produce a scientific report on his treatment methods and their results, this never eventuated either in written form as a publication or in oral form at the medical conventions he attended.

Discussions with well known oncologists led to their evaluation that Dr Brych did not know much about oncology in particular and medicine in general. Further interviews brought to the fore further suspicions through his evasions to answering questions. The continuation of his license to practice medicine was seriously given second thoughts.

At considerable expense, the New Zealand Medical Council, charged with dealing with such matters, investigated Brych's claims of having attended the Purkyne University, Brno and other aspects of Brych's life. The investigations and hearings were carried out on 23 November, 1976 under the auspices of the City of the Brno Court with representatives of the New Zealand Medical Council (Dr John Scott and David S. Morris, Lawyer), and Mrs Jane D. Anderson, Vice Consul of New Zealand in Czechoslovakia, in attendance. The hearings were presided over by Dr Miloslav Stefl, Judge. The evidence presented by a number of witnesses under oath exposed a story hitherto unimagined by those who heard it.

Olga Bartikova, Director, Industrial High School, Brno, remembered Vlastimil Brych for his bad grades and non attendance. Brych, who was born on 11 December, 1938, attended the school during the years 1954-1958. The witness reported that, year by year, Brych's grades became worse and worse, conflicts became greater and in the third year he failed to finish. He could not be classified because he was having psychiatric treatment for a mental disorder. Despite several invitations, Brych never again reported for studies. The documentation showed that Brych had missed a total of 420 classes and received a third grade for behaviour.

Further evidence for the same period was given by Jaroslav Kafka, Chemical Engineer, Brno, a former master while Brych was attending the same school. His evidence, though dealing with Brych's character from a somewhat different aspect, corroborated that given by Bartikova.

Robert Kavalec, a second hand shop owner of Brno, Meninska 3, gave evidence of events leading up to the attack made on him by Brych which resulted in a seven year imprisonment from 13 January 1959 to 25 October 1965. In his testimony he informed the court that Brych visited his shop several times, introducing himself by name and offering him things to sell. When this happened, Mr Kavalec reported, it was his custom to make out an identity card.

On 24 October, 1958, Brych visited him for about two hours at the end of which Brych asked him to show him a coat and, without warning, hit him over the head followed by two or three added blows. Kavalec reported he could feel the blood flowing from his head. Brych ran out of the shop with Kavalec running after him calling out, "Catch him! Catch him", but his calls were in vain. Charges of assault were laid and Brych was sentenced to 16 years in prison, but, at an appellate hearing, this was reduced to 7 years.

Jana Trojankova, Officer of Czech Commission for Scientific Degrees, Ministry of Education of Czech Republic, Praha 4, Kaplicka 20, was in charge of Defences of Doctoral dissertation theses, Notification of Scientific degrees, Legislation of Diplomas, and printing of diplomas for Doctors of Sciences. In performing these duties, he keeps lists of candidates of sciences and doctors of sciences. His evidence was needed to confirm Brych's claim that he defended his thesis in December 1967 and received the degree of Candidate of Sciences in 1968. The name of Vlastimil Brych could not be found in the records. Dr John Scott examined these records himself and confirmed that Brych's name or any similar name does not appear in the records.

Brych had produced a certificate of attendance at an Industrial Chemical school with a certificate of performance for a period of seven years, the same period he was serving a sentence in a correctional institution. Dr Jan Novotny, Director of the Policlinic in Brno, with qualifications in Internal Medicine and a specialist in Social Medicine, gave evidence that he had given a job to applicant Vlastimil Brych on 8 December, 1965. This was an attempt to give Brych a second chance. Brych lied to him that he was in gaol for the religious reason that he was a Jehovah's Witness and distributed tracts on its behalf. Brych withdrew this when faced with the fact that it was known that he was convicted for attempted robbery.

Although at first he worked well and was unwarrantedly obliging, later he worked with a Mrs Jakoubkova, and anomalies in the work started to appear in the exactness of laboratory reports and working time. Both were reprimanded. It was discovered that Brych was giving reports of results without taking the necessary material from patients. On 30 April, 1966, Brych's employment was terminated.

Having served his sentence for robbery was not the end of his criminal offences His brother-in-law Miroslav Dvorack and his wife Milada gave evidence, as did many others, of fraudulent activities for which Brych received money from friends for services which were never realised. In an attempt to escape from these, he was apprehended and served four years in prison. Later still he was imprisoned for 30 months for more criminal activities.

He has the following record in the penal register:

1. Peoples Court , Brno, 13.1.1959, 3T 242/58, paragraph 232/1 penal act 1952, seven years imprisonment, unconditional, sentence completed 25.10.1965, with loss of civil rights and forfeiture of property.

2. District Court, Brno, 5.10. 1967, 7T 52/67; paragraphs 248/1, 250/1a, 176/1, 8/1, 109/2, Penal Act 1960; 4 years imprisonment, unconditional.

3. Municipal Court Brno, 25.10. 1971, 7T 696/71, paragraph 109/2 Penal Act 1960, 30 months imprisonment unconditional with forfeiture of property.

The results of these investigations led to the removal of Brych from the New Zealand Medical Register. Milan Brych appealed against this decision, but withdrew when he realised the evidence was overwhelming. Despite this, he publicly claimed that he was being victimised and stuck to his story that he was a qualified physician.

* * *

Now Sir Albert Henry and Dr Joseph Williams, his Minister of Health, enter the picture in shining armour to save Brych from his "persecutors". In this they were ably supported by a vast number of the public. Joh Bjelke-Petersen (now Sir Joh), then Premier of Queensland, Australia, himself implicated in 1988 by the Commission on Corruption for the major role in massive, long term, statewide corruption, was one of them. These and a string of cancer patients and those who imagined they had cancer were out to save Brych from "victimisation by the medical profession." There were also some doctors of medicine in Australia in this queue of sympathisers.

It was probable that Sir Joh and most others were in this with a good heart and motivated by human compassion. Certainly Sir Joh had his personal experience with Sister Kenny, the Australian nurse who initiated the more intensive physiotherapy treatment of poliomyelitis paralysis. She had treated Sir Joh with apparent success. Sister Kenny's methods were at that time severely criticised by the medical profession. Therefore, it was reasonable that Sir Joh would see the Milan Brych episode as another unwarranted attack by doctors on someone who had something of value to offer. Others no doubt were lured by the possible miracle being promised. But I obtained the distinct impression that Albert was out to make this into another of his ploys to regain his waning political strength.

* * *

The information on the court hearings in Brno was made available to Dr Joseph Williams and Dr Archie Guinea, the then President of the Cook Islands Medical and Dental Association, the official body responsible for such matters in the Cook Islands. To my knowledge they all succumbed to the political forces to allow Brych to practise in the Cook Islands. I personally made an appeal to Dr Guinea, but was told that he and the Medical Council could do nothing about it.

By this means Brych was given the sanctuary of the Cook Islands to continue providing his "services" to the many patients from overseas who were afflicted and those who thought they were afflicted with cancer. Up to then, they knew they had few avenues of escape from the suffering and early demise associated with this condition. They could hardly be blamed for grasping at the hope that Brych cruelly offered them. To my knowledge, Brych never offered or was asked to treat a resident of the Cook Islands.

* * *

In 1976 Milan Brych was installed in Rarotonga. He was allocated accommodation by the government. A wing of the Rarotonga Hospital was taken over and renamed "Sir Albert Henry Hospital". This was the name used on Brych's letterheads for his hospital treatments. Recuperation accommodation was provided by the rapid construction of the Edgewater Motel, now the Edgewater Resort Hotel, and by a number of units constructed for the purpose by Cook Islanders.

These became an important part of the beginnings of our tourist accommodation industry. They did not see it at that time, but I was not loath to state publicly that when the Brych era came to an end, as it must, these units would become the beginnings of our tourism accommodation industry. Most regarded my statement as having no foundation in fact and truly believed that Brych's cancer industry was here to stay and were making long term investments in it.

Government nurses allocated to Brych were paid higher rates and various individuals, some of them key figures, received tangible benefits to affirm their support. His charming personality as well as the substantial money pouring in made him a charismatic figure for many of his supporters.

I had seen this type of medical phenomenon come and go several times both here and overseas. Whenever the medical profession is unable to deal with a problem, the way is open for faith healers, herbalists and medical charlatans to move in and promise sufferers a way out. Although the profession has made significant advances in the successful treatment of many types of cancer, it remains an unsatisfactorily resolved medical problem. This, however, cannot in any way be regarded as an acceptable reason for charlatans to ply their trade of selling false hope.

This phenomenon is also seen when the medical profession has a solution which is not being promulgated either through ignorance, maladministration or inefficiency. Charlatans of all kinds pop up out of nowhere merely because the medical profession is not doing its job properly. At this time of writing in 1989 and for the past year or so we have this situation in the Cook Islands again. A faith healer and dispensers of local potions and practices currently have a large following. It is doubtful that this situation can be resolved in any permanent way as long as government doctors in the Cook Islands are protected from litigation for malpractice.

* * *

To the naive, Brych's treatments were plausible. He used standard compounds used by the profession in the treatment of certain cancers. However, he and his cohorts used them indiscriminately and without concern for the type of cancer. He used them on patients who merely thought they had cancer. He used them on patients who had already been cured of cancer for many years. He used them on terminal cancer patients where they would have a deleterious rather than a beneficial effect. He talked terminal patients into taking more courses of expensive treatment when they would obviously not benefit from it.

The apparent success of his treatment was fortified by the short periods of dramatic relief from symptoms that is known to take place with such treatment, and then getting such people to fly home "cured", when in fact they died soon after their return.

Treatment with these drugs causes severe blood and immunological changes as well as constitutional changes. The rationale that they are toxic to cancer cells does not mean that normal cells are immune from their effects. The falling out of the hair of patients is indicative of their general toxicity. It is doubtful that Brych paid any more attention to the results of tests than he did to the tests he reported, but did not make, in the Policlinic in Brno. For the most part he used the agents with little regard for their toxic effects.

Later he pushed laertril as additional treatment for his patients. He had his patients cracking and eating apricot kernels, which contains laertril, said by some to be anti-carcinogenic.

* * *

The cost of a six week course of treatment was NZ$12,000 (about $35,000 in constant 1989 dollars). It included the cost of the few days of treatment in hospital and accommodation outside the hospital, but excluded air fares. Patients were usually accompanied by relatives. Our people, perhaps without knowing it, were getting a taste of a specialised tourism industry. Patients who died in Rarotonga were buried in a special plot across the road from the Airport. Locals called it the "Brych Yard".

* * *

At first the patients avoided direct contact with me. This was understandable as it was well known that I was strongly against the charlatanism being practised in a grossly blatant manner. The whole country, practically without exception, was caught up in the deception. They were publicly assured by Albert that it was a humanitarian act of saving lives and bringing great economic benefits to the country. Only jealous conventional doctors like myself were opposing it, he told them.

I never met Brych. He avoided me like the plague. Whenever I was present in a public place where he was also present, he would quickly remove himself. At first his patients also avoided me like the plague, but as time went on they actively sought my help and advice, usually surreptitiously, but sometimes openly. Those who came openly were mainly those who had been successfully treated by conventional means many years before, but feared a recurrence and had gone to Brych. They subsequently perceived the folly of having submitted to Brych's attentions but were caught in a web of financial commitment from which they would dearly like to be free.

Those who had been cured of cancer were commonly women who had had cancer of the cervix which is one of the most easily treated cancers. When I enquired why, after so many years of no symptoms and assurances from their doctors that they were cured, did they allow themselves to be inveigled into the Brych cure, they readily admitted their error, but they had at first felt they did not wish to miss the opportunity of a cure, just in case they needed one.

The doctors in the Cook Islands Medical Service should have known that the Brych treatment of these women at $12,000 a course was unwarranted and dishonest. Certainly the Minister of Health, Dr Joseph Williams, trained in Otago Medical School of New Zealand, should have. These women were being taken for a ride and ripped off in the process.

The other patients who sought my advice were terminal cases who knew their cases were hopeless. Often the patients themselves did not want to embark on a course of treatment, but their relatives had induced them to do so. When a patient realises that he or she is a terminal case, they resign themselves to their fate. Except for the associated pain, they quietly wait for the inevitable in a degree of personal peace, not easily understood by others.

I know because I have been a cancer patient and I had to wait four years to be certain that my treatment had been successful. I resigned myself to whatever fate had in store for me and carried on with my work as usual. I was one of the lucky ones. This is not the case with relatives, they grasp at every straw for their loved ones. Who can blame them? But it is deplorable when lack of ethics and charlatanism, with full knowledge of the circumstances, take advantage of the unfortunate for monetary gain.

The example of one patient in this category will suffice. She knew her time was near and had known this for some time. She had been induced by relatives to take the Brych "cure" and she had, when I saw her, just completed a six weeks' course. One of the doctors working with Brych visited her that very day to convince her and her husband that all would be well if she would just take another course. She rebelled and demanded to be taken home to Melbourne where she could spend her last days peacefully with her friends and relatives.

Her husband would not hear of this. She then ordered him to bring me to examine her and she would abide by my advice and made him promise that he would too. In examining her, I had no difficulty defining metastases in almost every part of her body. That she was still alive was amazing. Having concluded with little doubt that she had already made peace with her condition, and perhaps also with her God, I was perfectly frank with her and told her that another course of the Brych treatment would not do her any good and probably could do her harm.

Weak as she was, she turned an angry eye on her husband and said, "See, I told you I was right and knew what I was about." She then turned to me with a less wrathful eye, saying, "Tell this fool husband of mine to take me home where I can die in peace with my friends and children around me." They took the next plane out and as far as I know all her wishes and expectations came true in the only way she knew they could.

* * *

One would think that medical charlatans would not be much in evidence in the presence of a modern medical service. But they are. In small communities they do not usually last long. Sooner or later the public integrate the negative results of their endeavours and the charlatan is left with a dwindling number of patients. To have patients on a continuous basis, the charlatan has to have a large population where information takes a long time to disseminate or where dissemination of it does not take place at all. Every patient being a new patient is the ideal. In the Cook Islands, where it is said that if one breaks wind in Mangaia it is quickly known in Aitutaki, the failures of treatment are quickly known.

An old sage friend of mine used to say that a medicine man with false claims of a cure in the Cook Islands will practice for only six months, but the foremost faith healer operating in the Cook Islands has been going for three years using blessed tap water as her only cure for all ailments. Although she may have helped many (such as those who stopped excessive drinking of alcohol and coffee to drink her water instead), she has caused the deaths of many others. These have been in the area of cardiac ailments and high blood pressure for which there are effective medications. As a result of belief in her water cure, some abandoned their medications with fatal results.

In the United States, as best as I could judge, an ineffective cure has a life expectancy of about three years. There, it is the practising physicians who finally integrate their experience with an ineffective drug and come to that conclusion.

This was now happening to Milan Brych. After he lost his licence to practice in New Zealand, he also lost his New Zealand patients. In the Cook Islands, his patients were almost exclusively Australians. By early 1978 he had lost most of this following.

When I became Prime Minister, he realised that he was nearing the end of the line. Even though I never made any overt moves against him, there was no doubt in his mind that I might not tolerate him for long. He soon wound up his affairs and must have moved his money out of the country prior to this. There was no doubt about his affluence when he first arrived and during his time here.

Two cars and expensive household furniture were paid for by cheques regardless of amount. After he left and went to the United States, we were able to recover one of the vehicles and $17,000 in the Trust Fund.

Brych subsequently could not help but do his thing in the United States and ended up in prison for practising medicine without a license and 12 convictions for grand theft. The latest report is that he was paroled from a Los Angeles prison in September 1986 and that he is working in Switzerland with "one of the big drug companies" based in Geneva.

* * *

An ineffective agent used by a charlatan poses no problems unless it is toxic or keeps patients from existing efficacious means of treatment. In cancer this is especially a cause for concern when the charlatans use their product, without discrimination, on all cancers. The inclusion of treatable cancers prevents their timely treatment and puts such patients in jeopardy.

Several factors facilitate medical charlatanism. A high proportion of illnesses are self-limiting and any medicine prescribed as a cure in such conditions appears to be an effective cure. Both charlatans and poor physicians have good practices through this characteristic of many medical conditions.

Other medical conditions show periods of remission and exacerbation and it is easy to credit a natural period of remission to the curative effect of an agent. Some cancers exhibit these periods of remission and exacerbation to a marked degree. A charlatan can make much of the periods of remission as being due to his skill.

The placebo effect is a friend of the charlatan as it can make a person feel very much better as a result of being given something known to have no medical effect at all. Hypochondriacs are often effectively treated with nothing more than an injection of distilled water or the administration of a tablet of chalk.

* * *

In 1976 I had my own cancer problem. I should have attended to it earlier, but was waiting until such time as I went to New Zealand to have it attended to as the local medical scene was politically infiltrated and not conducive to my personal welfare. In the meantime it got away from me and required two surgical interventions by my friend David Rogers in New Zealand.

At the first sitting of Parliament after my return to duty, Dr Joseph Williams, the Minister of Health, made a blistering political attack. He informed Members of Parliament and all those listening on radio that I should take better note of Dr Brych's skills as he and his methods could most likely be the means of saving my life. He reminded everybody in the House and over the air that he was a Doctor of Medicine and gave the public a review of my cancer, adding that I would be dead within two years. It was a waste of time my being in politics and he urged the people at the next elections, if I was still around, not to vote for me or for my Party because I would soon be dead and they would have wasted their votes. I could not help feeling that he was right, but I resolved to carry on and do what I had to do without regard for the possibility he so lucidly projected. As I said, I was one of the lucky ones.

CHAPTER SEVENTEEN

Bribery and Corruption

It is important that you should have the reputation of being honest, otherwise no one will trust you. However, from time to time you will have to lie, and then you will have to carry it off with ease and authority. MACHIAVELLI

Suddenly the 1978 general elections were upon us. Though not due to be called until December, they were called on 11 January to be held on 27 April. We seemed to be in good shape and for the first time we were confident we would win. Whatever good things had happened for Albert and the Cook Islands Party over the recent past such as his knighthood, the opening of the International Airport and the Rarotongan Hotel, did not seem to be working in their favour as might have been expected. The Brych affair as a political vote-getting scheme, if indeed it had been that, was ill-timed and Brych's sensational value had already waned.

Just prior to the calling of the election, I had been offered the Vice Chancellorship of the University of the South Pacific (USP), an eleven nation university which has its headquarters in Fiji. The Cook Islands is a member country. I was honoured, and was seriously considering whether I should give up politics and accept the offer which was something I knew how to do. I was given plenty of time to make up my mind. Albert knew about the offer and some believed that he called an early election to force my hand into accepting the USP offer. This would have been good riddance of his problem. However, although there were other equally good reasons why he called an early election, it is in keeping with his character that he would not have missed an opportunity to have made this one good also.

Sir Albert, again with always an eye out for a ploy of some sort to augment his political position, made a strong public accusation that I was out to assassinate him. This ploy was built out of my being a pretty good pistol shot and having been invited to practice with friends at a pistol range near Christchurch. Surgery for my cancer had crippled my right arm permanently and I was recuperating with friends in Governor's Bay. Due to my infirmity, I shot using the doublehanded grip and could do no better than one off the possible while one of my friends, a policeman, was shooting possibles.

Albert got to hear about the episode and, during the pre-election months, made a great story out of my practising shooting and acquiring a gun to assassinate him. The scheme backfired and probably did me more good than harm.

Like Tim, my number 2 son, I am a gun nut. I have owned and used guns all my life and was a champion shot at Kings. At a tender age each of my children had to know all the safety rules of handling guns and using them, if they had a wish to as all of them did. During the war, when my 303 sporting rifle, which I had modified from a military Lee Enfield, was pressed into service (returned after the war in very good condition), I found and bought a muzzle loader which I used mostly for rabbits and game birds in Central Otago and the outbacks near Dunedin. I used toilet paper for wadding and, after each shot, I had to wait for the shreds of toilet paper mixed with the smoke of black powder to clear before I could ascertain the effectiveness of my shots.

I learnt a great deal about muzzle loaders and, when a movie crew were shooting a recent movie, one of the more recent versions of the "Mutiny of the Bounty" shot in Rarotonga, I was called in, as a known expert, to teach and supervise the use of the flintlock muzzle loading pistols and rifles required in the movie. Needless to say, this time, I used proper wadding.

Tim has a collection of 16 guns and whenever I visit him in La Porte, Indiana, we haul the lot to the nearest shooting range and bang away at targets until we run out of ammunition. The last time we did this was in 1987 when I was visiting him after I had visited John, my number 1 son. John had just undergone a quadruple cardiac by-pass operation. He took this in his stride and has done fine ever since.

In 1985 while visiting Napier with my wife Pa to meet some Cook islanders and have a look at the town and the place where she went to school at Hukarere College, members of the local gun club invited me for some practice. Detective Sergeant Bobby Matapo, who was acting as my Aide, accompanied me. Bobby, having never shot a handgun before, shot up the hill above and behind the parapets. This resolved him to go for his handgun marksmanship certificate when he attended the Police Academy near Wellington for a course and obtained his certificate with flying colours. His challenge to out-shoot me is still outstanding.

My innocent involvement in one of my hobbies gave Albert the chance of a lifetime to make accusations which many people believed, including some in authority in New Zealand.

* * *

The Democratic Party, with its loss of support in the exodus to New Zealand, should have been set back in the 1974 elections, but instead we gained a seat and broke Albert's two thirds majority. We felt that we had gained more support since then and our spirits were high. A win at the '78 polls looked like a pretty good bet if we could keep our act together. The "united we stand" attitude was very evident. Everybody put their best foot forward and we seemed to be doing everything right. When campaign time came around, we were ready for it and our timing for the start and build up of campaigning seemed to on target.

* * *

We again resorted to flying in voters from New Zealand with the strong stipulation that the flights were open to all voters regardless of their political affiliation and that they would have to pay their own fares. Our flights were organised almost immediately after the election announcement. To make these flights effective, I and two others did a whirlwind tour of New Zealand from Auckland in the North Island to the Bluff at the bottom of the South Island, meeting our people and informing them of how they could take advantage of their voting rights. To facilitate this, we explained, we were again arranging charter flights and setting up registrations at strategic sites. Our committees worked hard to enrol as many qualified Cook Island voters as they could.[37]

While our people were doing this, Albert decided that the Cook Islands Party would also fly in voters, and that they would do it in grand style. He was planning for 800 voters we were told. We did not think there were that many qualified voters overseas, but we started to think about where he was getting the money to do this. He was having a hard time finding planes to charter, but on March 12 the newspapers reported that Sir Albert had secured six charter flights with Ansett Airlines of Australia. We were now more than ever interested in the source or sources of his funds.

A great deal of publicity in the media was centred around this question. His answers were many and varied. He quoted sources. Around $50,000 from grateful relatives of cancer patients resulting from his association with Milan Brych. He cited an amount of $190,000 from Cook Islands supporters in New Zealand and back home. He arrived in New Zealand and displayed a brief case full of money. All of these to give credence to his claim that he himself was raising the money to pay for the charters.

Sir Albert needed about $300,000. Nobody believed that the Cook Islands Party had a fraction of this amount of money or could raise it within the Cook Islands. Who would lend Albert or the Cook islands' Party this amount of money without something in return of at least equal value? People were raising all kinds of sinister speculations. Some thought Sir Albert acquired the money by agreeing to sell or lease the island of Manuae. Some thought the Russians were putting up the ante. There was a plethora of other rumours and speculations, many of which did not make much sense. Even without all this speculation of money for flying voters, the campaign was the most expensive ever.[2]

It became obvious that Albert was offering free flights for his voters and was making sure that no Democratic Party supporters would get on the plane. We were able to confirm this by trying to obtain bookings for our supporters on these flights. They were firmly rejected. They were free flights, but only for Cook Islands Party voters. This, together with giving a feast when they arrived at the Rarotonga Airport, was tantamount to giving an elector "valuable consideration" to induce him to vote for the Cook Islands Party candidates. This was bribery under Section 69 of the Cook Islands Electoral Act 1966. On this basis we obtained an injunction that the flying votes would be counted separately and kept separate from all other votes.

* * *

When the polling booths closed, there was an air of hushed expectancy. There was quiet hoping. There were whispered assertions of confidence. There were no gatherings. Everybody seemed to have gone home to wait for the results to come over the air. It was a long wait. It seemed longer than usual. Waiting at headquarters, I could not see or recognise any clues which might have given me the feeling, but I could feel the tension mounting. It was tangible. Still we waited.

Still nothing happened. The tension was still mounting. If it increased further, it seemed something would have to give, but still we waited. Nothing gave. Occasionally the silence would be quietly disturbed by a whisper, a sigh or a quick intake of breath. Even the crickets in the dark outside were silent.

After what seemed ages, the first runner noisily clumped up the steps and our tensions audibly gave way. The first results he brought showed a clear swing to the Democratic Party. We were jubilant, but we remembered that the flying voters results had not yet been included. We also remembered that in 1974 we had an early lead, but the later results had overcome this lead. We also knew that the Cook Islands Party were staking their hopes on the flying votes of which they had so many more than the Democratic Party. The Democratic Party count still kept coming in ahead of the CIP and it was appearing to widen. Then late in the evening the flying votes came in and swamped us out and the Cook Islands Party again won with 15 seats to the Democrats 7. It was a severe blow. The Unity Party which appeared for the first time in January 1978, and the independents, got very few votes and no seats.

We did not give up. Because we had runners and were keeping better count, we were somewhat better informed than most listening into the radio and it appeared that we would have won if it were not for the CIP flying voters. Although we had never heard of it being done before, our injunction to separate out the CIP flying votes had been acceded to. If we could have these pulled out of the overall votes, constituency by constituency, it was on the cards that we could win. The usual way petitions worked was that, if a petition was successful, the winning candidate lost his seat and there was a re-election for the constituency in which he stood. A cursory look indicated that, if this practice was adhered to, re-elections could take place in as many as 16 electorates.

* * *

The final arrangements for the Cook Islands Party charter flights were for four flights on 25 March and two on 28 March. Each flight was able to carry 136 people and the Cook Islands Party expected 800 electors to travel to the polls. However, the organisers were able to muster only 445 voters for the three key electorates of Rarotonga. Nearly 300 persons not eligible to vote travelled on the free flights for the heck of it and to fill up the available free seats. In contrast the Democratic Party voters were required to pay for their own fares and had chartered two planes each with a capacity of 110 seats. Some Democratic Party voters had used scheduled commercial flights to do their voting.

A clearer analysis of the results at the polls showed that, without the 445 flying voters, the Democratic Party would have defeated the Cook Islands Party. On Rarotonga the Democratic Party would have won at least seven and possibly all nine seats as opposed to the total of only seven seats in the twenty two seat legislature.

Based on this analysis, the Democratic Party challenged the legality of the free flying voters in accordance with the Electoral Act of 1966 which required that this be done within 14 days of the declaration of the results.[53] The

Democratic Party Legal Advisory Committee, which eventually consisted of all the lawyers in the Cook Islands, participated in the filing of the petition and other subsequent legal activities. The disappointment of the Democratic Party in losing an election had shattered everybody, but their subsequent actions showed that they were still full of fight and had no morale problems. After all, they had been through this many times before. Nevertheless, I felt strongly they needed some reassurance that something was being done about what they saw as a clear case of strong illegal inducement for voters to support the CIP cause to win the elections.

Immediately after the elections everything was pretty dead. People talked furtively in little clusters here and there. Jokes fell flat. No guitars were playing. No song fractured the air. Even the CIP contingents were not their usual selves after a general election. No trucks were driving around the island singing campaign songs or shouting ribald remarks when they thought they were near supporters of the Democratic Party. What there was, was very much subdued and insecurely offered. Quite unusual, there was no drinking in overt evidence.

It seemed that many Cook Islands Party supporters were not proud of what had taken place. Their subdued and hushed reaction to their win perhaps reflected a possible feeling that they had won a hollow victory. However, when it became evident that the results favoured the Cook Islands Party, Sir Albert Henry made a speech over the radio in which he said, "I am quite sure it is because of His guidance and His decision that I again take the helm of your canoe." The leader of the Unity Party was invited to speak, but I was not. It was not till the next day that I was given an opportunity to say something.

Next morning the radio was full of Sir Albert's victory speech and his singing of the CIP victory song. He sounded drunk and tired. He granted a national holiday for the day. The shops opened as usual, but not many people went out and in town, where it is the custom to greet everybody with a hi and a smile. It was reported that there were a significant number who averted their eyes from those they did not want to greet, meet or speak to.[3]

The radio was filled for days with the reading of telegrams and letters of congratulations from Cook Islands Party supporters in the outer islands, New Zealand and from beneficiaries of the Party's power. There were also the standard ones from neighbouring governments. These were conspicuous by the delay of those that came and those that never came. There were bitter personal arguments. Family feuds were renewed and aired. Many punchings took place, but there were no serious confrontations.

The Cook Islands Party celebrated in one way or another for many days. There were dances. There were round the island convoys. Beach picnics were held. Feasts and gatherings were organised to bolster everyone into a feeling of a well deserved victory.

* * *

The first obvious adverse reaction to the results of the election was a lone placard reading, I LOVE DEMO, carried the next morning by Makiuti Tongia, one of my ardent supporters and committee members. Later in the morning he was joined by Michael Tavioni, a defeated Unity Movement candidate. Together they prepared a big placard with the words BUT FOR THE $300,000: DEMO 12, CIP MAKAIORE 10, (makaiore is the term for fruit that has withered and dropped from the tree). They mounted the placard on a frame on the back of a truck and drove up and down the main street for most of the day. This incited others. At a meeting at my home, it was decided that a round the island convoy of our own was in order. We dispersed and everybody took off to make the necessary arrangements.

We made two brief announcements over the radio for Democratic Party supporters to meet on the main road at the Social Centre next morning, but campaign organisers visited known supporters to enlist their support and prepare for the next day. Members of the Unity Movement also took part. Next day, a Saturday, a huge assembly of trucks, cars and motor-cycles formed themselves into the three districts of Rarotonga. The difficulty of communicating with the long procession was overcome by the use of walkie-talkies. Many of the demonstrators brought placards with them. Others were made on the spot. Even tee shirts were printed on the spot. A count someone made of the number of vehicles came to 381. A count made by someone of the number of persons in the cavalcade was 1,820, but many more vehicles and people joined the cavalcade as it went round the island. This was remarkable on an island of only about 4,000 adults.

* * *

The Democratic Party filed several petitions in the High Court, one for each constituency on Rarotonga. Another twelve petitions were filed on the final day allowed by law; three for each of the three constituencies in Rarotonga and three for the constituency of the Island of Mitiaro. The legal team then decided to file three extra petitions for these four constituencies. Each petition sought one of three alternatives available under the Electoral Act, namely that the successful CIP candidate was not duly elected or that the election was void or that the unsuccessful Democratic Party candidate was duly elected. All the Rarotonga Petitions contained the same allegations as to breaches of the electoral laws. All the successful Cook Islands Party candidates were named as respondents in each petition as well as the Chief Electoral Officer and the Returning Officers.

The Democratic Party and its legal advisors were faced with three important decisions: should a Senior Counsel be retained to handle the petitioner's case, could a suitable one be obtained in the short time available and could the Democratic Party raise the funds to pay for all legal expenses and fees. We had just emerged from a gruelling general election into which we had put our all and had no funds left. Raising more funds would not be easy and time was at a premium.

Eventually it was decided to approach Mr Paul Temm QC of Auckland to ask him to consider handling the petitioners cases and to give an estimate of the cost. At the same time the Democratic Party members were to raise what funds they could. We were all delighted when Mr Temm accepted and put his reputation and presence behind our cause. This greatly buoyed the bowed but unbroken spirit of the Democratic Party. There was now quiet hope. The Cook Islands Party employed Mr Lloyd Brown QC as their counsel to counter the petitioners' charges.

The petition relating to the constituency of Mitiaro, a small island 130 miles to the north-east of Rarotonga, concerned supplies sent to the island as a result of cyclone "Charlie" which had struck Mitiaro and other islands on 25 and 26 February. The supplies were sent as "hurricane relief." At the CIP campaign meetings over the radio in Rarotonga it was announced that the supplies would be sent by the Cook Islands Party to help the Mitiaro people. The supplies were sent to the CIP candidate and marked with his name and authorised by the Minister of Finance, Geoffrey Henry, and acquiesced to by the Premier. The usual method for sending such supplies was to address them to the Island Council to supervise their distribution. In this case the supplies were distributed by CIP officials. The Treasurer of the Cook Islands Government, on discovering this, advised the Minister of Finance, Mr Geoffrey Henry, to announce publicly that the supplies were government relief supplies. No announcement was made. The petitioners sought a finding that the successful CIP candidate was not duly elected and that a by-election for the Mitiaro seat be ordered.

The Rarotonga petitions covered a much broader area of misconduct which included bribery, treating and general corruption. 61 witnesses, 45 newspapers, 31 tape recordings, 5 television videotapes and many clippings, documents, telex messages and letters were produced as court exhibits. The hearings which spanned more than two months were heard in Auckland, Wellington and Rarotonga. These involved the provision by the CIP of free flights only for CIP supporters in New Zealand who were qualified to vote. Special efforts had been made by the CIP to ensure that only CIP supporters used these flights.

* * *

In Rarotonga, because of the small size of the official courtroom, the hearings were held in a building called the Nikao Social Centre, presided over by Chief Justice Gaven Donne, now Sir Gaven KBE. The Centre was situated on the beach and its numerous louvred windows gave good ventilation and a beautiful view of the foaming surf on the reef with the deep blue of the Pacific Ocean beyond and the multi-azured hues of the lagoon in the foreground where the gentle remnants of the crashing surf of the outer reef rode in and disintegrated with a hiss on the white sandy beach almost under our noses. When I attended the hearings, I paid more attention to the ever changing view through these windows than I did to the proceedings. I could not help wishing and imagining that I was out beyond the reef idly paddling in a canoe with an equally idle rod and line trailing behind, away from all this blossoming evidence of ambition and avarice for power and the corruption to make it someone's reality. I wondered whether, if my turn ever came, I would be as unwisely human.

In this centre the final act of an attempt to overturn the Government of the Cook Islands was being played out. The hearing of petitions alleging bribery and corruption was being vented through a justice system inherited from that nurtured, sculpted and continually honed over the ages far away in England. It was an alternative to what might otherwise have exploded into a scene unbecoming the serenity of this Pacific paradise.

* * *

In his opening submission, Mr Temm emphasised that the petitions were not from disgruntled candidates to upset a lawful election on legal technicalities. They were from hundreds of citizens whose votes, and those of many others like them, were nullified by a deliberate scheme to thwart their legal right to select a government of their own free choice. His presentation could not be heard without a deep sense of outrage.

He emphasised the major principles upon which the petitioners relied, among which were the casting of votes without undue pressure or intimidation or hope of reward or sense of personal obligation and free from any taint of corruption. Elsewhere, he said, the courts have acted so firmly and so strongly down the years that most politicians in sophisticated societies have given up attempts to influence voters unlawfully. If detected, all their efforts gain them nothing.

He stated that the petitioners understood that what they asked the court was one of the most remarkable applications ever to have been laid before a court in the Commonwealth. They knew of no case where a court has been asked to put a Government out of office.

* * *

In addition there was the matter of where the money to pay for the free flights came from. Was it from funds legitimately raised by the party or did it come from the public purse? Every indication from reliable sources indicated that the money came from one of the sources of public revenue, the Philatelic Bureau. Whether by design or naivete, one of the four Ministers who were signatories of one of the cheques on its way to pay for the flights, publicly over the air expressed his pleasure at having signed the largest cheque of his life.

This first cheque went to a Company called the Cook Islands Govt. New Projects Co. Ltd. It was for $337,000.00 and signed by the Manager of the Philatelic Bureau. The necessary travel to conclude these transactions was also paid by the Philatelic Bureau. The travels took the conspirators to Hawaii, New Zealand and Australia. Through the tenacity of the two lawyers, Vincent Ingram and Iaveta Short, who were themselves Democratic Party candidates in this election, aided by no more than good luck, we were able to intercept the cheque at one of the Auckland banks on its way through the laundering process. This was the clincher and from then on it was plain sailing to show that public money was used to pay for the flights. The American member of the conspiratorial team, the agent for the Philatelic Bureau, was considered to have broken the American Lockheed law which limited the financial involvement of Americans in foreign political engagements.

* * *

On 24 July 1978, Chief Justice Donne handed down his momentous decision. In the 40 page judgement dealing with the Mitiaro case he found "the dominant motive to have been the achievement of political popularity and not charity," and quoted another relevant judgement which said, "...it is really not charity, but party feeling following in the steps of charity, wearing the dress of charity and mimicking her gait."

In the Rarotonga cases, the Chief Justice disallowed the votes cast by passengers on the CIP charter flights as being tainted by bribery and corruption. That left all 8 CIP candidates without a majority and he declared elected in their stead, the 8 Democratic Party candidates. This gave the Democratic Party a total of 15 seats and the Cook Islands Party 7, with the Mitiaro seat to be recontested. This eventually went to the Democratic Party giving it 16 seats out of 22.

It was the first time in the history of the Commonwealth that a court ruling has changed a government.

* * *

Various judgements were passed down on the conspirators, who were convicted. Some received suspended sentences including the American who was judged under his own law and repaid the $337,000 dollars to the government.

* * *

In his judgement, The Chief Justice made some notable comments. In response to Mr Brown's claim that Sir Albert's motives were at all times proper, he said, "The matter of substance was whether what Sir Albert was doing was illegal. He was advised it was, but decided, as he put it, to take the risk..."

"...I find that there was unlawful conduct of monumental dimensions and there is ample evidence of a corrupt or criminal intention. The use of public monies was a means to an end, an illegal means, an illegal end...."

"...the enormity of the wilful wrongdoing is so striking....If I were to order new elections, there can be little doubt that many of the voters who paid their own way on the Air Nauru flights arranged by the Democratic Party would be unable to afford a further trip. In a new by-election they would be disenfranchised....in my judgement it is better that there be an unequivocal denunciation of misdeeds of the offending candidates and their agents than that by-elections be ordered which may allow transgressors indirectly to profit from their misconduct which...was of vast dimensions..."

* * *

That day, 24 July, I was requested to be on hand and was escorted by the police who remained with me at the Social Centre until I was needed. At last I was informed that the judgement had been handed down and I was required to form a government and was I ready to do so. I replied that I was. I was taken to room 208 of the Rarotongan Hotel where I was ushered into the presence of the Chief Justice who now was to play his role of Queen's Representative. He, in his turn asked me if I was ready to form a government. I named my cabinet of six besides myself and eventually we were all sworn under oath as Premier and

Ministers of the Crown. It was later that the title of Premier was changed to Prime Minister.

* * *

As a consequence of these events, a number of press articles tried to capture the meaning of them to the Cook Islands. It was touted as one of the most important events in the history of the Cook Islands. "It may be seen in the future as a milestone, the political 'coming of age' of the Cook Islands. Other nations with a Westminster type of government took decades or even centuries and countless election court cases to convince the populace and politicians that it does not pay to tamper with the polls. It has taken the Cook Islands a relatively short time, 13 years, to be confronted with this reality. The 300 to 400 people who packed the Court room during the hearing in Rarotonga were surely the basis of the famous 'coconut wireless', thus ensuring that a wider population - even the total populace - would be aware of what took place, though not necessarily the accuracy of what happened." (*New Zealand Herald*)

I am not sure that these predictions can be upheld in their entirety. Albert spent most of his life in New Zealand and was intimately involved in its politics and the rights and wrongs before, during and after general elections in New Zealand. What had he learnt from them that he would perpetrate these wrongdoings in his country of birth? I have noticed since then that it is the well educated who have been brought up overseas or born overseas with ample opportunity to be part of the Westminster system there, who are most likely to do wrong and create instability in the political scene here. They are also the ones most able and willing to interpret the power put in their hands as a mandate to subvert public property and finances to the benefit of themselves and their friends.

We are left with the inference that the difference in the behaviour of these same people under one set of political circumstances and not the other is the sophistication of the population in one and its naivete in the other. It seems to have little to do with the inherent sophistication or naivete of the politician. As Albert said himself, "I knew it was wrong, but I took the risk."

The hope is that the population is able to discriminate the right and wrong that a politician does and be prepared to act correctly on that knowledge. That is what is going to take the time. It would be nice if it happened in both the population and the politicians at the same time. The political events of 1978 may have pushed us further along the path of the kind of sophistication that will prevent bribery and corruption. However, the enormity of the transgressions were such that it is unlikely to be repeated. This should not lead Cook Islanders to believe that the occurrence of seemingly lesser political transgressions is a measure of the desired development of our sophistication in these matters.

CHAPTER EIGHTEEN

Economic Problems

A man is not poor because he possesses nothing but because he is out of work... The artisan who has given his children his skill for their inheritance has left them a fortune which is multiplied in proportion to their number. The case is not the same with him who has ten acres of land to live on and divides them among his children. BARON DE MONTESQUIEU

The steps to reach the stage where it was possible to do something positive had been tedious. At last the time came to put theory into practice. I believed that nothing social or political could be achieved without a healthy economy, which ours was not, with low productivity, ineffective incentives, massive dependence and apathy. Economic reform was the over-riding need of the Cook Islands.

Although not intended to be so, what took place could be regarded as a horizontal experiment in the economics of a small Pacific Islands state. It was a scattered community of under 20,000 people, used to a controlled economic system and isolated from the mainstream of the world.

* * *

My observations and skimpy readings had given me the impression that political theorists and historians tended to view political and economic theory as one, while economists viewed politics as a minor aberration on economic theory. Nevertheless, economists and philosophers might make better politicians than lawyers, not to mention doctors. In any event my instincts over the years concentrated on economic problems, their causes and consequences. The gnawing question was what economic model or theory best suited our circumstances.

Everybody said we were too small and lacking in resources to be an economic or political unit. This was a major problem and ordinary means were not going to be enough. To date they had not.

I had a broad idea of what was not needed. I also believed that whatever was needed to be done would be opposed. The concepts I had been unconsciously developing over the years had not been tried in their totality anywhere that I knew of. Implementing them in the United States, the accepted home of free market ideas, would have been difficult. The hurdles were greater, as was shown later, when President Reagan tried something similar. This does not mean that they would be easier to implement in the Cook Islands which had never seen anything but a state controlled economic system. However, the need for economic, social and political development was greater.

The specific way to deal with it still escaped me. This preyed less and less on my mind as I came to realise that in fencing, boxing, rugby, war or most other contests, one may have broad strategies and the learned skills, but it is in the arena that the specific method of attack, defence, retreat, counter and riposte is developed second by second as the foe reveals himself.

Many political theorists of the past had dealt with liberty and human rights in a general sense. Though startling at the time, they became commonplace in most western societies. For exercising that kind of freedom and rights, Tom Paine was persecuted out of England to France which also found him too hot to handle. He ended his days in America where he was not fully welcomed either. Economic freedom has not been achieved to the extent that any one of us can go into business without excessive licenses, regulations, lawyers to fill out the many paged, complicated application forms and a Board to tell us what we can or cannot with our own capital. That kind of human right was missing in the Cook Islands economic scene. It was missing in most other places too.

Being in business was not a practical option for most Cook Islanders. The existing economic prescription offered limited employment and about half the work force had no realistic opportunity to find or make work.

Two things became clear. A socialistic control type of economy, as was being practised, removed individual incentives and lowered productivity. I became certain that, if we were to develop a viable economy, this was not what our Third World underdeveloped country needed. Secondly, we also did not need a capitalistic enclave which favoured a few elite persons and kept others out, as was practised. What we had was a mixture of a constrained market system for most and a free market system for some. The beneficiaries of the system thought they had the best of all worlds. That this view could lead to economic mediocrity, if not to stagnation, was not believed.

Those who believe in a controlled economy do not realise the devastating effect it has on the ordinary person who is contemplating an economic venture, or might contemplate it in a better economic climate.

If the same view is applied to any of the human rights we now accept as a matter of course, the furore would be great. Yet as compared to these, the right to earn a living and attain a decent standard of living must be at least as important.

The barrage of deterrents that face a novice contemplating a career in business makes escape to the haven of doing nothing a welcome option. This leaves the field of commerce to the hardy, the ruthless, the egotist, the greedy and those well trained to assert themselves. One might say that this is well and good because those with the "right stuff" are going to make it. That would be fine if the market place and the economic well-being of a society depended only on the results of a contest. But that is not what is required. It should be a place where everybody who can make an economic contribution and raise the economic level of himself and his community, is given the opportunity to do so. No nation can claim to be rich if a significant proportion of its people are out of work.

* * *

There were numerous constraints and barriers to developing a viable let alone a workable economy. The people did not envision development as requiring improvements in roading, transport systems, energy, water, communications and amenities. Neither could they see that removal of constraints to individual economic activity was also important. Development was conceived of as higher incomes being derived within the existing facilities and constraints. Later, attempts to improve the infrastructure and overcome the obstacles were met with opposition, both in parliament and in the streets as a misuse of funds.

To this day much of this development remains uncompleted, such as the foreshore rehabilitation, sea walls, the second water reservoir, power, roads and others. Money gained for some of these purposes was considered by enough people as best used by distribution to the population in one form or another. "Kia kai tatou i te meitaki", "Let us eat the benefit," was a frequent saying. With the economic development that took place, the roads became inadequate for the proliferation of vehicles, the supply and reticulation of power was stretched to the limit. Tourist facilities and many private homes are providing their own power and water supply systems simply because we refused to accept a water storage reservoir system and an upgrading of electric power. As of the time of writing, the completed reservoir and the one nearing completion has been virtually destroyed by the present government.

In the outer islands, road development was seen by most, including aid donors, as useful in the development of agriculture. It was the major source of outer islanders' income. But, because shipping was poor or not the right mode of transport for the perishables they produced, these roads virtually ran from nowhere to nowhere.

The geographical distances between islands, each of which had somewhat differing economic problems, was exacerbated by difficulties of transport which we were not able to improve substantially and which became worse and currently leaves much to be desired.

The overall physical and population characteristics led experts to pronounce many times over that we had no economic future. We were, they said, always going to need outside grants. It was also the time of the rage for economies of scale. It was complained that our 15 islands are too small and scattered to form a cohesive economic whole. Their combined area of 94 square miles had no known mineral resources. Yet economic viability of the outer islands had been demonstrated in an earlier era.

After the 1929 economic crisis reached us in 1932, the fairly significant economy nurtured by a hard working private sector deteriorated into a controlled economy where government took responsibility for exports with inadequate shipping to make it worthwhile. In earlier years we had experienced the economic benefits of a free market system and many of my age group had been educated in New Zealand with the help of its benefits.

The experts said that because the total Cook Islands population was the size of a small agricultural town like Morrinsville in New Zealand, our thinking should be geared to that level. To us we were a nation with nationhood forced on us at the beginning of the era when it was fashionable for colonial powers to do so. We did not have the benefits Morrinsville had in good communications and short distances to markets.

Whereas getting our products to the market involved great distances, small quantities and many institutional obstacles, most services provided to Morrinsville people are provided from the national capitol in Wellington. A borough council was not going to meet our requirements, economic, social or otherwise.

We were prepared to overcome these difficulties as well as run a parliament and all the services deemed necessary for an independent country, but the dying economy[33] after independence seemed to be proving that all unfavourable evaluations and predictions were correct. If this has always been patently obvious, why offer us political independence with no possibility of economic independence? This was true for other small islands states, such as Tuvalu, Kiribati and others.

The obsession that advisors had with economies of scale and lack of natural resources put us, for them, in a category in which nothing could be done. That small operations could make a contribution to the economy, even where agriculture was concerned, received little consideration.

In the obsession for operations of scale, attempts were made to contrive them. Since it was considered that any orange plot less than 20 acres did not meet the requirements of scale, our existing small plots were put together to make up a unit of scale more like those of Australia, New Zealand and elsewhere. These looked good until the accounting of the first fruits was done.

After the costs of labour and the purchase, fuelling and maintenance of tractors, other equipment and fertiliser were deducted, what was left may have been a livable return for a one owner unit, but for twenty or so owners it was not. All the return was absorbed into overheads. On the other hand, a family can work an orange plot of one or two acres with simple equipment and make a go of it with time left over to earn other income.

Transport was always a problem and the overseas market sought citrus from other sources which could supply vast quantities at lower prices. This wiped our citrus and pineapple industries out during my administration.

* * *

Agriculture is an important part of the economy of most countries, but there are problems if it becomes the main economic base. The problem is not apparent as long as there is plenty of land for everybody to do this profitably and there is a market outside of the society to purchase the excess that will be produced.

There is no market within the society because all are farmers. All are doing about the same thing. If there is no outside market, agriculture becomes an uneconomic measure except for subsistence living. Education of the population will be of little value because wielding a hoe needs only a little of it. Under such circumstances a community will weaken and stagnate, regardless of its size. China illustrates the problem.

If the obsession persists, even in the circumstance that there is an outside market and all produce of the land is sold, the future of the society is assured only for two or three generations by which time the land cannot be profitably divided amongst all children. Montesquieu warned us of this, "The case is not the same with him who has ten acres of land to live on and divides them among his children."

This simple truth was a major cause of the dark ages, its problems, the lord/serf relationship, territorial wars, roving bands of plundering knights, ignorance and injustices to mention only some. It was also the cause of similar problems in Polynesian society. Sooner or later land cannot be further divided and all except the first born can profitably inherit. The others of the family are left with no prospects except a menial status, emigration, colonisation, banditry, serfdom and warriorship to fight the territorial wars resulting from the system. War under such circumstances becomes an alternative economic measure. The persistence of the agricultural dependent society prolonged the centuries of intransigence of the dark ages. It caused the wars of Europe, China, Japan and Polynesia to mention but a few.

An agriculturally dominated society can only survive without such problems if there is but one child per family, or if there is a perpetual availability of abundant new land. Paradoxically the impetus of an agriculturally based society is to increase its family size, not to reduce it. It needs workers and having children is the simplest way to solve that problem. But when it comes to dividing the land among them, the beginnings of strife is born. The inevitable end is a burgeoning population, a poverty stricken society ruled by an elite who have taken over the land, the wealth and the pursuit of offensive and defensive territorial wars.

Europe broke the chain of events by the Industrial Revolution. Polynesia, in the absence of any other means than migration, tried to solve it by controlling the number of children using infanticide of female infants as the means. That is why Captain Cook was out in his estimate of the population of Tahiti. He was right in his estimate of the number of warriors in the naval fleet of King Pomare, but he was wrong in ascribing six other persons to each of them. Most of the warriors in that fleet had no wives and few female children if they had wives.

Infanticide was a partial solution, but it was not carried out without some sensibilities. If, during the process of removal of the child, its cry was heard by its mother, the child was saved.[32] China is attempting the one child per family solution by means of birth control sanctions, monetary reward and punishment. In the past it also practised infanticide.

At the time I returned, we still had an agriculturally based economy, but poor transportation was inadequate to make it effective. We had a people who were highly educable and deserved all the opportunities that a good education could provide. Unless something was done, the only market to exercise the benefits of education was New Zealand, Australia and elsewhere. At considerable cost to ourselves we were educating our people for the economic benefit of other economies. Obviously our solution was to develop a place for our educated right here at home by expanding existing economic possibilities and opening up new ones.

For years eighty percent of our economic effort was in agriculture. When it was dwindling for the right reasons our leaders decried it as a backward step. For some time I had developed the notion that the right percentage of a work force in agriculture is ten percent or less. This is the proportion I thought would be provided with a good living off the land and which would meet our local and foreign market needs.

I always worked towards that figure for agriculture while finding other ways and means to profitably employ the remaining ninety percent of the work force. Activity in the division of land can be gauged by the number of land court hearings, and there are little pieces of land with as many as 300 owners. Absentee owners who refuse to allow others to work their inherited holdings and that perennial nigger in the woodpile, transportation, added to the confusion. Thus it was that only one tenth of the arable land was in profitable cultivation. In the eighties we were able to improve this to about thirty percent. Land by law is inalienable except by leases of up to sixty years. If it were not so, it is likely that the majority of the indigenous population would be landless. But there are still other ways we could make the system more productive and less conducive to dispute.

* * *

For large industrial economies, the availability of land, labour and capital in quantities usually in excess of the minimum needed are considered prerequisites. We, as a small Island state, are not blessed with much of any of these. We must try to create an economy which does not require them in quantity. We must also borrow or invent ways that can earn us a living that do not require large quantities of land, labour and capital. Our economic advisers have trouble seeing this viewpoint and see us as a lost economic cause. I was not willing to accept that evaluation at face value.

* * *

We were given a great deal of advice about what kind of economics would suit us, but it was all more of the same. The existing systems were considered right and all we needed was the right person to run them. The history of failures and farces showed that either the systems were no good or the people with the magic to make them work did not exist. What I thought we needed were systems that worked without finding people with qualities, which did not seem to exist, to operate them.

Economists from Victoria University in Wellington suggested that, if we returned to our traditional ways, the migrants who had left would be attracted back, solving much of the migrant and economic problem. They did not understand that emigration was due to our people wishing to escape their sterile and unrewarding traditional circumstances. Only a more fulfilling life at home could reverse this. Even the dismal, gloomy Malthusian and Ricardian models, born in the worst period of the industrial revolution, were mooted as having possible application.

Economic, social and political development were treated as unrelated entities. In this we were not unique. I believe that they formed an interdependent triad with relevant and appropriate social development following the natural course of events as an economy develops. In developed countries whose economic development is already in place, leaders may see it the other way around, but that is not yet the case in the Cook islands.

Programmes in business promotion, organised by the United Nations and other international and national organisations for developing countries, produced few trainees or recipients who became entrepreneurs worthy of notice. On return from their courses, most end up in a government department telling other people how to do business or, worse still, in an economic regulatory body whose primary aim is informing hopefuls why they cannot be granted a business license. This discouraging decision is usually assisted by the advice of those already in the business sector the applicant wants to enter.

If a person has gained entrepreneurial knowledge and acumen, he is faced with a barrier of antagonists who don't want him competing in an area they have reserved for themselves. They are assisted in maintaining the status quo by civil servants who pride themselves on passing judgement on an applicant's financial and other qualifications to venture his own money. If the applicant has to borrow to achieve his aims, the advice of the "wise" has preceded him. I do not believe this is an exaggerated picture of what Cook Islanders faced (and may face again). The legislative and administrative structure under the guise of economic development codes illustrates the picture I have painted.

* * *

All goods from New Zealand were import tax free, so almost all imported goods were from there. Goods imported from New Zealand but originating from other countries had New Zealand's own import duties imposed on them before exporting them to the Cook Islands. Such duties were recoverable, at a cost, under the drawback system on anything exported, but not everybody knew that and many of those who knew did not bother owing to the cumbersome procedures.

We are an import intensive country and virtually no attempt had been made to promote import substitution (producing our own products instead of importing them). Locals, in obedience to previous colonial influence, thought it was good for the economy to import from New Zealand. They never questioned whose economy, and my attempts to overcome these detractions from our own economy, were met with attacks that I was undermining it.

Our agricultural products assisted New Zealand in its shortages during the winter months, but we needed to give more priority to our own economic advantage. We can just as readily grow produce at any time of the year for other markets. Some products marketed to New Zealand ended up in Samoa or Tahiti, having been redirected there by the New Zealand companies importing our products. Profits from manufacturing of clothing and other goods for export from Rarotonga were taxed locally at full commercial rates and some premises had closed because of this.

As an import intensive country we imported the inflation rate of New Zealand, our prime source of imports. Other countries had been import taxed out of competition by the former New Zealand Administration. So our attempts to control our inflation rate had little effect. Even after thirteen years of independence, we had done little to change the colonial tariff structure. At this time the inflation rate of New Zealand was a high flying yoyo and we needed relief from it.

* * *

I spent time examining the structure of the main sources of revenue. There was a graduated personal income tax which started at 5 percent at the low income level and ended at 45 percent at the high level of $12,000 with a formula to extract more from incomes higher than this. The company tax on net profits was at two levels: 35 percent for local and 42 percent for foreign businesses. All categories of businesses were taxed equally. Import duties were complex and made little sense. The highest was 80 percent for all goods imported from foreign countries. Goods from countries of the British Commonwealth were taxed, some at 52 and others at 55 percent.

Despite company taxes of 35 and 42 percent on net profits, only 7 percent of government tax revenue came from the business sector. So many real or fictitious expenses could be claimed for exemptions that the miserable amount of taxes collected might be all that could be obtained from the private sector. The market place, where most of the money is eventually spent, should be the source of more than the mere seven percent it was providing. The problem did not lie with the percentage of tax on net profits. It was high enough and raising it would be unreasonable as well as counter-productive.

Import duties and levies contributed 63 percent and personal taxes contributed 30 percent. There was no structure for policing the collection of company taxes and it seemed that it would be uneconomic to do so. Employing a tax examination force to check tax evasions and continually pursue the private sector, would not pay for itself and would be difficult in a small economy where auditing skills were scarce, networks of personal obligations were wide and sympathy generous.

Agriculture and manufacturing, the only wealth creating industries we had, were tottering along. The clothing factories were having a continuously hard time. Agriculture was the best (or worst!) example we had of the deleterious effect of government interference in the operations of an industry. In its wisdom of controlled direction, we had a government-run Marketing Board initiated in 1936. Nobody could export primary produce except through its kind attentions. Produce trickled sluggishly through its sclerotic passages, narrowed further by inadequate transportation space and other impediments to export. Its mismanagement resulted in a write off of nearly $300,000 in 1979.

The most active segment of the private sector was import retailing. It was also costly to the economy. Every dollar paid for an import was lost to us. Certainly the net profit it made for the merchant and his workers was spent in significant part within the economy, but it was not an earned part of the economy. There was little adding to it from the outside to increase the internal pool, let alone maintain it. Only the limited earnings from agricultural and clothing exports, our limited tourism plus New Zealand aid were offsetting the cost of imports. The negative trade balance was about ten to one. This factor alone was dragging the economy downwards. It could not go on for too long. As I explained it to the public, a reasonable analogy is a home where nobody has a job to pay for the groceries, but the groceries still have to be paid for out of reserves, low income bearing activities and largesse from working relatives overseas who had troubles of their own.

Conversations with people in different walks of life indicated that there had been little understanding of this simple economic fact. When I spoke to retailers about the importance of being involved in the export trade to ensure that there was money to pay for the goods they were importing and would like to import, I was told that it was none of their business because government through the Marketing Board was handling that part of the economy. They also told me that there was nothing worth exporting or doing other than what was already being done.

Economic statistics to give us some idea of the state and trends of the economy, were virtually non-existent. The CIP government had made it plain that, since the reports on the economy provided by the Dutch economists, sent as aid by the Netherlands, were unfavourable, it was not interested in further probings into the economic state of the nation. It refused to publish their findings and recommendations.

* * *

The high proportion of the work force employed in the Public Service was a continuing problem which defeated us except in a small measure. The victory was small and it was hollow. At the slightest wavering of vigilance, it would bounce right up again.

Three ministers in my first seven man cabinet realised that the public service needed to be reduced. The others thought it was an area which they could use to reward their supporters and little else was foremost in their minds. In my last cabinet there were none who were prepared to reduce Public Service overstaffing. After my demise as Prime Minister in July 1987 and just before the general elections of January 1989, the members for Atiu and Mitiaro gave free rein to their wishes to influence the course of the elections by giving seemingly every able bodied person a government job. By doing this, they effectively removed them from productivity in the coffee and pineapple industries. A similar thing was done in Rakahanga, the constituency of Dr Robati who took over from me as Prime Minister. It also happened in Manihiki and Penrhyn.

At the current level of 11 percent of the population, our Public Service, including those on wages and ad hoc bodies, is large. To a degree this can be excused on the basis that what is provided for the small population is similar to that which has to be provided for a much larger population. Perhaps there is no direct relationship between population and the public service when we get down to small populations such as ours. We could double or even treble our population without increasing our Public Service much. It is one of the penalties of a small population.

To us it was a huge burden which should have been reduced to more equitable proportions, but with poor employment opportunities outside government, this was difficult to do without creating hardship. In 1978 only about 50 percent of the working population was putting in a personal income tax return. In absolute numbers this amounted to around 2600 persons of whom around 1800 were employed by government. This included wage workers and employees of ad hoc bodies. By 1980 our policy of reducing this number by attrition and replacement from within the Public Service reduced this to an unexciting number of around 1400.

The stranglehold of bureaucracy was epitomised by the large number employed by Public Works and Agriculture with most other departments running at a higher number than they should. At this stage, the Education Department had one salaried employee for every 12 students and was the primary reason for the high cost of education while its other needs were foregone to meet this staff payroll.

The Agriculture Department had a large number of field advisory officers. Most of them were planting as well as receiving their salary. Farmers said they were unhelpful in dealing with their problems. The Nursing Service, by churning out nurses from the School of Nursing, was overstaffed with nurses in addition to a substantial group of wardsmaids to assist them. There was a government health employee for every 65 persons in the population. The syndrome of overstaffing and lowered efficiency was evident.

Since I had worked hard to localise the medical service and established the Nursing School some thirty years before, I was personally abashed by the deterioration of the professional delivery of medical care as seen by the public. Fortunately my establishing a private practice surgery and its being taken over by two successive local practitioners, had alleviated the problem to a degree.

It seemed that the only way we could overcome the Public Service problem was to continue our plans for improving the economy so that employment opportunities in the private sector would increase. However, when this was achieved, we doubled the total number of people employed, but the number of public servants remained essentially unchanged. More recently with political changes of government the problem has increased.

There were areas where we could have reduced our Public Service without lowering its efficiency. We could have increased this efficiency considerably if we transferred a number of activities to the private sector (privatisation). But attempts to do this by whatever means were strongly resisted by ministers who held the particular portfolios. Since 1978, a strong private sector has developed and we could do without most, if not all, of the activities of Public Works with a considerable increase in efficiency.

The present Public Works budget of almost 4 million dollars would achieve better returns if the work they are supposed to do is tendered out to the private sector. This alone would reduce the Public Service by a significant amount and strengthen the private sector in the area of its operations.

Government ran a number of trading operations which directly competed against the private sector or prevented the private sector from becoming involved in similar operations. Nearly all of these were run at a loss with public revenue making up the deficit. Some, such as fishing and survey, were undercutting commercial operations with government salaries meeting wages and costs.

* * *

The Cook Islands have no social security or national pension plan. There is an old age pension and payments for the destitute and infirm paid out of the public fund. A superannuation plan run from New Zealand is available only for bona fide salaried public servants and nobody else. In general, employees of the private sector could look forward to an old age with no remuneration for their years of service. Despite a great deal of effort, we still do not have one.

* * *

A society is economically at its healthiest if all its people in the work force are able to be productive to their optimum capacity. Trite as this saying might be, individuals who are prevented from participating in the economy to the extent of their capacity are an economic loss. If the various capacities of individuals can be increased by education and training, the society as a whole is benefited. This is only true if we increase the opportunities for its use.

Constraints were hindering expansion of the private sector for more job opportunities. There was a need for individuals to be given equal, untrammelled rights to enter the market place to do what each perceives will be to his or her benefit. By so doing individuals will bring all their capabilities to bear on their individual economic problem. Most will solve it one way or another: some by becoming businessmen, some by providing professional services, and others by working for those who solved their problem in a manner which needs partners and workers.

The niches in such a society are numberless and there is a possibility for a place for everybody, but there will always be those who will prefer to watch it all go by. If they have been truly given equal opportunity and are not able to perform, we should provide for them in a sensible measure by sensible means.

We were not able to overcome a number of the constraints, but in spite of that, progress was achieved. To stabilise the gains into a workable national economic system and overcome the significant remaining barriers, would have taken more time. It is hoped that others will recognise and see a way to overcoming them. However, in spite of the things that could not be done, the economy went forward at a growth rate better than 10 percent per annum.

* * *

Aid was limited to New Zealand except for small projects aid for total packages of around $20,000. Other metropolitan countries which were giving aid to other Pacific countries had been convinced that, if they gave aid to the Cook Islands, they would be stepping on the sensitive toes of New Zealand. New Zealand denied this, but consistently we met with resistance to our attempts to share aid from other donor countries.

The Lome Conventions consistently denied us membership with the African countries being the most insistent in resisting our entry. In 1986 the Minister of Foreign Affairs failed to obtain membership for us in ESCAP (United Nations Economic and Social Commission for Asia and the Pacific) in which we have every entitlement.

I am still unsure as to New Zealand's attitude towards the question of our membership in international organisations. The then Prime Minister of New Zealand, Mr David Lange, made it clear that he was not pleased with our independent views towards developing economic and other relationships with other countries unless they passed through and were condoned by New Zealand's Department of Foreign Affairs. Rob Muldoon, the previous New Zealand Prime Minister, had quite the opposite view with regard to our international diplomatic and trade efforts, but I think New Zealand officials did not share this generous view.

In time we were able to surmount obstacles to a sufficient degree by developing enough credibility with other countries to pursue our own destinies with them. By the end of my time as Prime Minister we were formally members, as a sovereign state, of six United Nations international agencies and eight regional organisations. We were also accepted de facto as a sovereign by many others, such as USA, France, Japan and a number of other international agencies.

Aid from New Zealand had its ups and downs. In the mid seventies it was as high as around 40 percent of government revenue. In 1978 it had decreased to about 26 percent with a high of 30 percent in 1984 and a present low of near 16 percent. It was divided into Project and Budgetary Aid with the major part of it going towards Budgetary Aid. In my time, as soon as our revenues improved, it was all, except for about 8 percent, moved to development projects, but still passing under the guise of Budgetary Aid. It was of great assistance to us in the period of our most rapid economic development.

* * *

Although Cook Islanders of both European and indigenous extraction did not comprehend the philosophy and sometimes paradoxical concepts behind the economic policies, I never had any doubts of their ability to meet the demands they would make on them. Lazy is one thing a Cook Islander is not. Although the philosophy and theory behind policies may be a mystery, comprehending a practical problem and overcoming it in practical terms was what they did best. Over and over again in the past they had followed policies which led them nowhere and came out worse off, but smiling. Therefore, I had no doubt that when the step by step implementation was put in place they would give it an honest try. The problem was going to come from those who thought they knew better or considered it a threat. I hoped that the successes of the policy, if there were any, would bring understanding.

A difficult aspect of my new status was the loss of friends. There were many facets to it. Time to pursue the requirements of the job was the most important. Life was no longer a lackadaisical movement of the day from one relatively unimportant hour to the next with frequent breaks to enjoy the company of friends and smell the flowers on the way. The responsibilities of government involved long hours of concentration, interruptions and trying to meet the pressing demands of both job and people. At the end of the day I was glad to get home to recuperate.

Even then there were reports to read, reports to write, personal and official mail to answer. People who would not have given me the time of day before were now demanding answers to letters they wrote. There were letters from stamp and coin collectors who must have known that a bureau existed to deal with their requests. I inherited staff who could not or would not redirect these. They were almost all brought to my personal attention.

People wanted to meet me, groups wanted to pay courtesy calls. If all could not be fitted in, there were unpleasant repercussions. It seemed everybody who had a vote had voted for me personally and wanted me to spend time with them personally and to do things for them personally. That was why, some argued, they voted for me. The time was not available and their personal demands were difficult, if not impossible, to satisfy. Those who thought their vote meant that I was now their personal servant, soon became political enemies and some publicly declared themselves as such with unfavourable embellishments.

Spending time on someone whose project was of national importance, but whose vote was thought not to have been for our party, was an unforgivable sin. The smallness of the country and the network of kinship and association was such that not only did everybody know everybody personally, but they expected personal contact and commitment. This made the job seem more demanding than might be the case in larger countries.

I tried intermediary staff to deal with these demands and to have them directed to the ministers or departments relevant to the personal problem they wanted dealt with. This was another unforgivable sin. It implied that I did not care for them.

I inherited Albert Henry's Secretary to Government. He was supposed to deal with the mail and make the simple responses to the numerous letters that kept pouring in. He was unable to put a letter together or even to classify material according to its importance and redirect it to the proper quarters for response. I now understood why in the past my letters to government were never answered. During my nine years as Prime Minister I had only one person, a Cook Islander, who could handle this job well. He was whipped away to a much more highly paid position with the South Pacific Commission in Noumea, New Caledonia. In the meantime I coped as best I could, but never could find the time that I once had to meet friends and relatives and smell the flowers along the way. It made me despondent. The loneliness of leadership made itself evident in this respect and many others.

The demands of Cabinet meetings, the wranglings over what to do and how to do it were time consuming, especially when the way to deal with most problems was obvious and should never have been brought to Cabinet. Priorities were foreign to the thinking of many. All things were important they said. The love of Polynesians for meetings and talking would have taken a great deal more time, if I had not limited it. One or two ministers in my first cabinet would rather talk about problems than deal with them. In my second and subsequent cabinets, the numbers increased. In their minds, talking about a problem was the solution to it. My first Cabinet consisted of two doctors of medicine, two lawyers, one engineer, a schoolteacher and an ex-shipping agent from a local business firm. I should have been lucky. I had the most qualified cabinet in the Pacific.

When the concepts underlying the economic policies were not understood or not considered worthy of consideration, I adapted myself to the proposition that these were facts of life I had to live with. I had had to live with similar attitudes in my other endeavours, so it was not a new experience.

My marriage to Pa Tepaeru Ariki in 1979 greatly alleviated the loneliness that goes with being at the top. Sharing some of the problems with her made them easier to bear and made others easier to solve. It would be difficult to convey the depth of her assistance to me in the tricky matters of state that plagued us. Since our marriage, Pa, as President of the House of Ariki, had problems of her own in that role as well as in her role as Paramount Chief of the district of Takitumu which encompasses over one third of the island of Rarotonga.

There were always problems of land tenure, investitures of titles, settling of clan and inter-clan problems, and advice on numerous matters which might include naming of children and where the dead should be buried. However, she handled these roles and her role as First Lady with seeming ease and aplomb.

CHAPTER NINETEEN

Economic Solutions

"It is not from the benevolence of the butcher, the brewer, or the baker, that we expect our dinner, but from their regard to their own interest. We address ourselves, not to their humanity, but to their self-love, and never talk to them of our own necessities but of their advantages. Nobody but a beggar chuses to depend chiefly upon the benevolence of his fellow citizens." ADAM SMITH

... It is enterprise which builds and improves the world's possessions ... If enterprise is afoot, wealth accumulates whatever may be happening to Thrift; and if enterprise is asleep, wealth decays whatever Thrift may be doing.
JOHN MAYNARD KEYNES
The state in organising security should not stifle incentive, opportunity, responsibility; in establishing a minimum, it should leave room and encouragement for voluntary action by each individual to provide more than that minimum for himself and his family. LORD BEVERIDGE

Although there were modifications to suit our particular circumstances, the free market system followed was that advocated by Adam Smith in *Wealth of Nations* published in 1776 when James Cook was sailing the Pacific Ocean. I have not read all of this enormous work. I am not an economist by trade, but have gleaned where I can. The distillations found in the writings of Robert L. Heilbroner[40] J. K. Galbraith[36] Milton and Rose Friedman[35] and many others have been more than useful in this respect.

Where possible, we remained true to the basic concepts of the free market system. I did not deviate from them due to arguments of other economists, except to fit it to the special circumstances of our milieu. In simple terms I followed the economic model that self-interest is the primary motivating force that drives the system which, if left to itself, will be largely self-regulating with regard to quality, price and quantity of goods and services.

In considering this approach, the boom and bust periodic episodes so characteristic of the free market system described by Keynes was kept in mind. However, in our circumstances, this was a minor consideration compared to the need to improve the economy by the best means possible.

We can perhaps view an economy by its position on a continuum with one end represented by an economy with only a small proportion of its people having the opportunity to operate gainfully within it and the other end represented by a free market system with everybody having an equal opportunity, but not necessarily an equal capacity, to operate and gain within it.

If this be true, the economic health of a country is related to the proportion of its citizens involved in entrepreneurial activity. This ensures that there is adequate competition to provide goods and services of the highest quality for the least price in the quantities demanded. If left to itself it will be largely self-regulating in both quality and number. The less efficient having fallen by the wayside.

Therefore, I believed that the economic health of a society is in proportion to the number of its members who are permitted the opportunity to exercise their creativity, their competitive spirit, their inventive nature, their artistic qualities, and their urge to better themselves. The economic, social and political well-being of a society is the net result of these urges and the degree to which they are constrained or encouraged to operate in the economic process.

The profit motive in the broad sense of deriving benefit is the motive force. It is not exclusive to the moneyed system except in the narrowest sense, which fails to recognise the urges in our nature. They drive us in any society, in any epoch, in our economic and social development to exhibit our wish to own and command the things of value, to display our status in the dominance hierarchy of our particular society.

The advantage to both the individual and to the community was the motive force of the food gathering and hunting economy. Not necessarily to the specific profit of anybody, but also to the preservation of the group and support of the differentiation of the various levels of the hierarchy.

Profit in the broad sense was the motive force of the farming community which soon developed into a highly organised hierarchy of dominance, land ownership and serfs. It is the motive force behind the economics of communism as it is in the elite system of South American countries, Haiti, the Dominican Republic, the Phillipines, and some Pacific, Asiatic and African countries. Few were not driven by the desire for advantage in material things; to be the best and to live the best. One real difference between systems lies in the opportunity for the greatest proportion of the population to generate benefits and to share them.

The economic activity of a society is in proportion to the number of its members who are permitted the opportunity to exercise their creativity, their competitive spirit, their inventive nature, their artistic qualities, their urge to better themselves. The economic, social and political well-being of a society is the net result of these urges and the degree to which they are constrained or encouraged to operate in the development process.

The fact that economic participation is available to everybody brings about a natural grading of capabilities to perform in it. We may be born with equal opportunity, but we are not born with equal capacity to respond to it. It is through this mechanism of equal opportunity, but different capacities to respond, that each of us can find a comfortable niche in the system. The arenas in which individuals may perform are as varied as there are inventive ways to exercise personal and collective abilities. Some may not wish to perform at all, but that choice should be for them as much as is the choice to perform is for others. It is when this freedom of choice is thwarted that the drives of our human nature become troubled and distorted into behavioural patterns that are not socially or morally acceptable as the available economic niches become limited.

When the economic system is a controlled one in which the government takes a strong hand in what people within it should and should not do, most people and especially our peoples of the Pacific will sit by and wait to be told what to do. There is a level of dominance suppression of these behavioural charac-teristics beyond which nothing is worth doing and apathy is the chief characteristic that comes to the fore. Awakening breaks through on occasion, exhibiting its own characteristics of disordered aggressive behaviour.

There are economic and other penalties which accompany a society that suppresses these urges to near or absolute extinction in the majority of its members. Under such circumstances, poverties develop and resentments or even wars are conceived, born and nurtured. The cudgel or the nuclear bomb are but incidental to this main issue.

* * *

Government's role in the free market system, I tried to engender, is to create a climate within which its citizens can operate in the best way possible - freely, easily, naturally and open to everybody. But it should not end there. Government must also assume the role of disciplining our urges so that they do not run riot and threaten people, animals, natural resources and the environment. It does not have to interfere unduly with the market system to do this.

Although the formula says that a free market system, if left to itself, will be self regulating, there are some positive aspects to the imposition of regulations to direct the course of market development and to strengthen weak and soft spots in the economy. The formula, in its bid for minimal regulation, reduces the restrictive and other regulations which interfere with the free aspects of its operation, especially those that regulate the number of businesses in an economic sector and those which set up regulatory bodies which decide on an individuals' fitness for the venture upon which he wishes to spend his own capital and personal effort.

Free as we may want to make it, the system must operate within the general laws of the country. A free market system cannot operate outside the criminal laws. It gives no license to murder, steal or sell harmful narcotic drugs in pursuit of an economic base. Neither does it give rights to subvert the codes of moral and ethical behaviour.

In the interest of improving the economy, it may be expedient to introduce regulations to aid the process of economic development. In our circumstances it was expedient to do away with the majority of import taxes, reduce corporate and personal taxes, and drastically reduce taxes in the wealth-creating industries of manufacturing, agriculture and internal transportation. It was a positive expedient to repeal or by-pass regulations with restrictive components, to introduce an excise tax which has a broad base and ease the burden of personal income tax.

* * *

The basis of the economic theory that I felt fitted our needs was to promote the exercise of the characteristics inherent in our human nature as the motive force to develop our economy. It is more than just self-interest. It is also display of power, wealth, achievement rivalry and, in its least aggressive form, just trying to make a living. We can refer to these in a variety of ways to include the profit motive, greed and covetousness. Some would even include altruism based on a wish to serve. Whatever we might call them, they are powerful motivating forces for driving any economy.

With self-interest as the primary motive force to drive the economic system, left to itself, one would think it would run wild and the poor consumer would be overcome with high prices, shoddy goods and unprofessional services, but the very fact that the market is free to all to enter puts the controlling aspects of the system in place.

Any successful market venture soon has individuals vying to have a part of the action it creates. The original instigator of the venture soon finds others arrayed alongside him competing to produce a better product at a better price. The more successful a business venture, the more competitors it will attract. On that basis consumers have the best possibility of receiving goods or services of the highest quality, at the best prices and in the right quantities. This may be unfair to the innovator, but who said life is fair?

This was the heart of the economic model that I believed would awaken the economy and develop Cook Islands out of its third world status. If allowed to operate freely without hindrance or unnecessary control, it should increase productivity in each sector. Government must do its part in providing the economic climate, the infrastructure and an empathetic aura for its propagation. These were, I thought, the most important ingredients in the prescription for improving our economy.

Once developed it would no doubt take on the personality of active economies with ups and downs which might need the kind of regulatory preventive measures that Keynes conceived. But for now they had to be relegated to the far background. The over-riding need was to incite the minds of everybody to doing things that would give birth to a viable economy. Whether it would wear pink or blue or need a particular formula to nourish it later were secondary considerations.

Because many more individuals in a free economy than can ever be available in a control economic system are seeking every potential avenue to engage in a profit-making enterprise out of their own resources and the resources of their environment, the variety and number of business ventures soars to unimagined limits. This does not exclude the development of the arts, the material and moral culture, the social and cultural structure, and the physical and mental capabilities of the community. On the contrary, it is a stimulus to creativity and human development.

* * *

Real and abstract enemies of the system are always lurking in the background. Economic planners, beloved of the control system, are always waiting to skew the market to fit their own biases to seek government subsidies to achieve their skewed ends. The planners who are particularly dangerous are those who plan for products rather than operational means to reach economic objectives.

They subsume the poignant minds of entrepreneurs who are honed to a sensitivity not only by the profit motive, but also by the need to succeed and maximise the utilisation of effort and capital expended on their ventures. They should be much more aware of the possible gains or losses to which their capital can be exposed. They are better equipped to gauge the potentials of the market. They stand to gain or to lose - not the planners. By judicious tax restructuring in addition to other measures, the numerous minds at work can be exposed to an area of the market which government perceives as needing their consideration.

* * *

Long term planning is basically part of a command type of economic system and is often doomed to failure because the more important conditions that planners themselves demand can only be found in a free market economic system. Usually these cannot be satisfied, at least, in the Pacific Islands' communities.[33]

"The planning process needs the proper atmosphere," they say. "Government needs to provide the infrastructure and to pursue the broader goals in education, health, income distribution, regional balance of development and many related objectives of society as a whole," they aver. "Planning must avoid the character of a straight jacket; it must be rather the creation of a whole environment in which growth is made possible, stimulated and assisted," they insist.[33]

What they have just described are characteristics found only in a free market society. But their actions and recommendations imply, "Although this is difficult in a highly socialised economy, it is impossible in a private enterprise economy". Most plans in the Pacific not only do not have the ideal conditions described, but they also do not have the transportation in place to deal with the products of the plan and neither do they consider market changes that are likely to trample their forecasts underfoot before the plan has matured. A cyclone or a drought in the Phillipines have a greater effect on copra prices in the Pacific Islands states than any well laid plan. Similar forces apply to citrus, bananas, pineapples to name a few.

In the societies we South Sea Islanders live in, the best plan is for a truly free market system in which entrepreneurs can operate freely. The most that government can and should do, besides attending to the infrastructural support systems, is to reduce taxes where a particular economic sector needs to be assisted. I also know no better way to increase the revenue of government, a paradox which few believe in enough to put it to the test. The question is one of behaviour, not accounting.

It was not blind belief or courage that made us entertain and use these measures, it was more a case of desperation as we could not make the situation worse than it was. It can be said that this is a form of coercion similar to those in a command system. It is, but the freedom to exercise the tax incentive or not is for the entrepreneurs who may have more valid reasons not to accept the challenge than the government had for offering it.

Another group of enemies of the system are the government regulatory bodies and the Ministers of the Crown who create them through the most extraordinary belief that they can best direct economic activity as opposed to the multitude of minds creatively and intensely bent on economic ventures into which they have put their hearts, minds, capital, families and property in the hope of success, survival and a decent living.

A parliamentarian is no different a person the day after an election than the day before. As an MP, he is no better than his record as a person. A public servant who receives regular pay each fortnight is unlikely to be an economic genius in determining the destiny of a citizen's economic plans and aspirations. And, if we accept all they say about their deciding why we should or, more likely, should not receive a license to go into a business, we deserve no better, if knowing better, we do not rise up and complain with a firm, loud voice. It is a citizen's inalienable right to make a living within the limits of good ethics, morality and the general law.

Even more inimical to the system are regulatory bodies which include members from the private sector to advise on who should or should not be granted business licences. These members are unlikely to be impartial especially when a license is for a business in their sector. They are even more dangerous than purely government regulatory bodies because they in concert with government tend to emanate an aura of impartial authority which they do not have. Instead, they can manipulate decisions to reduce their own competition and increase their own advantage. They can be awesomely arbitrary, each having the cloak of the other to aggrandise the false appearance of wisdom in their judgements on our behalf.

Monopolies and mergers maximise a position in the market place and disadvantage the competition. Their power to fix prices need not be doubted. However, in a truly free market system, their size should not protect them from competition, for if successful, they are as likely to be copied. It may be more difficult, but the incentive to overcome difficulties is there. It is when the market is not as free as it should be that their influence is greatest against likely competitors in the making. Antitrust laws are probably useful in preventing monopolies gaining this advantage, but, in a truly free system, they may not be necessary.

There is the general belief that large conglomerates (large companies dealing in a variety of widely differing products) are evil as are multinationals (companies dealing with either a single or many products in many countries). If efficiency is enhanced by size and quality, and prices of goods and services are competitive to those produced by other means, and there is freedom to choose, then the requirements of a free market system is satisfied. Many people shop at J. C. Penny, Sears and large supermarkets because they feel that quality and price are comparable to or more favourable than those produced or sold by smaller concerns or Ma and Pa shops.

Moreover, there seem to be enough conglomerates and multinationals in competition with one another to ensure quality, price and quantity of goods and services coming out of their portals; provided they are not in collusion as sometimes occurs, to control prices. It is the responsibility of governments to keep the market truly free.

The large conglomerates of IBM and AT&T, just two examples of many, are continuously plagued by their former employees setting up on their own and becoming competitors. Attempts to deny them choice by the imposition of contracts to enslave them and the products of their active minds have, as ought to be expected, not succeeded. In a much smaller way, but a no less valid example, many of the new business activities now carried out in the Cook Islands are by former employees of the established larger ruling companies who were supported by former regimes devoted to a controlled economy.

Subsidies may look a good way to prop up faltering or plainly unwanted products, but they distort market trends which suffer the subsidised products or services only because of their low price. If they had to sell at their real value, they would no longer exist. In the Cook Islands our citrus, pineapple, banana, copra and other industries have been subsidised in one form or another. The right thing to have done was to let the market place show whether they are needed and, if they are not, let it show other avenues where a profit can be made, even with the same products. If entrepreneurs look hard enough, they will find them. If they are diverted by subsidies, they will never look.

BUILDING
in constant 1987 dollars

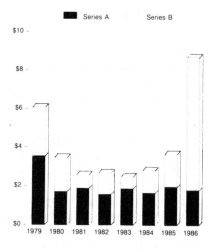

A: RESIDENTIAL, B: COMMERCIAL

The word Capitalism, coined in the era of potentate expression of the market system, is probably no longer the right word to describe the free market system adopted here and to greater or lesser degrees practised by Western countries today. It may have flaws, but it works.

Maybe we can keep on using the term Capitalism only because the use of capital in the form of investment is still part of the system, but this can be a relatively small factor in the operation of a free market system. In the Cook Islands between 1981 and 1985, we were denied capital for development. We could not raise capital from the one bank in the Cook Islands or any of the banks in Australasia. It was at the very time we needed it most, but we had to do with what we had. It was said that this economic "squeeze" we were put under was a punitive action because of our attitude towards the break down of the ANZUS pact and our international economic activities which Mr Lange found unbecoming our free association relationship with New Zealand.

During this period, although our commercial building activities were at an all time low, our GNP (Gross National Product) and GDP (Gross Domestic Product) continued to soar ahead in the face of a decreased commercial building program. Where there is a will, there is a way and expansion needs were met by one method or another including bringing into operation unused buildings, regardless of their state of disrepair. Therefore, irrespective of the economic system, what counts is the creative effort and the adaptability of man to get on with the job. Investment capital would have made things much easier and allowed us to develop and expand in the approved fashion, but it was not essential to the productive development of the economy. We needed capital for inventories and expansion, but the lowering of corporate taxes assisted in this area.

* * *

Since the system depends on individual capability, the upgrading of educational facilities and opportunities was an important part of the economic policy. Before 1978, few scholarships were made available for tertiary education to New Zealand and there were less than ten at the University of the South Pacific. Passes in the University Entrance examinations were few. We were able to increase this very quickly to more passes and more scholarships. Although we supplemented the financing of scholarships from the public purse as well as shifting nearly all of New Zealand's project aid to supporting this increase in funding requirements, the number qualifying for scholarships outdistanced the number of scholarships we could finance.

Qualifiers at lower pass levels were financed by another much smaller fund from the public purse to supplement financial support provided by parents (Student Assistance Scheme, SAS). The University of the South Pacific was supported in setting up its ancillary facilities in Rarotonga. Most people have forgotten this vast increase in providing a higher educational level to their children and continue to criticise the inadequacies of our educational system. And that is perhaps as it should be. In real terms (constant 1987 dollars), expenditure on education increased by 49.7 percent between 1978 and 1987 despite a static population. This increase in funding and improvement in educational standard was achieved in the face of a decrease in overall staffing and does not include funding provided by project aid nor that for the Students Assistance Scheme.

According to our economic method, the market is its own driving force, its strictest taskmaster and, to a large extent, its own guardian. There are doubts that even large companies can disregard market forces, at least in the long run. In any event large size was a small factor in the economy of the Cook Islands. We were going to put our hope on individual effort which had been struggling to emerge in our economic scene for some time. Only the economic indices would show whether it was successful.

* * *

We might take a little time to review what was done to achieve a self-motivating and self-regulating and perhaps self-perpetuating free market system in the Cook Islands:

1. In August 1978, the public was informed that any citizen was free to make a living by any means he (or she) considered would be of benefit to himself, his family and his friends. This amounted to a right to enter the market, a right to succeed and a right to fail.

2. An earth satellite station was inaugurated in 1979 and improvements in inter-island radio communications were instituted.

3. In the following years, airstrips were built in all the islands of the Southern Group and some of the Northern Group.

4. Internal air transport increased from one to five planes and from one to two operators, while external flights increased from one to eight per week.

5. A number of government trading activities were abolished or passed over to the private sector.

6. In 1978 and 1979 and subsequently, major reductions were made in import duties and levies.

7. In 1979 corporate taxes were reduced: the corporate taxes of import retailing and service industries were reduced from 35 percent for local companies and 42.5 percent for foreign companies to 20 percent and 27.5 percent respectively.

8. In 1979, corporate taxes for the wealth creating industries of manufacturing, resource development and exporting were reduced from 35 and 42.5 percent to 5 percent.

9. In 1980, the Turnover Tax on gross sales was put into effect at a rate of 4 percent for all retail sales and services and 1 percent for intermediary services, internal transportation and agriculture. Recently it has been increased to 10 percent at the retail level. In the face of other tax considerations, this is high.

10. Later the graduated personal income tax was reduced by altering the maximum tax of 45 percent at an income of $12,000 to a maximum of 35 percent at an income of $20,000. Later this was altered to a maximum of 35 percent at an income of $30,000. This now should again be adjusted to the effects of increasing inflation and increased earnings.

11. In 1980 wages and salaries of the Public Service were adjusted to cost of living changes on an annual, and later, on a twice annual basis. With it a

promotion system was introduced. Industrial wages and salaries tended to follow suit or, in some cases, were increased to higher levels.

12. Where politically possible, restrictive legislation, regulations and practices were abolished. Where this was not possible, they were ignored. With this went active encouragement of individuals who showed signs of starting new business activities.

13. Education was upgraded so that more people were better equipped to take advantage of the system.

14. Tourism, although it had shown its most rapid growth during the period 1974 to 1979, did not contribute to improving the economy which during this period had continued its downward trend. This was altered by increasing local participation in the accommodation industry, appropriate retail development of goods and services and other less obvious involvements of the Cook islands people in tourism. This could not have taken place without 12.

15. Efforts were made to give support to the main areas of the wealth creating sector of the economy represented by agriculture, fishing, manufacturing and tourism.

16. An international financial activity was introduced in 1980 along lines that existed elsewhere such as on the Jersey Islands, Bermuda, the Bahamas, the Cayman Islands and, in the Pacific: Vanuatu, Nauru and the Marshall Islands.

Government's role, apart from instituting the system step by expedient step, consisted of the creation of a favourable economic climate for the operation of the system, protection of the market from irrelevant interference, upgrading the infrastructure, taking care of ancillary requirements to facilitate the operation of the system and streamlining requirements for entering the market. Once the system was in operation, government's direct involvement in the market was passive because, as hopefully predicted, it moved of its own accord and, in sectors where enough participants developed, showed positive signs of regulating itself.

* * *

In 1978 and for a considerable period before that, our rating on the GDP scale tended to vary from one economic reviewer to another. This was to be expected since it was the policy of the government of the time to discourage any attempt to assess and have a running review of our economic status on an annual basis because they were not flattering to the administration. Flattering or not, it had little impact on the majority of the voting population which either cared little about such matters or had little idea of their economic import.

Most in the private sector were naive about economics and attributed most of what happened to chance, God and archaic economic ideas. This is not a criticism, but a statement of fact to indicate my inability to communicate economic policies. Although they were mostly unconscious that a new system was in operation, their effectiveness in contributing to its improvement was unimpaired. Attempts to discuss economics with them led to my quickly abandoning this approach. It was even more unrewarding with members of the general public or my colleagues. It was a lonely economic policy.

Economic thinking at the academic level within the region seemed even more remote from my own. Press comments, except for only one that I know of, gave me the impression that it was over their heads. On a personal basis many were downright antagonistic and demeaning. If it were not for my own certainty of the rightness of what was being done and the irrefutable accumulating evidence of its success, I would have been more downhearted than I already tended to be. It was similar to the feelings I had during the five years it took to experimentally demonstrate the reality of non-shivering thermogenesis to unbelievers. It was, therefore, most refreshing when, on a visit to Washington in 1988, I was given an opportunity to address about 200 US economists and others who seemed to know of our efforts. Their enthusiastic response was heartening and made me realise that I was not alone.

* * *

The effectiveness of the operation of the system speaks for itself in the economic results obtained. When the population develops an appetite for it, it is my fond hope that it will resist any who try to degrade it. A better understanding of it has to take place before that will eventuate, but when people's pockets are hurt and they see the unnecessary reasons why, it may not take long.

* * *

I must diverge here because what took place in the political scene is relevant to the economic picture. In March 1983, I, along with others in the Democratic Party, lost our seats and the Cook Islands Party won government by 13 seats to 11 with Geoffrey Henry as Prime Minister designate, waiting to be confirmed by Parliament as having the confidence of the majority of its members. This may be an unusual requirement, but it is demanded by the constitution.

At that time Geoffrey was assured of the support of his thirteen members, but, for some inexplicable reason, instead of accepting the existing procedure for confirmation and getting on with the job, he challenged the constitutionality of it on the basis that, in the original Westminster Parliamentary system, his being the leader of the winning Party should make him automatically the Prime Minister without such confirmation. His challenge led to an injunction in court which took some months to resolve.

This delay gave opportunity for the Spoiler, Vincent Ingram, then the leader of the Opposition, to sow the seeds of discontent, at which activity there is nobody better. Only Norman George, "the bull at a gate" exponent is a near equal. They have the talent to divide but not to rule. They lay poison as they sow. In sowing the seeds of discontent, he had his ever-present designs on the Prime Ministership. To facilitate his cause, he persuaded Tupui Henry, a son of the former Prime Minister, Albert Henry, who was then in Geoffrey's government, to put himself up for Prime Minister and push Geoffrey out.

The seeds of discontent fell on fertile ground because Tupui, since his father's death, had nursed the grudge that he should have been chosen to lead his father's Cook Islands Party instead of Geoffrey, his father's cousin. In addition Tupui did not condone some of the political practices which Geoffrey tended to favour.

In any event Tupui became convinced of the rightness of Vincent's conspiratorial notions. So after the court over-ruled the injunction, three names were thrown into the ring - Geoffrey's, Tupui's and, lo and behold, Vincent's. Day after day, when the votes in support of each candidate was called in turn, the result was a three way tie and no one could obtain a majority. This undemocratic way of becoming a Prime Minister failed.

The Queen's Representative had no choice but to call a general election because the debacle taking place was in breach of what the people had been led to vote for. So, during the year, there was my government up to March of 1983. Then there was Geoffrey's government until the confirmation debacle. Then there was a government by edict where the Queen's Representative took over because no budget could be passed. This was followed by a caretaker government after parliament was dissolved for new general elections to be held early in November and, finally, there was my second government of the year, when I and my party won these elections, 13 seats to 11. During the period of my holiday from politics I built myself a fishing boat and was in process of adapting myself to the joys of retirement.

The Spoiler seemingly had outwitted himself again, but in my new government he was up to his old tricks to spoil my confirmation as Prime Minister. He was discouraged by Democratic Party supporters turning up outside Parliament with firm orders for him to desist. His unhappiness with me grew and finally he and his shadow, a member from one of the constituencies of Mangaia, physically separated themselves from the Party, while still publicly claiming to be staunch members of it as members of the real Democratic Party which Vincent Ingram referred to as the Democratic Tumu Party, Tumu meaning source or root to give the impression that he was the founder of the Democratic Party. A few were gullible enough to go along with it, or it suited them to do so.

* * *

During this year, the disregard of parliamentarians for their democratic responsibilities to the voting public had adversely affected the economy. Between 1970 and 1978, GDP had decreased in real terms.

On first assuming power in 1978, we were able to almost immediately turn this around and, except for the dip in 1983, GNP and GDP moved forward at a very satisfactory rate in real terms. This dip in 1983 coincided with the five governments debacle. Recovery was rapid, but did not make up for the losses incurred that year.

Personal spending which had paralleled the increase in GNP and GDP also reflected this 1983 dip in the economy.

Again in real terms, income per capita had increased from $892 to $2000, an average annual increase of 13.8 percent over the nine year period.

The real annual average increase in per capita income of 13.8 percent was associated with a near doubling of employment.

Phenomenal economic growth was achieved in Rarotonga, which contained 55 percent of the national population and to a moderate extent on Aitutaki. Our failure to obtain similar results in the smaller islands was due almost entirely to

GDP & GNP
In Constant 1987 Dollars

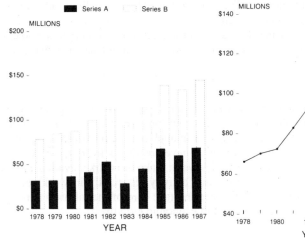

Series A   Series B

MILLIONS

A: GDP. B: GNP

SPENDING
In constant 1987 dollars

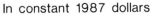

MILLIONS

EMPLOYMENT
Internal Revenue Returns

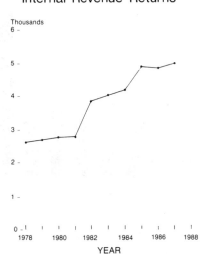

Thousands

INCOME PER CAPITA
In constant 1987 dollars

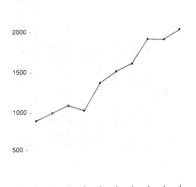

DOLLARS

our failure to improve transport sufficiently. Air transport improved greatly and Aitutaki was the main beneficiary from that. Sea transport remained a bottleneck.

Nevertheless, the national average for purchasing power of individual income earners was maintained. This was facilitated by cost of living adjustments in the Public Service, which, together with increases in the minimum wage, was the easiest way to influence the wages and salaries of the country as a whole. In any event the private sector wages and salaries moved satisfactorily in the right direction.

* * *

The application of the free market economic principles were specific to our circumstances and in the bounds of what could and could not be done. In certain areas, there were significant difficulties in applying the measures which were thought necessary. Therefore, some were never instituted. In brief, the measures taken to conform with these principles were: make the market available to all; restructure taxation to incite economic activity, especially in weak sectors; create a favourable economic climate; and take care of the infrastructure and other ancillary requirements to support economic growth.

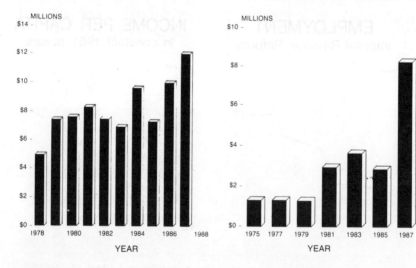

EXPORTS
In constant 1987 dollars

CLOTHING EXPORTS
In constant 1987 Dollars

There are paradoxes in the measures applied. Reducing taxes is one of them. To the legal and accounting mind, the question is how can this measure move the economy out of stagnation and, much more baffling, how can it increase revenue? On the surface, the measure is illogical. In the mind of a behaviouralist, it is logical in that it will increase business activity (and honesty with revenue contributions) and this increased volume of activity will increase revenue. In our case this was very well demonstrated in the effect of reduction of taxes in manufacturing represented by the clothing industry export figures for which we have records before and after the measures were instituted.

In real terms total exports increased from 4.9 (1978) to 12 million dollars (1987). Since then it has decreased to 4.2 million dollars(1989).

Lower personal income tax will increase spending, thereby increasing the revenue from turnover tax which is applied after the economic multiplication factor has had its effect. It is easy to see that total spending far exceeds total earnings (about $120M as against $35M), therefore, taxing earnings is getting one's share at the short end. At the other end, a little tax goes a long way. Sensible as this may seem, new measures arouse extraordinary resistance. So some measures could not be instituted, but enough was put in place to demonstrate that the free market system is self-motivating, self-regulating and, if government does its part in creating a favourable climate and taking care of the infrastructure, self- perpetuating.

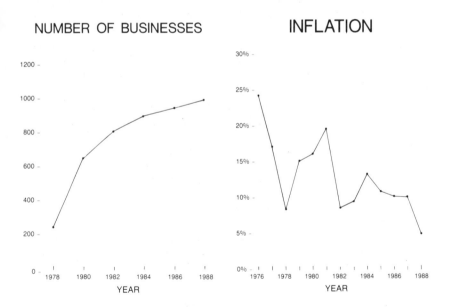

Opening the business sector to everybody increased the number of active businesses (those filing tax returns) in Rarotonga from about 150 in 1978 to 761 in March of 1988. In the outer islands the figure increased more modestly from about 100 to 226. The total of 987 as of March 1988 (Inland Revenue Department figures) is at a ratio of about 1 business for every 18 persons in the population.

In review, the following gains can be enunciated:

GNP, measured in constant 1987 dollars, increased from $77.5M in 1978 to $144M in 1987, an average annual rate of increase of 9.55 percent.

GDP in 1987 constant dollars increased at the annual rate of 12.16 percent from $31M in 1978 to $67.8M in 1987.

Real personal spending increased at the annual rate of 10.26 percent.

Real income per capita increased at the annual rate of 13.8 percent and employment did so at an annual rate of 10.04 percent.

Reduction of import duties and levies seemed to have had the expected salubrious effect on inflation rate.

Not only did the economic cake expand, but its distribution improved. The number of people with their own businesses increased five-fold, the number of people with regular employment nearly doubled, the basic wage increased from 31 cents to $2.00 in current terms and 63 cents to $2.00 in real value, the old age pension increased more than two-fold in real value while the destitute and infirm allowance multiplied three-fold.

Where once there was no traffic problem, one now exists, mild as this might be in comparison to other places. Where once there was incipient malnutrition and apathy evident in our children, there is now robust health, bursting energy and increased mental agility.

These were the good economic things that took place. They did not take place by accident. They were worked on with purpose, kneaded here and massaged there to shape the system to achieve as close to a free market system as was feasible in the time and the context.

The system was being tested in a society whose people were considered most unlikely to respond to economic forces. I did not believe this. The forces upon which the system depended were fundamental in all mankind. Once set in motion, it was self-motivating and self-regulating, needing no more than a gentle hand on the helm, complemented by the introduction of judiciously helpful regulations to nurse it in the right direction, past the reefs and through the storms it was bound to meet. It also needed the high literacy rate that already existed in the population and the rapid and substantial improvement in the educational system for people to seize and make a success of the opportunities provided by the economic policies introduced by government. Even those who one would not have believed could take advantage of the opportunities, did so.

* * *

Besides the good economic things that took place, good social and cultural things grew with it or out of it. Economic matters had sorted themselves out in a manner which was more organised than they had been before, but far different from that which would have been envisaged by planners in a control system. People were earning better wages and salaries and had money to buy more of what they wanted. They had less need to be their own market gardener, butcher and fisherman to eke out their earnings. Although there was not much real increase in income per taxpayer, the number of people with incomes high enough to pay taxes, doubled.

From 1980 on, a division of labour has been possible in that income earners could concentrate more on their primary earning occupations while farmers, fishermen and other specialists could work full time on their occupations because it was now worthwhile to do so. They had a local market. More money and leisure time now allowed more social activities and voluntary services to take place.

Proponents of a control market system do not seem to view an improvement in economic indices as a reason to change their economic views. To them the ideology of a control system has an emotional content not easily altered by facts. It is from these that persistent resistance continues.

* * *

The household expenditure survey showed that the outer islands were not as well off as Rarotonga from a cash in hand point of view, but they were able to put more time into agriculture for home consumption, or for sale to Rarotonga and even overseas. In comparison to Rarotonga, this was small due to failure of our efforts to improve shipping. Installing an airstrip on every island in the Southern Group and some islands in the Northern Group, brought marginal overall improvement, but significant improvement in medical, administrative and personal services.

The island of Mauke took advantage of air services and marketed a significant amount of their farm produce to Rarotonga and beyond in a plane quite unsuitable for the job. Atiu and Mangaia were unwilling to give up their pineapple industry which could no longer compete overseas against the products of Malaysia and Australia.

* * *

Most of what happened socially was spontaneous. By 1978, sporting activities had dwindled to the mainly two struggling codes of rugby for the men and netball for women. In a very short time the gamut of sports which could be indulged surged into place. Tennis, cricket and golf which had been the preserve of a privileged few, became accessible to ordinary citizens in large numbers. Athletics, rugby league, martial arts, darts, soccer, jazzercise, fitness clubs, and others were added.

Sports fields and sports facilities were upgraded and extended. For the first time we became a force to contend with in the South Pacific Games and earned the right to compete in the Commonwealth Games. In 1986 we became part of the Olympic Games fraternity, competing in Seoul for the first time in 1988. By 1986 we were sixth equal in the world in netball and have improved this to fourth place in 1989. When we consider that we draw most of our athletes from the 2000 or so youth of Rarotonga, these are outstanding achievements.

* * *

At the same time, adults were giving attention to their ideas of what was important to them. Community halls, church halls and churches were renovated and, where none existed before, new ones were built. The intensity of these activities were such that in one Christmas message, I praised them for what they had done for their communities, for their children and for posterity, but said it was perhaps time they should direct their energies towards upgrading their home environment which was as important an aspect of the well-being of our communities. I felt they had tended to neglect this.

In Western communities, the home plays an important role as a status symbol. In Polynesia a person sees his contributions to community and social efforts as being important in establishing his status. The open display of contributions in cash, food or personal effort is far more important as a symbol of social status and he often sacrifices home and family to this end. Where he gives freely to these community ventures and obligations, he seeks other means, the main one of which is to hold government primarily responsible through the granting of subsidised loans to establish an acceptable home for himself.

As the economy improved so did the employment of school leavers. The proportion in the population with higher education continues to ascend. Emigration slowed visibly from the high net losses of 4106 for 1972, 1973 and 1974 to first ever migration gains of 205 for 1983 and 214 for 1985.

* * *

Our failures were manifold and I must take a major part of the responsibility for them for they were failures in my ability to communicate the concepts behind my policies to my colleagues and to the people. My only excuse is that in most cases there was no point of reference which I could use as a common starting point. The concepts of my economic plans and plans for the infrastructure were new and strange to my colleagues and to most of the population and even the region. When I introduced the word "infrastructure" in Parliament everybody roared with laughter that such a word could exist.

I was utterly unable to transfer the vision so clearly in my mind even to my colleagues who boasted in parliament at the increased number of automobiles as a sign of economic improvement under our administration. I was unable to have more than a few kilometres of road improved and was unable to have one kilometre of new road established by Public Works, and I failed entirely in communicating the economic rationale which allowed the economic improvements to take place.

I have referred to our failure to give the outer islands an effective transport capability to have them participate adequately in the benefits of a burgeoning economy being enjoyed mainly by Rarotonga. Sea freight was abysmal. Nobody wanted to pay the freight rates that should have increased with increasing inflation and no one on the outer islands showed interest in working the ship when it arrived. Sometimes no one would come out to work the ship until two to even six hours after its arrival. We improved facilities for air transport by putting in the airstrips, but interest by the newly developed local airlines was for passengers and, in this, Aitutaki received most of their attention because that is where the passengers wanted to go. However, rural areas of even the most advanced countries provide a picture that is comparable. Perhaps that is the way things are.

I abandoned several plans for an airfreight plane because it aroused so much controversy. Now the failure has gone further and there is no outer Island shipping except that which can be done on a catch as can basis and at high cost. Public Works had to be ignored for the building of the water reservoirs and it was done by a private contractor who used equipment he had salvaged from the beach in front of Public Works, which had been discarded as no longer serviceable. The reservoir was completed in less than a year. Finally after my demise, when Public Works took responsibility for the second reservoir, it was left to crumble away, uncompleted. The first reservoir has been wilfully destroyed.

* * *

The universal superannuation scheme had been conceived in 1978 and honed to a workable level and prepared as a bill ready for parliament not long after. Both sides of the House were fully involved in working it up, but it could not get past several unrelated hurdles. As is customary in this part of the world, many could not accept it being in the hands of a private insurance company. Since Vincent Ingram was involved with one of the insurance companies with a proposal, many felt that his support of the scheme was purely monetary. The Public Servants who were the only recipients of any superannuation scheme were against it on the basis that it might receive a few dollars less than the New Zealand government scheme they were on. A clause in the bill that guaranteed no loss to Public Servants in the existing system, did not dissuade them from their relentless opposition.

Finally the bill was presented to Parliament in 1986 and it was immediately moved for it to go to a select committee to be chaired by Geoffrey Henry, Leader of the Opposition and, since January 1989, Prime Minister. Since, as it transpired, he is opposed to the measure, a national superannuation scheme is not likely to eventuate. Accordingly, of the total work force, only Public Servants have a retirement scheme.

* * *

Then there were the things viewed as the bad things by the people. People all over the world interpret the economy as it affects them personally. Most of us believe we are worth much more than we are or can get. A fundamental human assumption is that any improvement in one's economic status, once it becomes a reality, is never enough. This is so strong a drive that the one who has brought about the improvement is likely to be in trouble for not providing more.

If one asks people, regardless of their income, how much more income they need to live in reasonable comfort, the answer is likely to be around one third more than that being received. Therefore, when a government improves the economy, its efforts are seen as having achieved a shortfall of about one third at all times.

Recently I was accused of having made the people of the Cook Islands poorer and that the price of things was outrageous. The accuser was leaning on his shiny Datsun pickup outside the supermarket. Not long before, they had never owned a vehicle other than an overworked Honda 50 motorcycle. He and his wife had raised a limited range of vegetables, chickens and pigs for their own use because they could not afford to buy them and there was no supermarket. Many like them had to do this as well as work eight hours a day for a wage or salary, if they could get a job. A home telephone was an unheard-of luxury.

They were not aware that the increase in their income was more than the inflation rate and that they had shifted from a precarious and irregular subsistence to a stable cash economy with a household expenditure average of around $14,000 per annum. Neither did they remember that a short time ago their kids were suffering from incipient malnutrition, attested to by their pot bellies. Their eldest was now at school overseas, which would not have been a remote possibility for them up to 1979. His wife came out of the supermarket with their two younger kids loaded with goodies. She kissed me and asked her husband whether he had changed the video tapes and paid the telephone bill. No doubt he filled her in about how he had told me off for having kept them in a state of penury.

A young and successful businessman whose success had been achieved entirely during my administration recently informed me irately that he was one of the few of the 200 businesses paying Turnover Tax. I ought to do something about the others. Not many of the other business men were any more aware than he of what had been taking place. My own efforts to publicise the economic gains were met with yawns of disinterest. When I explained to him that as of March 1988, there were 987 businesses paying turnover tax based on gross sales of around $120,000,000, he told me I did not know what I was talking about. He later told others that Papa Tom was having economic delusions.

Another citizen informed me how lucky it was for me to have been Prime Minister during the time of the Cook Islands phenomenal economic and social development. At least this one admitted that economic and social improvements had taken place.

Several citizens have complained that I complicated their lives. I never asked anyone to do what they were doing. Others said I had moved the economy too rapidly, but, I replied, I did nothing to the economy except hand it over to them to move at their own pace. I never set any pace or economic programs or targets. I never said do this or do that. My economic policies did not believe in programs or controlled economic targets set by government. However, my government or I personally would help those who set their own targets even if only with a word of encouragement.

There were those who said that my economic policies were destroying our culture. It did not occur to them that much of our ancient culture had already been changed by Christian teaching, commerce, technological advances and travel, and by their own changing aspirations. If it were not for tourism, the revival of some aspects of our culture would not have taken place. There was inadequate comprehension of cultural development as a dynamic process or that social and cultural values were the result of an ever-changing and enriching process which was not necessarily deleterious. The culture of 50 years ago was far different from that of today, and from that of 100 years ago. Only certain themes make it recognisable as the same root culture.

I relate these few of many incidents to demonstrate the political hazards of improving the economic lot of a nation. But they also demonstrate the tremendous power of the system we brought into being in that it could be made to operate without the people understanding or being interested in how it worked, or even having to know that it was taking place or having any special qualifications to make it work.

CHAPTER TWENTY

The Pacific Neighbourhood

Imperialism is not just foreign trade nor just foreign investment. It is these plus political interference, economic exploitation, military force, and a bland disregard for the interests of the poorer nation by the richer.

ROBERT L. HEILBRONER

The economic views of the Pacific countries were little different from those held by my own. The private sector were considered thieves and they sometimes were. Where there was insufficient competition or where there was collusion, their mark-ups were horrendous. Their role in the economy was not recognised either by government or by the private sector itself.

Our resources were not enough to do much about economic development. Agriculture and fishing, both traditional family food sources, were not considered business occupations. Countries which had mineral and other natural resources like Papua New Guinea and the Solomon Islands could not seem to get self sustaining development off the ground. However, Australia and the United Kingdom, in their time, had not done very much about them either. France, which had developed the nickel of New Caledonia, the tourism of Tahiti and the reef fishing capabilities of the Tuamotu atolls, was considered beyond the pale.

There was an attempt to address the economic problem in 1966 by the formation of the Pacific Islands Producers Association (PIPA). It was primarily a Ratu Sir Kamasese Mara innovation supported by other leaders of the Pacific neighbourhood. Although its aims were in the area of economic development, it followed the pattern of other Pacific regional organisations in failing to come to grips with economic problems.

In 1971, the heads of independent islands' governments, plus New Zealand and Australia, began to meet annually in the South Pacific Forum. The secretariat of the Forum was, interestingly called SPEC, short for the South Pacific Bureau of Economic Co-operation. But, in 1989, in realisation that its economic endeavours were not very successful, the name was changed to the Forum Secretariat.

Except in things like SPARTECA (South Pacific Trade and Economic Co-operation Agreement) and the Forum Shipping Line, which was separately managed, SPEC's activities were for the most part non-economic in nature. Many economic studies and programmes were instituted, ranging from a Pacific Islands Common Market to a common currency, but with little success.

The development of the Forum Shipping Line was typical of the thinking of governments which formed the Forum, that is, governments can do better than the private sector. It persisted in the face of losses by New Zealand positively picking up the tab. Australia very reluctantly followed suit. The European Community supplied free containers. We of the Pacific Islands States did what we were told. Finally we succeeded in running some privately run shipping lines off these routes.

This was an area where Rob Muldoon and Malcolm Fraser, Prime Ministers of New Zealand and Australia respectively, disagreed with heat. Malcolm was against spending so much money for the losses of the Forum Line. He thought that much smaller assistance to private shipping lines would have solved the Pacific's shipping woes more cheaply and effectively. His view was a cry in the wilderness. Now the Forum Line has fewer competitors and is surviving as a monopoly on some routes owing to heavy subsidies of its ships (mainly provided under foreign aid), its containers (likewise) and other commercial assistance. Although its freight rates are now as high as its competitors, it proved to the socialists of the region that government monopolies worked. They do if someone pays enough.

* * *

SPARTECA was concerned mostly with tariffs and quotas of goods between New Zealand and Australia on the one hand and member countries of the Forum on the other. These negotiations highlighted the protective attitude of Australia, New Zealand and the Islands States towards their products. Our products imported by them were so minute in comparison to their exports to us that the extensive negotiations that went on at the official level seemed unwarranted and ludicrous.

The aura of the tariff problems between George III and the American colonists was there in its stark pettiness. My own tariff problems with Mr Robert Muldoon and New Zealand officials reflected the same attitudes, but we came to an understanding that the minute economy of the Cook Islands could not possibly threaten the, by comparison, gigantic economy of New Zealand. The general attitude seemed to be one in which, if sacrifices were to be made, the Pacific Island States were the ones to make them. They were used to seeing it that way and we were used to accepting it that way.

Because we believed it when we were told that small Pacific Islands States could never make a go of it without largesse from their former colonial masters, we did not try very hard to see the possibilities from our own points of view which had to be quite different from theirs. Theirs were based on large farms, large manufacturing concerns and natural resources of large land masses with large populations. The absence of these, especially in the small Pacific Islands States, made it difficult for them to see that there might be other avenues of economic development. We, therefore, accepted largesse as a right, without questioning the matter any further and without the thought that some day it may not be forthcoming.

* * *

We lived with some interesting hangovers from colonial history. The Dutch in West New Guinea, by the end of their colonial era, had decided that the ideal training for their administrators was in anthropology. The top six persons in government had PhDs in it. Next door in Papua New Guinea, the Australians regarded anyone with any university education as suspect, and hired "practical men" with little formal education. The British in the Solomon Islands, the New Hebrides, Fiji, Kiribati and Tuvalu required their men to be trained, preferably with an honours degree from Oxford or Cambridge, in the classics, philosophy, Latin, history etc. The French in New Caledonia and Tahiti, emphasised training in law. Each was convinced that its approach was right and the proven path to the proper government of Pacific Islanders.

* * *

We did not equate constitutional independence with economic independence and we became members of the right regional and international organisations and spoke at these with equal standing. Albert Henry at one of these meetings put forward the resolution that each of the metropolitan countries should put 1 percent of their Gross National Product towards the support of the Pacific island countries. It is too easy for hopeful recipients to specify what gifts they would like and from whom. This never eventuated and would probably have spelled finis to any thoughts of taking economic development seriously. We could have lived high on the proceeds without doing anything about economic development.

Previous efforts by predecessors in both government and opposition, I noted, had put much emphasis on social and cultural development. This pattern had emerged as the principle objectives of other Pacific Islands States also. Regional bodies, especially those formed by the regional governments and regional organisations, tended to emphasise social development. The South Pacific Forum, of which we were a charter member, was composed of Prime Ministers, Presidents and Premiers of the South Pacific Islands States. Whatever else it did, it gave economic development little priority as a subject for serious consideration, despite the rhetorical claim that this was the primary interest.

Our economic problems were seen more as social problems and fitted a category for other regional and international arrangements to solve. We were still in the era of Pacific history when economics as a discipline was suspect and man's problems centred around social and traditional structures to which economics clung for a precarious Cinderella type existence. In the Cook Islands the government banned the publication and distribution of reports by the Dutch economists whom the Netherlands government had sponsored for our benefit in the 1970s.

The relationship between economic and social problems seemed to escape us. The South Pacific Forum saw itself as a watch dog of other people's political problems (but the politics of any member state of the Forum was avoided) and arbiters of what should and should not be done in the region by metropolitan countries in, around and beyond the region. Attempts to bring up the subject of our economic development were received in silence and from this notably silent silence we passed on to other matters where members could orate loudly and clearly. Often it was about the sins, real and imagined, of one or other of the metropolitan nations, which were not present. Some of it was justified, but without positive action on our part, it amounted to no more than a hill of beans.

Next to social development, but low in the list of priorities, came political development with thoughts about whether the systems of government bequeathed us by our former colonial masters were appropriate. The subject popped up now and then, but never got to a stage where we could come up with something better or even something which formed a basis for continued discussion. Perhaps the Rabuka coup in Fiji, the emergence of Libyan connections and other episodes, indicative of political unrest, uncertainty and instability, may have been practical demonstrations of what was being thought but not expressed.

We still seemed not to have as yet shed autocracy and the practice of privilege that went with authority, characteristic of days of yore. Dynastic rule, the untransferrability of land for economic use, subsistence farming, fishing, handicrafts and bartering still lingered obviously among us. Earnings and material needs were small and precluded the development of a dependable worker-consumer force for higher standards of living.

More than any of these, the Forum concerned itself with the doings of the metropolitan countries. France and the United States received the lion's share of criticism. France for its nuclear testing and the New Caledonia question; USA for its nuclear warships and its multinational corporations which were given ogre-like characteristics. The Soviets shooting down a passenger airline received little attention as compared to the criticisms brought down on these countries for the potential evils they might cause.

Preservation of the environment was high on the priority list and led to some useful resolutions and a Pacific nuclear free zone, though there are problems with superficial notions that they contribute much to world peace and security. We all at one time or another put in resolutions requiring the French to move their testing from Mururoa atoll to France.

The Nuclear Free Zone was pushed hard by New Zealand and modified by Australia. If examined only a little more carefully, the treaty allows any of its signatories the right to allow nuclear vessels to enter its waters and other nuclear devices to be installed within its national boundaries, but not to allow weapon systems to be installed in the region on a permanent basis.

* * *

New Zealand's strong anti-nuclear stand had a more serious effect on its economy than is generally realised. New Zealand by its previous efforts had built a strong trading relationship with the United States, England and Europe. This was made relatively easy because New Zealand and Australia were considered ramparts of the Western ideology on the other side of the world. New Zealand's trade relationship with these countries was equivalent to it being allowed to carry coals to Newcastle. The United States and Europe needed meat and butter like they needed a hole in the head. They had much of their own and many other willing suppliers. But because New Zealand was small and a distant rampart against the assumed evils of the East, this trade was tolerated and it grew and prospered.

I was resident in the United States in the 1950s when the trade with the United States blossomed. I was aware of the resentment of the US farmers to the importing of New Zealand meat in direct competition with their products. They were quietened by the administration of the time on the basis that these imports were relatively small. The same thing had happened in Europe even earlier and, with time, New Zealand strengthened her trading position. Where in the 1950s there were just over 30 million sheep, this number has increased to nearly 70 million. Although the trade could be considered still small, to the farmers of the United States and Europe, it had been too large for too long. Because of New Zealand's unique position, the trade was still tolerated, but with stronger winges from its opponents. New Zealand's search for new markets was successful in only a few places because sheep, cattle and butter are common products of many large countries where worthwhile markets can be expected.

In any event, because of New Zealand's and Australia's unique position as ramparts of the Western way of life in the far away corner of the Pacific, near the backyard of where trouble might be expected to erupt, the ANZUS defence pact was born. This further strengthened New Zealand's trading position, not only with the United States, but also with Western European countries because they were relieved to a degree of worries about an adequate watch dog for their back door. Everybody who mattered was happy and New Zealand could continue carrying coals to Newcastle almost as much as it liked despite competing farmers' feelings against it. There is more to international trading than hunger for each others products.

David Lange's antinuclear programs flew in the face of this "defence of the West" plan. The American eagle was angry as was that of the Germans. The British lioness lashed her tail. The French smiled and said, "We told you so."

The farmers of these countries saw their chance and no administration needed to urge them to act against New Zealand produce. New Zealand was in the cold. The foundation of her economy was seriously eroded. The New Zealand farmer was now told by his government that he virtually had to live on less or give up farming for it saw no relief for his dilemma and the fault lay with their former foreign markets.

New Zealand was forced into a financial market strategy without visible props which resembled the US economy before the 1929 crash with similar results. New Zealand businesses as well as farmers went out of business one after the other. Our Cook Islands' policy of reduction of import duties and levies resulting in diversified import markets now paid off by insulating us from the brunt of its effects to a significant extent.

Bob Hawke played his own game, caught between the tendencies of his own antinuclear group and the far left and the need to preserve his relations with the West. He has the rapidly growing 190 million people of Indonesia next door, with their military government with expansionist tendencies. All of this seemed of little importance to David Lange. Hawke watered down the Nuclear Free Zone Treaty of Rarotonga on the basis that, if it was too rigid, not all the Forum countries would sign. He, Mara of Fiji and I would have had difficulties with a more rigid treaty. Tonga still refuses to sign even the watered down version.

Bob Hawke and I had long term good relations with the United States and Mara had recently developed the same. None of us, and may be others too, wanted to jeopardise this. Australia had more to lose because it had uranium ore to sell, which it did to the French soon after signing the Treaty of Rarotonga. Since 1978, I had supported ANZUS as a protective umbrella for the Pacific Islands States because there seemed no other military way of doing it. Its near demise and New Zealand's insistence that it alone could defend us created some problems between us because I claimed that it could not defend itself let alone us.

For the sake of some anti-nuclear protesters, who based their ideas of peace on the existence or non-existence of weapons, we were put through a great deal of trauma and circumvention and New Zealand's economy was adversely affected. Peace is based on much deeper values and principles than the presence of the cudgel or the nuclear bomb. As long as we are influenced by those who think that they can blame the weapons for our shortcomings, we will never get down to the nitty gritty of what peace is all about.

* * *

The relationship between the Cook Islands and New Zealand is based on three areas. The first two are in the Constitution Act of 1964. One states we are New Zealand citizens and the other says that New Zealand shall be responsible for our External Affairs and Defence after consultation between the two Prime Ministers. The third is the Aid it gives us. The total relationship hangs on these three. At times New Zealand makes much more of this than we think is warranted and in a way that is not to our economic advantage. We also have a Letter of Understanding which implies that we must abide by the values that New Zealand deems important. With our increasing economic independence, our increased trade and other relationships with other countries, and with New Zealand values deteriorating in some areas, this document has come to mean less and less. We can at any time change this relationship by a two thirds majority in Parliament and a two thirds majority in a referendum of the voting population of the Cook Islands.

The relationship is seen by our people to be a good one for us. Unlike other Pacific Islands States, it gives us free access to New Zealand and Australia and we are not in a hurry to change that. We are less dependent on their aid than ever, but it is still much the largest source of external assistance. The demeaning and enervating aspects of it are to my mind unacceptable and the economic drive of my administration was to free the country of it or bring it down to acceptable proportions. In any event Prime Minister Lange started to reduce it at an annual rate. If we were not such a profligate people it would not matter.

In external affairs and defence we developed activities and views which resulted in strained relations with the Lange Administration. We developed our own Foreign Affairs capabilities where this has been important to us and I must add that New Zealand Foreign Affairs, though showing signs of a reserved attitude, have always come to our assistance when we have needed it. We are most grateful.

In the matter of defence, our views have starkly differed with the Lange Administration. ANZUS (Australia, New Zealand and United States Council) I viewed as important to the security of the region. None of us in the region including New Zealand, Australia and the larger Pacific Islands countries can in the foreseeable future have an armed capability to care for ourselves militarily. With this reality staring us in the face, when I was asked for an opinion on the break up of New Zealand's role in ANZUS, I stated truthfully that I thought it was a pity, especially since in 1978 I had given our support to the pact and offered what services and facilities we could render, meagre as these may be, if a confrontation should ever take place. It incited a reaction from Prime Minister Lange far out of proportion, I thought, to the simple remarks I had made.

In any event the scattered nature of our islands states will not allow us to individually or collectively raise an effective force against an organised foe. I do not think that we are in any imminent or even distant danger but, if we are going to play soldiers, let us play it with good sense. In my view the best defence the Pacific Islands States has is to put our efforts into the context of world peace. We have no other. I do not mean that we should put our efforts into superficial activities like protests and incomplete disarmament drives. It only takes one nuclear bomb. There is a need for a profound and in-depth look at the world peace problem.

* * *

The military coup of Fiji came as a surprise in that its cause had been festering for decades with nothing happening. Experienced Fijians were in charge and we had come to believe that nothing would happen. Viewed from the outside, Ratu Sir Kamasese Mara's handling of the problem over the years was exemplary in that he kept the festering racial problem under control for seventeen years. It is likely that nobody else could have done it so well. From inside, the ordinary indigenous Fijians considered that they were being left out of sharing in the benefits of independence and that the Indians were being favoured.

The Indians who had been brought into Fiji as indentured labour, like the Japanese of Hawaii and the Chinese of Tahiti had, with changing times, prospered by participating in the economy as businessmen and on the land by renting and working it. They also multiplied and for decades outnumbered the Fijians. Added to this is the fact that Fijians and Indians, like water and oil, do not mix. It was a prescription for racial problems. Indian emigration since the coup has reduced their proportion of the population to 46 percent.

The Indians did not want trouble and hoped that it would never come, for they were doing fine. The Fijian chiefs did not want trouble either because they were also doing fine from the rents from the land and other gains due to Indian participation in the economy. The Fijians who were discomfited were not prepared to cause any real trouble as long as the chiefs did not want any major change in the status quo.

To understand the problem further, a brief look at a little history, apart from the Indian question, might help. Fiji has been for some considerable time composed of an aristocracy of Polynesian descent in a population of Melanesian descent. Several centuries ago and several times, the Polynesians of Tonga invaded Fiji and dominated much of it. In the 1800s the most recent wave of Tongan invasions under Ma'afu again conquered much of Fiji. They would have conquered it all had the Fijian chiefs not asked the United Kingdom to take over the embattled country in 1874. These invasions changed only the content of the Polynesian-derived aristocracy, not the Melanesian proportion of the society.

The Indian question was no problem as long as the Indians remained as farmers and businessmen. However, as the population of Indians outgrew that of the Fijians, the Westminster system of government would sooner or later assert itself in the matter of political representation. This happened in 1987 when the newly elected government was composed of a majority of Indians. This meant that the Council of Chiefs could no longer be assured that their perceptions of Fijian interests would be protected. There was only one thing to do - stage a military coup and appoint a government which would continue to serve Fijian interests.

Out the window went democracy which up to that time had been something of a facade anyway. It was an elite system before contact, it was an elite system during the Westminster system of government and it is an elite system now. Democracy in Fiji can take place only when Indians can be accepted as having equal socio-economo-political rights. But it is likely that for a time the future will be more of the present system established since the coup. A democratic system does not operate well in a controlling inheritance type elite society as we should know by now. And while it is relatively easy to operate in a diverse multi-cultural situation, it is very difficult in a country with just two major races equally balanced in population and radically different in religion, language and culture.

The response to the coup from outside the Pacific Islands States region was that of people concerned with loss of democracy and a good economy. This had little meaning to Fijians, the majority of whom were not getting much out of it.

Australia and New Zealand considered using military force to straighten out the Fijians who had somehow gone astray and needed the help of the big brothers. This was insensitive to the heart of the problem. Fortunately the Fijians were strong enough to make it clear that they would actively resist interference and the naval ships of the two countries in their waters were kept at bay. Had they not been, it would have made matters worse.

I happened to be in Auckland at the time and when approached by the media, I told them that the Fijians would handle the matter themselves. They did not seem very happy with this stance. The remarks made by Mr Lange were particularly insensitive and the Fijians will not quickly forget them. What the Fijians needed most from us was understanding and consolation which would have had a calming effect. Nearly all the Pacific Island States took this view and we sent messages to that effect.

The insensitivity continued into the Forum of August that year. Mr Lange, who had been taken to task for his earlier insensitivities, was quiet about the issue. However, Mr Hawke and Tupuola Efi worked hard at having the Forum agree to a resolution of theirs to send a delegation to Fiji to solve their problem and restore democracy. Most of us disagreed to such a move as we all felt that Fiji needed to be left alone to lick her wounds and work out her own solutions with our sympathetic assistance as they might request it. After three long after-hours sessions, we were unable to dissuade the minority to desist. With no consensus reached, a telegram was sent to Sir Penaia Ganilau to alert him of a Forum delegation to deal with their problems to be led by Mr Hawke. The offer was firmly rejected.

It is a characteristic of Pacific Islanders that keeping silent about a proposal does not mean acquiescence. Generally it means the opposite. In our cultures, it generally means reservation or opposition. We consider it rude to openly oppose our equals or betters. Therefore, silence is preferred and should be read as such.

The most vocal in the Forum were Australians and New Zealanders and it is no exaggeration to say that they verbally dominated our meetings. Our silence encouraged this domination. However, sometimes, our silence was because we had nothing to say on an issue. By most of us, the difference can be sensed.

On the Fijian coup, our silence and attempts at verbal discouragement of intentions on behalf of Fiji was one of disagreement with them. This is not a criticism of individuals, it is a statement of fact about our cultural differences. Our frankness and abusive behaviour in parliament is abnormal, but is done because it is deemed a necessary part of the trappings of the political structure we have inherited. Our House of Ariki has the same Standing Orders as parliament, but so far, as equals, they have not found the need to use them.

* * *

Where the Polynesian Society is still made up of a traditional elite group and the majority of the population is under their control, as is the case in Western Polynesia (Tonga, Samoa, Wallis and Futuna), there is limited capability for progress as was the case in Europe when it had a similar socio-politico-economic structure. For differing reasons, the traditional system in Eastern Polynesia has lost this elite control and everybody in the population is individually and collectively more free to exercise control over their socio-politico-economic destinies.

It is mainly for this reason that rapid economic, social and political gains have been possible in Eastern Polynesia, from Hawaii to French Polynesia to the Cook Islands. The barriers to progress are no different from those in a Western provincial township elsewhere and for similar reasons. Therefore, it is difficult for the South Pacific Forum to act in concert in dealing with one another's economic problems when its components: Australia and New Zealand, Melanesia, Western Polynesia, Nauru, the Cook Islands, and now Micronesia are at different levels and follow different pathways of existing and potential development.

* * *

The Melanesian wish to help their Melanesian brothers, the Kanaks of New Caledonia, towards a visibly difficult independence, led to a series of incidents and situations which did not resolve the problem as seen from their point of view. The main difficulty in this kind of move towards independence is that the Kanak population is in a minority to a combined variety of other racial elements which do not want independence from France. These racial groups consist mainly of French Colons, Tahitian and Wallisian Polynesians and Asiatics many of whom have been in New Caledonia for several generations and are well established in the economy of land and business. They no longer have strong ties to the origins of their forebears. Again a large proportion of the problem was the inability of these racial groups to mix with the indigenous Kanaks, a problem not seen in Polynesian communities.

Aided by the urgings of newly independent Melanesian brothers in nearby states who naturally wanted independence for the New Caledonian Kanaks, the problem seethed and was not assisted by the prejudices that the Region had against the French. Any dialogue that might have taken place, did not. The little that took place did not have the immediate desired effect. The sinking of the Rainbow Warrior did not help either.

The French were not receiving a favourable hearing at the Forum meetings for their plans for eventual independence for New Caledonia. A delegation headed by Mara went to Paris and came back with a plan which, though supported by the delegation, was unacceptable to the Melanesian Bloc. The difficulties of putting any plan into operation were receiving little consideration from Forum members who had no plan themselves for a way of doing it other than for the French to pack up and leave New Caledonia. This would likely have resulted in a blood bath with the Kanaks coming out of it very much the worse for wear. A Kanak blood bath of its own is not unlikely and the assassination of Jean-Marie Tjibaou, the leader of the largest Kanak political faction and the cave murders, are manifestations of this possibility.

The Melanesian contingency in the Forum were for more direct action and the attempt by some of them to form a regional peace keeping force was believed to be for this purpose. The move was not supported. Others of the Melanesian group, principally under the aegis of Vanuatu, were in contact with Libya to have terrorists do their stuff. Some were sent to Libya to learn terrorist methods. Whether or not the incidents where lives were lost were the direct result of these terrorist efforts never surfaced. As of the past year or so, the New Caledonia question seemed to settle for some months until the murder of Tjibaou by his own Kanak colleagues brought back the realisation that it will not be solved by simple decolonisation.

The dissatisfactions of the Melanesians with the handling of the New Caledonian question and other issues by the Forum has resulted in their forming a Melanesian Bloc of their own, but still remaining members of the Forum.

* * *

In French Polynesia there is always a group for independence but, so far they seem to be in the minority with only two members in a 42 member Parliament favouring immediate independence. It is doubtful that there will be, in the foreseeable future, any serious moves to break away from France. France has over the years worked towards a "free association" type of relationship with French Polynesia and for some years now it has been internally self-governing. The ease with which Caucasians mix with Polynesians, who are said to have some Caucasian origins themselves, makes the potential problem more difficult to arouse and easier to deal with when it raises its head.

The Polynesians of French Polynesia probably have a much stronger historical reason for wanting to be free of the French than do the Kanaks of New Caledonia, for the wars they fought against French domination, in the hope for a British Protectorate, were fierce and bloody.[5]1

We in the Cook Islands have a close family relationship with the Polynesians of all the main inhabited islands of French Polynesia. There are few Cook Islanders, especially those of the Southern Group, who do not have relatives in French Polynesia, from the Australs through the Society Islands, the Tuamotus to the Marquesas. The prejudices within the Forum towards the French included the Polynesians of French Polynesia and caused some embarrassment to us when we had to stand up and declare that they should receive the same courtesies that other indigenous inhabitants in the Pacific receive.

Because of our close familial relationship with the Polynesians of French Polynesia, we also have a workable relationship with the French and were able to arrange for scientists from New Zealand, Australia and Papua New Guinea to visit Mururoa, make on the spot tests for nuclear radiation and take biological and other samples away for more exacting tests. No samples showed a positive test for radiation. More recent investigations by Cousteau resulted in the same conclusions.

Forum members still hold the view that nuclear testing should be done elsewhere. There are claims that levels of radiation in water are high, but I know of no verified evidence of this. I find it irksome to be accused of being pro-nuclear because I am unable to find concrete evidence to fight the problem. I have openly declared that I will fight if the evidence is there to support it. The promise of such evidence from as far away as the Marshall Islands and as close as Tahiti and my own country has never eventuated. That declaration is still in effect. To join the rank of protesters supported only by a strong emotional content, is not my style. I am not unaware of the dangers.

Promises of safety with no future problems developing in past nuclear testing for military purposes have proved false. On that basis alone we have reason not to believe what is now promised and assured especially in testing for destructive military purposes. Similar promises have been made with regard to nuclear energy for peaceful purposes. Europe in large measure, up to eighty percent, is dependent on nuclear energy for power. The Chernobyl accident, as others that have occurred before it, warns us of the possibilities. In other respects it has admirable characteristics: it causes no pollution, it produces a small quantity of waste for the amount of energy it gives out, and, important for the future, it frees countries from dependency on oil producing states. These are only some of its good features.

Tragic as they have been, past accidents have taught us lessons how to manage nuclear energy. We are able to absorb road accidents at the rate of near

60,000 per annum for the US alone. This is a far greater rate per population than all the nuclear accident deaths put on the same basis of populations deriving benefit from it.

The oft-quoted assertion that the island of Mururoa is breaking up has not held up so far. It has been said that it might bother us in about 500 years from now. During an underground nuclear explosion, the intense heat generated turns the surrounding matter into solid glass which is said to prevent the escape of radiation. The evidence so far suggests that the nuclear tests are not producing higher levels of radiation than background.

The US/UK nuclear tests on Christmas Island increased radiation levels in the Cook Islands significantly, the French atmospheric tests were barely perceptible above background here, and the French underground tests not at all. Nevertheless, we should be aware that there are dangers. How one deals with this question until after the event is the question, but I do not believe we need to panic.

I personally deplore nuclear testing or dumping of nuclear wastes in our region, but in the absence of concrete evidence, there is little anyone can do except complain and that is all that anybody, including myself, has done to date. Only with concrete evidence can the matter be taken further.

* * *

Besides the South Pacific Forum, the South Pacific has been blessed with a number of organisations formed from outside and from within the region. The South Pacific Commission (SPC) was the first, having been formed in 1947 on the model of the existing Caribbean Commission. It held its first meeting in Fiji in 1950. Australia, under the leadership of William D. Forsyth, was its prime instigator supported willingly by New Zealand. They were able to obtain the co-operation of the United Kingdom, the United States and the Netherlands without difficulty. Obtaining the co-operation of the French was more difficult. It was finally settled on the basis that the headquarters would be situated in Noumea, New Caledonia. It will be recognised that these six countries had colonies in the Pacific. The Netherlands, having no further interests in the Pacific, once it withdrew from West New Guinea in 1962, is now out of the picture.

The purpose of SPC was to assist the dependent island territories of the Pacific Basin in the development of the economic, social and health elements in their societies. Political development was not included because, although four of the member countries favoured it, two refused, so the future independence of these territories was not considered at that time.

Makea Nui Teremoana Ariki, Albert Henry and I, as three of several of the members of the delegation from the Cook Islands, attended its first South Pacific Conference at Nasinu, Fiji, in 1950. Out of all the delegations from the Pacific Islands, the King of Tonga, Malietoa (the present Head of State of Samoa), Robert Rex (the Premier of Niue), Makea Nui Teremoana Ariki and myself are now the only five surviving members who attended that meeting.

Even though it has tended to reflect the views and wishes of its sponsors rather than its member South Pacific Islands States, the organisation has served the Pacific Islands well over these many years, The SPC technical assistance to the islands states has been of value.

The combination of solutions to the combination of problems were to be dealt with as the sponsoring nations saw them. Some of these did not fit the ideas of elected and traditional leaders of the Pacific and there is still dissatisfaction with SPC on this basis. The fact that our economic problems continued in the same old way with the same bottlenecks of transportation, markets and production, seems to support this dissatisfaction. SPC has not done badly in health, but we are still muddling along in matters pertaining to our economic development.

The South Pacific Forum was formed in part because there was a natural need for such a body and in part because of the dissatisfactions that the SPC was not fulfilling its role the way the leaders of the newly independent Pacific Islands States thought it should. In practice the Forum has become an organisation more concerned with the political affairs of the region and has not replaced or supplemented the role of the SPC.

For many years now, a Single Regional Organisation, SRO, has been proposed to include the SPC and SPREP (South Pacific Regional Environment Programme) and others to come under the control of the South Pacific Forum. This proposal has been put before the Forum on several occasions with only lukewarm reception from the majority of its members. A compromise has now been reached whereby the institutions remain separate, but their heads meet once a year to co-ordinate plans and avoid duplication.

Another organisation which came out of the Pacific Islands Conference held in Honolulu in 1980 is called the PIDP (Pacific Islands Development Programme). Unlike the Forum, which had a membership limited mainly to the island states which were independent enough to make on the spot decisions without reference to a metropolitan authority, it included all Pacific Islands groups from the width and breadth of the Pacific Basin. It too was to supplement or overcome the real or imagined shortcomings of the SPC. Although it went off with a good start with every leader expressing the needs of his country as he saw it and with a programme drawn up to meet these expressed needs, it has now, like the SPC, come under the spell of a sponsor, the East-West Center in Hawaii, which now directs what it believes is best for the Pacific countries.

If we include other organisations which the Pacific Islands States have formed, or aligned with, we can include CCOP-SOPAC (for mineral development), SPTC (for tourism development), ESCAP (for economic and social development), LOME (for development cooperation with Europe), the arms of the United Nations and many more. This constant probing for ways to meet our problems indicates that the Islands States do not clearly perceive and define problems and, when we do, we are unable to come up with our own solutions. But neither is anybody else. Therefore, I was more than ever resolved to find our own solutions to Cook Islands problems. They could not be worse or less effective than those offered us by others.

Since Pacific Islands States achieved independence, our political development has not been good. At the beginning when it was all new, we felt our way gingerly and behaved ourselves. In the past five to ten years, politicians have taken advantage of the loopholes in our constitutions, as well as whatever we can get away with in other ways, to disregard democratic principles.

The reversion of Fiji into a government not elected by the people is considered by others to be a backward step and it probably is. Although the Westminster type of government that it had for seventeen years may have been a facade to some extent, it was probably a step in the right direction. One cannot disenfranchise a minority in a society without trouble, but to effectively disenfranchise more than fifty percent of the population is to ask for a great deal of trouble which will not lie down easily.

* * *

In the Cook Islands, The CIP government that won the elections in January 1989 has improved its position from a tenuous 12 to 13 seats in a 24 seat parliament making conditions for threatening moves to upset the stability of government less tenable.

As might be expected many of the features indicative of a controlled economy that existed before 1978 and were neutralised during my administration have returned since the cessation of my administration in 1987. The reversion gathered pace under Dr Pupuke Robati's administration, and its effect on the economy is now apparent. Exports dropped to pre 1978 in 1989. Tourism arrivals have declined, there is a drop of 10 percent in the number of businesses. and gross retail sales (on which turnover tax is derived) have considerably reduced.

The Prime Minister, Geoffrey Henry, has publicly stated that there is a financial crisis. During the relatively affluent years up to 1987, our people made financial commitments with regard to improving their standard of living in many ways. These are becoming more and more difficult to meet.

Members of Parliament believe that what being in office allows them to do, makes it legal for them to do what amounts to a breach of the public trust vested in them. The Prime Minister of the Government which took over from me has allocated ownership of public property to himself. Geoffrey Henry, the present incumbent, has gone one better by using government funds to rebuild his wife's ancestral home.

Votes of no confidence have become a game played in most islands states. Loyalty to oath or principle or party has diminished, even Governors General join in the fray, quite out of line with the spirit of our respective constitutions and to the traditional understanding of their role. If a government is bad, it is not too long to wait for the next general elections in order to change it. A Head of State should do his level best to see that a government completes its term of office except in the most extreme circumstances. After all, it was the people's choice and he should use his influence to insure the stability of that government. The changes being made midterm throughout the region have little to do with obtaining a better government or promoting the principles of democracy. They are crude bids for power by those who were not voted into it, exploiting the unfamiliarity of constituencies with the democratic process, and the susceptibility of politicians and aspiring politicians to temptations of personal gain.

* * *

The cold war between the West and East that has its central confrontation at the line running approximately north/south between East and West Berlin, became our cold war also. The Pacific is the no man's land between the back door of Eastern ideology and the backdoor of Western ideology, the United States of America. The massive fixed armamentarium that guards the Eastern front door of the West has its equivalent in a massive floating force ranging the Pacific ocean with fixed bases to complement it. The United States of America and the Soviet Union operate freely in the no-man's-land that is the Pacific. Similar naval and fixed forces from both sides do the same thing in the Indian Ocean, keeping an eye on the under-belly of the Asian continent.

The force protecting the back door of Western ideology is supplied by the United States with perfunctory assistance from Australia, New Zealand and now Japan. The countries of the Pacific and its Western rim are not as up tight as the United States is about the Eastern ideologic threat. The Pacific Island states are no more than the grass that grows in this common no-man's-land and, if the elephants choose to fight in it, they will trample the grass as if it had no meaning at all. Any Pacific Islands state which thinks otherwise lacks understanding of how insignificant a part they play in this confrontation and potential open conflict of these or other Titans.

The two main actors in this drama believe in their individual ideologic causes to the extent they are armed to the teeth with megatons of nuclear weapons. In the light of what we know about what one megaton equivalent did as a result of the Chernobyl accident, this is unreasonable. The situation is not new. Montesquieu said over 200 years ago:

"A new disease is spreading over Europe; it has seized upon our princes and induces them to maintain an inordinate number of soldiers. The disease is attended by complications and it inevitably becomes contagious; for, as soon as one state increases what it calls its forces, the others immediately increase theirs; so that nothing is gained except mutual ruination."

Elsewhere he prophetically says:

"Ever since the invention of gunpowder...I continually tremble in case men should, in the end, uncover some secret which would provide a short way of abolishing mankind, of annihilating peoples and nations in their entirety."

Since we passive actors in the Pacific are as likely to be hurt as badly as other minor actors, we should do something positive about it. What are the possibilities and the options and alternatives? What we do best is not notice it, or not make it our business and do nothing about it, which is our usual response.

We could take sides, but our understanding of the ideologies involved alone does not allow us to make an easy decision. But in practice we can weigh the historically recorded benefits to those who have made such choices in the past. There are historical walls restricting freedom on the one side and substantial historical freedom and personal economic benefits on the other. So many people are trying to escape the controlled systems that there are arms, soldiers, walls, passes and other devices to prevent them.

We could play one side against the other. This is a dangerous game and history does not record many long-term successes in this approach. To hope for success by this route, one must be at least nearly as strong as the opponents being played one against the other.

Another choice concerns the activities of Mr Mikhail Gorbachev to move the Soviet Union to a free market system. As he chose to consult me personally on this move through his ambassador Mr Vladimir Bykov in 1986, I admit to having a personal interest in Mr Gorbachev's second "Russian revolution" as he referred to it. I must, however, confess that my interest, besides seeing it as a benefit to the peoples of the Soviet bloc, lies in the role of the free market system in the promotion of world peace. In my opinion such a move would be a significant step in the right direction.

This option that could deal with the question of our unwitting involvement in being a no-man's-land and possibly again a battle field for other people's disputes. That the leader of one side has made a public commitment which could bring the confrontation to an end is important to Pacific Islanders. Through his proposed internal economic reform policies, Gorbachev could bring his country into trade partnership with the West in a world which needs all the help it can to overcome its social, economic and political woes and meet the coming millennium with a clearer understanding of where we are going. Such a partnership could end the confrontation. The best defence for us Pacific islanders, being few in number and scattered over a large ocean we cannot defend, is peace. Any alternative could mean extinction.

New Zealand, by the annual displays of its tiny military force among us, Australia by its offer of patrol boats, USA with its wish for us to approve of visits of nuclear vessels and USSR with its offers of aid and wish for deeper involvement on a range of fronts, all seek our approval to sanction our front yard as a potential battlefield to settle their ideological and other disputes. But if the Soviet Union joins the fraternity of trade as did Japan and Germany after World War 11, we could save ourselves from another trampling.

Gorbachev's plan is not unanticipated. Kruschev considered it and it makes too much sense for it not to have been contemplated by a significant number of people in the Soviet Union. It needed one Soviet leader who believed in it enough to do something about it. As Mr Bykov stated to me, the plan is to introduce a free market economic system similar to the principles we were following in the Cook Islands. The free market system in the West today bears little similarity to the harsh cruel capitalistic system which Karl Marx, Engels and Lenin experienced and which influenced the development of the socio-economic system of the Soviet Union. It is an outmoded system which must be replaced. The sooner the better for everybody, including us Pacific Islanders.

In my little involvement in his plan, I have seriously tried to assess whether it is a clever ploy to split NATO which has stood together at great cost for nearly fifty years, as some have claimed. I doubted it because that would hardly be worth the unpopularity the plan might cause Gorbachev at home.

The problem of implementing the plan is due to the unfamiliarity of the administrators of the Soviet bloc with this strange thing called freedom. The force that motivates such a move, once started, is powerful. But there must be decentralisation of political power as well as a development of political freedom, for a free market economic system would be difficult, if not impossible, in a highly centralised and controlled political system.

If Gorbachev's plan succeeds, the cause of world harmony will have taken a quantum jump. But it could cause the Western economy serious problems which would impact on us in the Pacific. The obvious one concerns the redundancy of the military deterrent forces which has increased to unrealistic proportions, and of the industries that have burgeoned around them. New employment opportunities take time. The need for military forces and the industries supporting them would largely disappear, provided that the Arabs, the Indonesians and others can be persuaded to reduce their forces at the same time.

If the Soviet Union enters the world market as Germany and Japan did after World War 11, it could cause havoc, unless appropriate adjustments are made. A positive effort to move the Third World from their present stifling economic systems would increase their demand for goods as well as their ability to supply goods and services. That they will be competitors with developed countries is probably much less of a threat than that they will continue to increase in population and dependency and be the places from which discontent and strife will emanate if they do not develop. Fears of this nature are often based on a natural tendency to assess the future on the assumption that what exists will remain static. This will not be the case. If the Soviet politico-economic plan achieves its objectives, the world will never be the same again. Other control economies, which have much to do with their being classified as Third World states, will sooner or later follow suit.

This is not to say that the free market system is a panacea for the woes that beset the world. Far from it. Some will choose to stand and watch it all go by and others will not be able to perform in it for one reason or another. Nevertheless, it gives the greatest opportunity for as many of even these to find a comfortable niche in the system. For those who cannot, the system is profitable enough to accept the burden for their basic care and assistance.

The success of this basic care and assistance is the responsibility of governments and the keepers of our consciences, the religions. Both need a great deal of upgrading of attitudes and philosophies to face the modern world and understand its needs more adequately. The path open to us for our materialistic needs is full of pitfalls and temptations. It is the price of our social, economic and political freedoms. Only the quality of our ethical and moral standards and our spiritual consciences can smooth the way of our going.

One would think we had enough regional troubles without dreaming up new ones. The warming of the Earth and the inundation of our coral atolls and other low lying land areas through the Greenhouse Effect is one that we can do without. Do without it we probably will. The theory upon which predictions that the ocean level will rise about 1.4 metres by the end of the next century would seem to have some flaws. There are arguments and one 58 year set of temperature observations which tend to discount the prediction that there is a serious warming taking place and that, if the ocean level was raised to the extent stated, the atolls would become inhabitable.

Much of the information upon which the predictions of a warming and inundation of atolls and other low altitude places is based, is suspect and scientists have divergent views on it. We will confine our interest to such bottom line questions as, "Is the earth warming?" "Will it raise the ocean level at the rate of 1.4 centimetres per annum?" "Can the atolls survive if this should happen?"

In the popular media, I find only predictions. Some of them probably could not stand up to the light of serious scientific scrutiny. The claim that the atolls will be submerged is one of these. The atolls are in the main formed by the prolific coral polyp in association with the storms which deposit coral rocks and rubble on the coral reefs so formed. Coral growth stops just below the mean tidal level at which point it grows sideways. As soon as the ocean level moves permanently up the 1.4 centimetres per annum predicted, coral growth will follow it.

As a result of storms and hurricanes, coral debris will be deposited on the new coral growth and the atoll will keep pace with the rising ocean level. During my youth, the area where the wreck of the Yankee sits was a shallow lagoon, full of live coral. When I returned sixteen years later, it was as it is now, a solid sheet of dead coral, strewn with coral boulders and debris. It is that way only because it had reached the upper limit of its growth, the mean ocean level. Few remembered it the way it was.

This also takes place on the high volcanic islands and coral fringes. This was clearly demonstrated during Hurricane Sally in January 1987 when Rarotonga's land mass was increased significantly. Instead of being endangered by the predicted rise in sea level, the coral islands could become havens of refuge for those threatened on the non-coral lands of temperate and cold climates where the coral polyp does not grow. However, we can offer standing room only. If the predictors are wrong in this instance, are they right in their other assumptions?

The use of fossil fuels has been going on for a long time, therefore, the warming of the earth should have been taking place for a long time. Moreover, the warming effects ascribed to it could be lessening as the industrial nations have converted in large part to nuclear power. However, to some extent this is being offset by developing nations increasing their use of fossil fuels.

This rise in ocean level is also ascribed to the expansion of the ocean due to the rise in temperature which is still debated. All predictions are based on a considerable rise in atmospheric and ocean temperature, as high as 10 degrees

Celsius. The reasons for the predicted rise have been around for a long time and this includes the Ozone Hole, because the time of its discovery is not necessarily the time of its creation. That the hole can be favourable only to the proposition that heat gain through it will raise the atmospheric temperature, ignores the fact that there is heat loss through it to the absolute zero of space (-273.15 Celsius) during the dark hours about equal to that gained during the sunshine hours.

Long term temperature measurements of the air should give us some clues as to what is actually taking place and to verify the predictions. Since Rarotonga has air temperature records for the past 58 years, I examined the information and found a mathematical trend increase of near to 0.5 Celsius over that period. I subjected the data to the mathematical test of the probability that this trend was not due to chance alone. This mathematical test depends almost entirely on the degree of variability of the data. If there were no variability, there would be no need for such a test. A probability level of greater than 20 to 1 was taken as the cut off point.

The calculations resulted in a probability of 50 to 1 that the trend seen over the period of 58 years was not due to chance alone. Therefore, there is a temperature change taking place, but its rate, at less than 0.01 Celsius per annum, is both small and slow enough for a great deal of compensatory changes to take place. Shorelines are well known for dynamic changes in their configurations. To make long term predictions about them as though a rise of ocean level had taken place suddenly, is unacceptable. It takes 3000 cubic centimetres of air raised one degree to raise one cubic centimetre of water one degree. It will take a long time for the oceans to be raised in temperature to the extent where its expansion will be of significance.

The data from this one location may be insufficient to make a firm conclusion. Observations from other locations need to be examined and mathematically tested for probability that any changes observed were not due to chance alone. This will go a long way towards the reality of what is now no more than assumptions.

I believe there is no immediate cause for alarm and the coral growth of the coral islands will keep them safe from the dire predictions that they will disappear below the sea.

CHAPTER TWENTY-ONE

Hurricane

Blow, blow thou winter wind,

Thou art not so unkind

As man's ingratitude. WILLIAM SHAKESPEARE

The year 1987 was the Year of hurricane Sally. Hurricane is the word we use for cyclone. It is the same thing. For me it was not the only hurricane of 1987.

Hurricanes that come our way become recognisable as a threat at about 8 degrees south of the Equator at about Longitude 170 degrees to 180 degrees west, near enough to the date-line. The co-ordinates lie in the triangle made by lines connecting Kiribati, the Phoenix Islands and Tuvalu, about 1300 nautical miles north-west of Rarotonga. Near the classical path they usually take, they pass the Samoas and Tokelau, heading directly for Palmerston Island which gets the brunt of most of our hurricanes. Polynesians avoided inhabiting it for that reason.

It took an Englishman, a Captain William Marsters, to inhabit it with progeny from his Penrhyn wife and her two sisters. There are now literally thousands of Marsters, but the population of the atoll during my lifetime, before and no doubt in the future, has not often exceeded 70 nor been less than 60. It was 66 when I was first there in 1946, it was 66 when I was last there in 1983 and there is no reason to believe that it is not 66 at this moment. The three families from the three original mothers are jealously strict about their boundaries and their rights. There must be three of everything. How they regulate the numbers who remain on the island and leave it is a mystery. They are great sailors and generally do everything well that they put their hands and minds to. They can be found in every corner of the world.

On their way to us, hurricanes can, but may not, do damage to the Samoas or to Tokelau, but generally they do not intensify until they pass them. When they slow down and playfully jiggle around doing side steps and circles in one place, they usually build up strength. When they continue on their course they intensify some more. Auntie Sally, as she became known to us, did some of these things as she headed inexorably towards Rarotonga. Once she made up her mind to head in our direction, after she had done a couple of pirouettes, she did so leisurely, but in a beeline. High waves came to us straight from her centre from the north-west while the wind came directly from the north-east. They never wavered from this pattern, both indicating that her centre was coming directly for Rarotonga.

From the beginning the seas were high, but they became even higher. They crashed on the north-west coast in huge evenly formed waves which started to lift their crests high above the horizon well out to sea. From there they crested in rows one behind the other becoming steeper and steeper as they rushed in with their tops and fronts curling over more and more until they crashed and seethed in over the reef, tumbling and spurting jets of white water high in the air. They defied the wind cutting across their awe-inspiring, foaming tops.

While watching the waves, I was grateful for the reef that encircled Rarotonga for it visibly tamed these monsters. Where the waves marched towards the reef in awesome manner, their crests reaching high into the sky, they flattened to low tumbling foaming masses hissing wildly in frustration as they headed for the shore. Above the noise of their coming, one could hear the rumbling, rattling sounds made by the rolling, tumbling coral rocks, broken away from their moorings, being driven shorewards.

Even before the release of satellite weather reports, we were aware of Sally's coming four or five days before she hit us with all her wrath of wind and sea made worse by high tides. She started to affect us the day before New Year's eve, more with high seas created at the fiercely whirling centre than with winds which at that time were around 30 Knots. This wind crossing the waves at right angles made no visible waves of its own and, if it did, they were insignificant to the monstrous ones coming directly from the centre.

Waves spawned by a hurricane's centre travel at speeds around three to five times faster than the speed of movement of the hurricane itself. Therefore, they arrive at destinations in which the hurricane is travelling well before it does. In the southern hemisphere, the winds of a cyclone circle the centre in a clockwise direction. At any time the direction of the centre can be determined by facing the wind and stretching one's left arm directly out at right angles to the direction one is facing. The direction in which the outstretched arm is pointing is the direction of the centre. If this is repeated at intervals, the movements of the hurricane can be ascertained. In the Northern Hemisphere it is exactly the opposite. In Sally's case, she never deviated from her seemingly designed purpose of assaulting Rarotonga with all the violence she could muster.

Some said it was the worst hurricane since 1968. Others said it was the worst we have ever had in recorded history. Our 50 years of statistics on hurricanes say that we have never had a hurricane before December nor one after March, we have a significant one every 10 years and a really bad one every 20 years. Give or take a little, Sally was on schedule. It amused me to see the insurance companies put their premiums up and become reluctant to sell hurricane insurance immediately after Sally. This was the time to do the opposite because premiums are going to be coming in for about twenty years with no damage from hurricanes to speak of or pay out on.

At this time the wind conditions were not intrusive and many people I noticed were, like me, fascinated with the play of the big waves coming almost directly into Avarua, finally dissipating themselves almost at our feet as we stood on the banks of the foreshore, level with the main road. They were not as yet doing serious damage. On the opposite and lee side of the island, the reef and lagoon offered an aspect no different from that of a normal day. In fact there were people fishing in the lagoon and on the reef as though nothing abnormal was taking place.

They were not the only ones enjoying a day on the reef. Back in Avarua, the children of all ages from 5 or 6 years to 15 or 16 years of age were having the time of their lives surfing the big ones. Although we used to do the same in my childhood, I felt some apprehension for their safety, but not nearly as much as was being demonstrated by visitors to the island. They called the police who came, nodded their heads, said a profound word or two and left. We tried to assure the strangers that the kids knew what they were doing and would not get into trouble if they were not interfered with. This was hard for them to accept. The looks of concern never left their faces.

I also noted how the children picked the areas where there was no current or condition that might cause them difficulties. By this means, and over the years of growing up with "children's waves" every summer, the children would gain a knowledge of the forces of the sea and surf and be always able to handle them. This might explain why we have had only one loss of life recorded in a hurricane, and that was a European who was trying to save some agricultural records during the hurricane of 1935. On the evening when the worst of the storm was starting, I watched the children with renewed interest, surfing on the waves coming around the breakwater of Avatiu harbour.

The next day, the seas built up and so did the wind, both always from their own respective directions. The wind was now screaming. In Avarua the seas were gnawing at the waterfront, eroding it away up to the pavement of the road and taking away some of that too. The seaside park was under water and suffering from the sweep and backwash of the waves. At high tide, the seas were coming over the road and bringing with them the coral rocks that they had torn from the floor of the ocean beyond the reef. They rolled them over the reef and were now depositing them on the road, across the road, in front of the business buildings and, in many places, through the buildings into the backyards.

I have watched this build up of land in hurricanes and storms many times and am amazed when the "Greenhouse Effect" scientists predict that the atolls will be the first to be inundated. Instead they will grow from coral rocks and rubble brought ashore as well as from the upward growth of the prolific coral.

Public Works and people with appropriate machinery were out in force and were keeping roads clear while linesmen kept the wires for power and telephones in operating order when opportunity afforded. They kept this up during and after the hurricane, keeping communications open without let up. Happily they were helped and relieved by linesmen from Tahiti and New Zealand who flew in as soon as they were able.

Fortunately, none of the large boats from overseas nor the inter-island freighters were in port before the onset of the hurricane, being safely elsewhere at the time. The small fishing boats in Avatiu and Avarua harbours were, as was the practice, lifted out by cranes. Nearly all the small boats had been towed away on their trailers by their owners. The Torea was already in her cradle on the wharf before the hurricane. No one believed that she would not be safe there. But a huge wave came into the harbour, rose high over her and crushed her beyond repair. The same thing happened to the brand new restaurant, Trader Jack's. An eye witness described its demolition by a wave curling over the top of it and thundering down on it. The same wave demolished the building immediately behind Trader Jack's. There were two boats still in Avatiu harbour moored by several lines to various points on the surrounding piers. One of them was the government fishing boat, the 55 foot Ravakai, and the other was a yacht of around 30 feet being single-handed around the world.

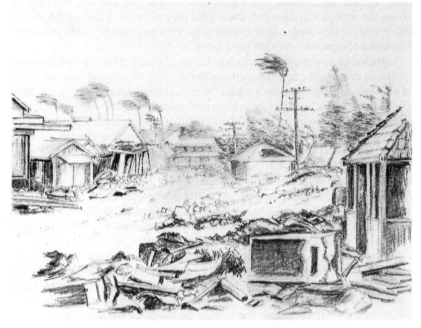

Both chose to take their chances in the harbour and it was not a bad choice, if a series of events had not taken place through the inexperience and carelessness of the officials in charge of the harbour and other matters of a marine nature that came under their sphere of responsibility. It was not the first time they had neglected their duties and absented themselves during emergencies. Fishermen were occasionally in trouble with motors which give out on them and often storms come up from the north causing vessels in the harbour problems necessitating their help. These officials are to my knowledge never available at these times. They also disappear with the keys to the repository of equipment needed on such occasions. It was no different on this occasion. The last time I looked, the two vessels and their respective crews were riding comfortably in the harbour where there were no breaking waves to bother them.

During the night of the worst part of the storm, the unsecured barge onshore at the water's edge floated into the harbour and played havoc with the mooring lines of the two vessels, holing them in the process. It was only with great difficulty that the crews managed to save themselves.

The high seas and the high tide flooded the area around the Administration block and the Banana Court with surges moving into depths between ankle and knee to waist deep. The low areas behind the business centre were under water and families in homes in the area were evacuated. The Earth Satellite Station looked like a floating island.

We were always well prepared for hurricanes and, every November, people were informed through the press and radio of the precautions that needed to be taken and what to have on hand to protect property and themselves. Inundations and de-roofings were standard damage to homes. Places of refuge were designated for people and families requiring them. These were usually church or community halls. People in different areas were told which ones were designated for their use.

Homes on the shore side of the residential area to the west of Avarua were inundated by the seas and packed with coral rocks and sand carried in by them. However, damage was miraculously minimal although a great deal of excavation was needed to bring these homes into full view again.

The outlets of the drainage systems in the north-west, the north and north-east shores were blocked with coral rocks and sand. Fortunately this was one of the few hurricanes which was not accompanied by heavy rain. However, it is possible that, if it had rained more, the flow of water would have kept the offshore debris from accumulating in the drains the way it did. Trees were being undermined and uprooted one after the other. Their foliage was stripped and many of the hardy ironwood trees had no greenery left on them.

* * *

On the third day, during a night when high tide was around midnight, Sally caused most of the problems after which her centre passed over Rarotonga. It was around mid-morning when the noisy turmoil that goes with a hurricane ceased. There was a sudden hush. The silence was damply oppressive. It was unnatural. The leaves left on the trees hung limp, especially the coconut leaves which were broken, split and bedraggled. The fallen debris, which had been on the move constantly, lay about in a sad, still and sodden state. In Avarua, the seas continued to surge over the road which now seemed constantly under water. The harbour facilities were under water with the cargo sheds showing their insides, now bereft of the cargo previously stowed in them. The area was littered with the debris of damaged goods. The centre of a hurricane is an area of raised water level caused by the low pressure in it and this, combined with high tides, raises the sea level to abnormal heights.

In the belief it was all over, people came out to take in the sights. They wandered around downtown examining the damage and picking up damaged goods on the way. The youth were in great prominence and, for most of them, this was their first bad hurricane. They were obviously enjoying the experience as were most people. Hurricanes are a break from the humdrum of life. It is exciting and, rather than causing apprehension, it seemed to have the opposite effect. It was new, different and exhilarating. At least that is the way we appear to see it and I was reminded of my first hurricane when I was about 9 years of age. No one nor the possibility of punishment could have kept me home. I walked to Avarua during the height of the hurricane and had a wonderful and exciting day that I will always remember. Nobody seems to worry unduly about the damage hurricanes cause. There is enough time later for that. Its all part of life. This was coming out in the breathless stillness of the "eye" of Hurricane Sally. The visitors, or most of them, joined in this spirit of 'not to worry'.

Through the clouds high above, patches of blue sky showed and the sun shone on the still and silent scene of unbelievable debris and desolation made up of uprooted trees, coral rocks, bits of wood from demolished structures, sheets of roofing iron, some wrapped tightly around trees and posts. Only the moderate hiss of the surges from the ocean rippling through this conglomerated mess, the crackle of a motor cycle wading its way through the debris, and the sudden outburst of giggles and laughter from wandering bands of children and teenagers broke the silence.

At home, my wife, Pa, who also thought it was all over, asked me to help her start the cleanup. I did not want to do two cleanups, but it took some convincing that it was not over and that the wind would be coming in from the west and the south-west at an even greater velocity than we had so far experienced. And it did.

After about four hours of this unearthly silence, seemingly without warning, Sally made her second coming known. We were at home and I again made sure that enough windows were open. This is always necessary because the natural reaction of people is to close everything up tight. It is the surest way of causing damage to a building. The negative pressure created outside buildings by the passing of a high velocity wind is so great that, if the high relative pressure within a building cannot be relieved, the building literally explodes or, at the very least, loses a window or so or a roof as well.

We had sent the house girl home to take care of her own hurricane problems, so Pa and I settled down to await Sally's second coming. When it came, we had only a few moments to appreciate that the onslaught was on its way.

The wind came with a crashing, throbbing rush down the slope of the hill behind our house, rattling the trees violently as it came. It had come over the steep slopes of the 2000 feet peaks of Te Manga and Te Atukura and its ridges, rushing down at our house in a fury. These were not enough to weaken its onslaught. The noise of its coming was awesome and, almost as soon as we heard it, it struck the house with a sickening violence. I was pleased that I had designed my house to withstand such violence, but, for a tangible moment or two, I doubted that I had really achieved that purpose. Anyway there was nothing to be done but wait it out.

* * *

My thoughts went to the people on the west side of the Island, because, if on the lee side we were getting what we were experiencing, they must be getting it in far heavier doses. I made a note to visit them as soon as conditions allowed. Up to now that side of the island had escaped the brunt of Sally's power.

At home, apart from the screeching of the wind and the slapping rattle of the remaining foliage, the bangings coming from the roof was the only other noise and that was not very welcome because it could mean a lot of things, none of them comforting. It later turned out to be a couple of loose roof tiles flapping in the wind. It was the only damage.

In passing over Rarotonga, Sally deposited more rocks on the properties near the north-eastern foreshore and caused damage to residences situated there. The football field of Matavera Village was strewn with coral rocks of all sizes. By early next morning, the worst was over.

In this second coming, the winds came from the opposite direction to that before the arrival of the centre. this second wind of hurricanes is stronger, for its strength is now often aided by the speed of movement of the hurricane itself. So after the centre passed, the west side of the island, which had escaped damage during the first part of the hurricane, received the brunt of these much more violent winds. Where there were any weaknesses, they showed themselves. Roofs came off and sheets of iron and aluminium roofing became hazardous missiles, flying through the air and brought to a stop only when they hit an obstacle around which they became firmly wrapped like passionate lovers.

Trees in the village of Arorangi which had withstood the force of previous hurricanes for a century or two, were ripped from the ground. Those which did not suffer this indignity, had their limbs torn away and flung carelessly down wind. Most of the tourist accommodation is in this area and, except for the removal of a couple of roofs at the Edgewater Resort Hotel, accommodation here and in other parts of the island suffered little or no damage. This did not prevent one of our officious officials in the Cook Islands Consulate in New Zealand advising tourists not to travel to Rarotonga. It was a costly action by someone taking advantage of a situation to appear important.

After it was all over, we examined the damage, the rubble of rocks, the debris and the uprooted trees, to assess what was needed to clean up the mess. The leaders, traditional, appointed and elected, were there to organise and supervise the cleanup in their respective areas. Traditional leaders always do community efforts of this kind well. My apolitical working committee in my constituency had the matter quickly in hand although there were difficulties in the sharing of available machinery to assist in getting the job done.

* * *

Throughout the nine years of my administration I had kept good diplomatic relations with the countries of the Pacific and beyond. Whatever differences they had with each other, I avoided taking sides and I made it clear that this was my policy. In the battles between the countries, I tried to see both sides of the problem and, if requested, I did my best to bring these to some mutual understanding. However, many of the reasons causing these rifts tended to reach emotional proportions and logic was not often accepted as playing any role in resolving them.

At the beginning of my administration, many of the Pacific countries had very little time for the metropolitan countries. In addition, New Zealand and Australia played a game of one upmanship with each other on many issues. Malcolm Fraser was a strong right winger while Robert Muldoon, head of the conservatives in New Zealand, paradoxically, was socialistic in many of his views. This created some real opposing views in the Forum. As already mentioned, the French and the United States were considered beyond the pale.

My stance of disregarding these international feelings and treating with all in a manner suitable to the occasion and the subject in question seemed to have paid off, for, after Hurricane Sally, assistance poured in from these countries. But it was more than that. The people, who had now achieved a state of relative affluence, became tourists themselves in their own particular way. Our people do not believe in doing most things unless there is a purpose. They reverted to the traditional way they toured in ancient days and that was as a group and for a purpose.

The purpose then was a little different in that it was to renew family bonds and arrange suitable marriages to widen the genetic pool, to eat their hosts out of house and home and generally to have a whale of a time. Where appropriate, as when touring New Zealand and Australia where Cook Islanders reside, these purposes are present in modern form. The eating is still there, but the purpose of travel to new countries is to challenge the hosts in sporting events in many cases and, in some, they went on a tour to entertain. On more rare occasions, it was no more than to see the world and have a good time. These groups are ambassadors extraordinary in all cases and have made friends for the Cook Islands everywhere in the world they go. So it was not surprising that when the World heard of our problems with Auntie Sally, it responded with the extraordinary generosity of friends and not just strangers helping someone out.

* * *

The French Foreign Legion, linesmen and private Tahitian groups were the first to arrive. The Government of French Polynesia, on their own volition and with the blessing of Prime Minister Jacques Chirac, came by a beach landing craft disgorging directly on to the land, bull-dozers, front-end loaders, several trucks, chain saws, ropes, chains and all the paraphernalia one could think of that would aid the clean up. President Gaston Flosse flew in personally to see that everything arrived and was off-loaded safely.

They also came by planes with light gear and people who knew how to use them. In the El Nino period of 1982 and 1983, French Polynesia, usually an area free of hurricanes, suffered five bad hurricanes. Some atolls were nearly wiped out of existence. Tahiti also suffered extensive damage.

Therefore, our nearest neighbour was well versed in what was needed to clean up the effects of a hurricane. These groups with their machinery combined with our people with our machinery to do the clean up. In one day the roads were fully cleared. Uprooted trees and those severely damaged were removed and piled in available open spaces outside the villages. In two days electric power and communications were fully restored to all areas. Gangs of carpenters made temporary and permanent repairs making damaged homes and buildings livable. On the third day the business area was back in full swing. Thereafter, those who came to Rarotonga, could not believe the veracity of the reports that Rarotonga and especially the capital, Avarua, had suffered serious damage.

New Zealand came in a Hercules air freighter with more linesmen, materials, chain saws, food and clothing accompanied by the Minister of Police. Canada and Australia sent money while the UK gave a significantly generous donation to be used in kind for whatever was needed. The Japanese came with donations and engineers to assist us in planning the protection of our capital from future assaults by hurricanes. Later they offered assistance to renovate and improve the waterfront and the roading system to assist the traffic problem which had reached undue proportions and promised to become a greater problem. They also later agreed to pay for the extension of our airport.

Auntie Sally, by wreaking the havoc it did, gave us the opportunity not only to repair the damage, but also to improve our capital and make it a more worthy place for this purpose. I had voiced this in conversations with Gaston Flosse and to New Zealand officials, both of whom had indicated a similar interest. The French had asked what finances we needed to improve Avarua. We discussed how such a plan could be put into effect. New Zealand came up with a plan to upgrade the Government Centre. This included the renovation of the original government building which was now hardly recognisable because of the additions of lean-to annexes in a most haphazard manner.

These shanty lean-tos had swallowed up the original government building. However, it was still there intact and, if the numerous additions were removed, the original building would require little work to bring it back to its original glory. It was a structure of architectural charm and full of Cook Islands history. To accommodate the staff occupying the lean-tos, the New Zealand proposal was to build a three storey structure. The first storey was to be left open for parking. The New Zealand plan was to include the upgrading of the now opened area including the unused Avarua harbour wharf area into a sizeable market and gardens overlooking a marina for which there already were private bids. It was a beautiful plan.

The French Plan we worked out together was to cost NZ15 million dollars. $9M was to go towards new commercial buildings to be built on government property on the main road of the Avarua business district. Before Hurricane Sally there was a shortage of office space and retail outlets. The number and variety of these were inadequate as attested to by the fact that only about 50 to 60 cents of the tourist dollar was remaining in Rarotonga. After Sally, this shortage became even more acute. Therefore, it seemed sensible to put some, if not all the government offices now occupied by public servants on prime commercial land, into commercial buildings with retail outlets on the ground floor and offices on second and third floors.

These were to be rented out at standard rates for repayment of the loan and to add to the revenue of government for all time. This in time would have allowed relief, particularly of personal taxes which for some time has been in need of further relief. Public servants from this prime commercial area were to be moved to the New Zealand planned Government Centre and to government areas of no particular commercial value. This was also part of the plan and $6M was put aside for it, making the total loan $15M, the bulk of which was to come from Caisse Centrale at very favourable rates of interest and repayment. Cabinet approved the plan and it was to be signed in September of 1987.

The Japanese showed its interest in rehabilitating the waterfront and harbour development. It was explained that the harbour development was in the hands of New Zealand and Australian assistance. However, they came up with a plan for the waterfront rehabilitation and roading to relieve congestion. Cabinet approved the plan. With all the equipment on hand we began to put the plan into operation as we conceived it and the protective rock sea walls were completed except for the one on the east side of Avarua harbour. Even though they are not completed, their worth was demonstrated during hurricane Peni in 1989.

In the meantime, I visited Japan for the meeting of the Asian Development Bank in Osaka where I voiced our need to upgrade our international airport in Rarotonga. Over a period of some time, we had researched this with pilots flying in our tourists in DC10s and Boeing 747s as well as others knowledgeable in the field. The information we gleaned indicated that our airport was substandard only in the matter of its length. The runway at under 8000 feet was uncomfortably short for take-offs in which emergency aborts may be required. Another thousand feet, or better fifteen hundred feet, they said, would make all the difference. As it was, the planes could not take off with a full passenger, cargo and fuel load. It was getting away with the runway as it was because of the short haul to Auckland in which case they carried a small load of fuel. However, a full flight to Los Angeles non-stop could never be a reality unless the runway was lengthened.

This bothered me as the future of our tourist industry had to conceive of North American tourists becoming part of it. The possibility of direct flights as part of through flights, as were taking place through Tahiti and Fiji, might enhance this taking place. I felt that we could not continue with tour packages out of Auckland and have a tourist industry worth very much. Through-flights via Fiji and Tahiti airports often had labour and other problems. The Rarotonga International Airport could offer a viable alternative, greatly increasing its revenue as well as bringing visitors from North America and beyond. Therefore, there were good and valid reasons for extending the runway. In mid July, I received word via the Asian Development Bank that Japan had agreed to fund the project. I was happy. It only needed approaching the landowners, most of whom were my own family, for their views. I might add that being family did not necessarily make the job of obtaining their agreement any easier. As it was, within a week, I was no longer Prime Minister and the project has yet to eventuate.

The signing of the French loan was done on the due time of September by the Prime Minister, Dr Pupuke Robati, who took over from me. However, nothing much seemed to happen and it seemed that my former cabinet had scrubbed the proposals we had prepared with the French and had not agreed upon an alternative proposal because, I was informed, Cabinet Ministers were fighting over how the money should be spent. The new Prime Minister wanted it spent for the Northern Group, Minister Norman George wanted it spent in his Island of Atiu and the new Minister Matepi Matepi wanted it spent on his Island of Mangaia. The plan to repair and upgrade our capital which had been devastated by Hurricane Sally had gone by the board.

I kept in touch with the French about the progress of the loan and was told that the new proposals they were waiting for never came and that was still the situation as of the change in Government in January of 1989. However, the new government of Geoffrey Henry has not been able to reactivate the loan. Altogether, the government which took over from me, lost fifty million dollars in loans and grants. This had been planned for expenditure over a five year period and would have kept us in good economic working condition, furthered the progress of our economic development and given us a presentable capital.

* * *

On the diplomatic front, Gaston Flosse and I had discussed plans with other Polynesian leaders concerning the formation of a Polynesian Economic Community. This was favourably received by all, not the least by the King of Tonga, who supported a meeting in Rarotonga for our first discussions in September of 1987. Originally we had intended this to consist only of the recently independent and self-governing Polynesian countries of the Pacific, but soon the Hawaiian Polynesians and the New Zealand Maoris wanted to be part of it.

It was our particular answer to meeting our needs without having to expend the inordinate time being spent on political issues at the Forum meetings. The New Caledonia question and the Mururoa nuclear testing took up about 90 percent of our meetings year after year. In addition, the Melanesian countries had formed a Melanesian Spearhead group to deal with them and their own internal issues. After my ousting, the economic plans, the loans and grants and the regional plans evaporated - hopefully on a temporary basis only.

* * *

Since early 1986, my own hurricane was brewing. It ran hot; it ran cold. Vincent Ingram and Geoffrey Henry had made their bid during this year, but it was abortive. Then Norman George started to work on his campaign to take over leadership using all the dissatisfactions that came to the fore, associated with my refusal to use public money in the unauthorised way they wanted. Dr Pupuke Robati was to be used as a front to achieve his purpose. It backfired because Pupuke received the support and became Prime Minister instead.

I had firm rules about how public money should and should not be used. One of these was that it could not be used for personal reasons other than that established for sickness, emergencies and catastrophes and then only after approval by cabinet.

This my colleagues tended to view in a sense much broader than I could reasonably accept. Nearly all of it for personal reasons. Constantly there was a cry for increased allowances for members. These covered travel, personal automobile mileage, repairs and maintenance, members representation allowances and, of course, salaries. We had overhauled salaries so that in the Pacific we were better off as parliamentarians than any other Pacific Island state. Furthermore these were inflation protected, but the truism that, no matter how much a person receives, he always wants one third more was proving itself again true.

Borrowings by one or two parliamentarians from the Development Bank were being made for personal needs far in excess of that allowed normally. It had been the practice that parliamentarians did not use development bank funds for their personal ventures, but as Norman George said loud, clear and often, "We have the numbers and that is what counts. We can do anything we like." He was voicing the feelings of nearly all of the members in government.

Dr Pupuke Robati took over for himself as personal property the government owned house he occupied as a minister and later Prime Minister. He firmly believes that this is not a breach of trust. He also aided and abetted the misuse of the copra stabilisation fund and tried to have me as the Minister of Finance approve it after the fact. The Crown Law Office was unable to determine whether this fund was public money or not.

The member for Penrhyn invited Penrhyn Islanders living overseas to visit Penrhyn, assuring them that I would guarantee a loan to do this. When it was brought to cabinet, I pointed out that they had lived in New Zealand for many years and could see no way they could repay the loan or a valid reason for it to be allowed and, if they thought their request was reasonable and proper, it would be more fitting for them to have made the request to Roger Douglas, the New Zealand Minister of Finance, or Mr Lange, the Prime Minister of New Zealand.

Norman George brought a request to cabinet to guarantee a loan to a travel agent friend of his who was not able to meet the payment for the prepaid tickets of his clients because he had misappropriated $10,000 of the prepayment. The bank who got wind of the proposed request called me to warn me that this person had no hope of repaying a loan of any kind.

Norman George used my refusals to acquiesce to such requests to sow the seeds of discontent which culminated in a motion of no confidence in me as Prime Minister. The budget was used as a reason for bringing it about, but after the deed was done, they simply continued to pass it without change. The Opposition, including Vincent Ingram and Geoffrey Henry, made much of the inadequacy of their reasons for moving the motion and the fact that they were passing the budget they used as a reason without putting up a budget of their own. In the general commotion, there were interjections of "et tu Brute" etc.

The Opposition demanded that the proper thing to do was to call a general election, but in the planning for my ousting, the Queen's Representative was absented and returned on the morning of the day the deed was to be done for his part in the conspiracy. During his absence, Norman George was in radio contact with him to ensure his co-operation and this also involved a promise to renew his term. Inatio Akaruru, the Deputy Opposition Leader was also a passenger on the boat where these radio conversations took place and reported their context.

The Queen's Representative's response to my personally delivered note to call a general election on the basis that nigh on four years of the term had passed was received in a manner which left no doubt that he went along with the conspirators.

The next morning I turned up for Parliament as usual and took the lowest seat in government amid shouts from my former colleagues for me to take my usual seat and that I was still a Minister of the Crown. This was received by the Opposition with loud shouts of "serve you right," "You now have nobody to lean on and take the blame" and similar epithets indicating that government now had no one to control their questionable practises.

At the break, the new Prime Minister asked me to continue as Minister of Finance or as Minister with any portfolio of my choice. This I refused. The day before, when the motion was moved was such a relief to be free of the practices they wished me to condone, that returning to a position which would continue such involvement was abhorrent. Also having passed a motion of no confidence on the excuse of non-acceptance of the Appropriations Bill and then asking me to continue as Minister of Finance was not seen by them as ludicrous. It indicated that their action against me was personal and had nothing to do with my performance as Prime Minister or Minister of Finance.

The Opposition made much of this and several times demanded guidance as to what the policies of the new government were. The answer they received loud and clear, and without a blush, was that there would be no changes from the policies that I had laid down. The Opposition then demanded that if they were going to follow the budget I, as Minister of Finance, had brought down and were going to follow the policies that I, as Prime Minister had set, then why did they move a motion of no confidence. They had no answer, except to say that I had become too authoritarian. To which the Opposition responded that I had to be authoritarian to curb their questionable practises and stupidities.

Although I was grateful for the supportive efforts of the Opposition, there was no doubt in my mind that they were just as happy to get me out of the way and their votes went the only way they could in usual Opposition style. I made no attempt to defend myself. It struck me as demeaning to do so. If people believed I had not performed as I should, that was their problem not mine.

From the beginning of 1986, I felt the increasing weight of the increasing improprieties of my government and had talked with them about it in the vein that, if we continued these flagrant acts, we would have no chance of continuing as government at the next general elections. They took this friendly advice from their Prime Minister and Leader of their political party as an insult and my days as Prime Minister were numbered. When it came on 28 July 1987 with practically no warning and no reference to the party, I felt a great weight fall from my shoulders. I was now released from further responsibility for practices I was unable to condone.

The action was traumatic, but I felt that to have acceded to their requests against my judgement of what was proper, would have been more traumatic in the final analysis. I and my wife, Pa Ariki, would have lost what reputation we had gained over the years of honesty and working always for the benefit of the people within our capabilities and within the remuneration and privileges prescribed by law and no more.

At the general elections of January 1989, the Coalition Party broke every principle of party politics. As typical of Pacific history, everybody wanted to be boss. Dr Pupuke Robati put up candidates, Norman George as well as Dr Terepai Maoate each put up their candidates all for the same "party". In addition others who also wanted to be at the top either formed new parties or stood as independents. They all believed that the position at the top was now open to them. They seemed not to realise that they were vying for the same votes and were going to give the elections to Geoffrey Henry and the Cook Islands Party. My admonition in this respect was ignored. Analysis of the results showed that if they had put up one candidate for each constituency, they would have retained government hands down. But Pacific history was repeating itself.

   As far as I was concerned that was the end of my political career. I had spent over six years as leader of the Opposition and nine years as Prime Minister. This averages the usual quota of time in the different endeavours of my lifetime. I have left an economic formula that worked under the circumstances in which it was used. It is likely that it will not continue to be used, for those who follow the command formula will do so regardless of negative economic results.

   Now I can concentrate on the things I have always wanted to do, but put aside in the interest of doing what was needed of me. I will concentrate on cultural endeavours and perhaps research if the interest moves me and I can afford it. Already I have had an exhibition of my art work and have written a dramatisation of the history of a particularly interesting part of our history circa 1000 to 1350 AD. At seventy three, a little fishing, designing and building a sixty foot replica of our most famous canoe, the Takitumu, and other simple interests, I am enjoying myself immensely. However, because I am convinced that poverty, disease, ignorance and threats to world peace are in large part due to the application of poor economic thinking and the vain flailings of human weakness at the top, I will fight that fight at every opportunity to the bitter end.

Bibliography

1. Batley, R. A. L., Ngati Rangi, The J. of the Polynesian Soc., vol., 82, 1973.
2. Crocombe, R., Money and All That, in Cook Islands Politics, Polynesian Press, Auckland, Mew Zealand, 147-158, 1979.
3. Crocombe, R., and M. Crocombe, The Saga of Tension, in Cook Islands Politics, Polynesian Press, Auckland, New Zealand, 243-260, 1979.
4. Cullison, J. W. and T. R. A. Davis, The Isolation of Enteric Pathogens At Barrow Alaska, U.S. Armed Forces Med. Journal, 534-538, 1957.
5. Davis, T. R. A., Control of Filariasis in the Cook Islands, N. Z. Med. J., 48: 363-367, 1949.
6. Davis, T. R. A., and J. Mayer., Imperfect Homeothermia in the Hereditary Obese-Hyperglycemic Syndrome of Mice, Am. J. Physiol., 177: 222-224, 1954.
7. Davis, T. R. A., and J. Mayer, Use of High Frequency Electromagnetic Waves in the Study of Thermogenesis, Am. J. Physiol., 178: 283-287, 1954.
8. Davis, T. R. A., and J. Mayer, Failure of Thermogenesis and Effect of High Frequency Electromagnetic Waves in the Hereditary Obese-Hyperglycemic Mice Syndrome, Fed. Proc., 13: 454, 1954. (Abstract)
9. Davis, T. R. A., and M. L. Davis, Doctor to the Islands, Atlantic, Little Brown, Boston, Mass., 1954; Michael Joseph, London, 1954; Paris Soir, Paris, 1954; Bonniers, Sweden, 1954; BBC, England,1956; Oswald Sealy, Ltd., New Zealand, 1962.
10. Davis, T. R. A., and J. Mayer, Nature of the Physiologic Stimulus for Shivering, Am. J. Physiol., 181: 669-674, 1955.
11. Davis, T. R. A., Demonstration and Quantitative Measurement of the Contribution of Physical and Chemical Thermogenesis on Acut Exposure to Cold, Am. J. Physiol., 181: 675-678, 1955.
12. Davis, T. R. A., and F. T. Elkins, Cold weather Test of the Evacuation Bag, Milit. Med., 120: 125-129, 1957.
13. Davis, T. R. A., Hydatid Disease in Alaska, Am. J. Med., 23: 99-106, 1957.
14. Davis, T. R. A., An outbreak of Infectious Hepatitis in Two Arctic Villages, New England Journal of Medicine, 256: 881-884, 1957.
15. Davis, T. R. A., D. R. Johnston, F. C. Bell, and B. J. Cremer, The Regulation of and Nonshivering Heat Production During Acclimation of Rats, Am. J. Physiol., 198: 471-475, 1960.
16. Davis, T. R. A., Shivering and Non-shivering Heat Production in Animals and Man, in Cold Injury, Transactions of the Sixth Conference, Josiah Macy, Jr., Foundation, New York, pp. 223-269, 1960.
17. Davis, T. R. A., Man Alive in Outer Space, Atlantic Monthly, March, 1960.
18. Davis, T. R. A., and D. R. Johnston, Seasonal Acclimatisation to Cold in Man, J. Appl., Physiol., 16: 231-234, 1961.
19. Davis, T. R. A., Chamber Cold Acclimatization in Man, J. Applied Physiology, 16: 1011-1015, 1961.

20. Davis, T. R. A., and Robert, J. T. Joy, Natural and Artificial Cold Acclimatization in Man, in Biometeorology, Pergamon Press, New York, 286-303, 1962.

21. Davis, T. R. A. Davis, Effect of Heat Acclimatization on Artificial and Natural Cold Acclimatization in Man, J. Appl. Physiol., 17: 751-753, 1962.

22. Davis, T. R. A., and R. J. T. Joy, Cold Injury and Cold Acclimatization in Man, Army Science Conference, 1: 173, 1962.

23. Davis, T. R. A.,The Influence of Climate on Nutritional Requirements, Am. J. Public Health, 54: 2051-2067,1964.

24. Davis, T. R. A., S. P. Battista, and C. J. Kensler, Effect of Cigarette Smoke, Acrolein and formaldehyde on Pulmonary Function, Fed. Proc., 24: 518, 1965.

25. Davis, T. R. A., H. S. Nayar, K. C. Sinha, S. D. Nishith, and R. M. Rai, The Effect of Altitude on the Cold Responses of Low Altitude Acclimatised Jats, High Altitude Acclimatised Jats and Tibetans, in Biometeorology 11, Pergamon Press, Oxford, 1966.

26. Davis, T. R. A., Contribution of Skeletal Muscle to Nonshivering Thermogenesis in the dog, Am. J Physiol., 213: 1423-1426, 1967.

27. Davis, T. R. A., S. P. Battista, H. J. Bronstein, and C. J. Kensler, Mechanism of Respiratory Effects During Exposure of Guinea Pigs to Cigarette Smoke, Irritants and Non-Irritants, Arch. Env. Health, 15: 412-419, 1967.

28. Davis, T. R. A., Physiological Adjustment to cold, in Physiology and Pathology of adaptation Mechanisms, Pergamon Press, Oxford and New York, 1969.

29. Davis, T. R. A., S. N. Gershoff, and D. F. Gamble, Review of Studies of Vitamin and Mineral Nutrition in the United States (1950-1968), Journal of Nutrition Education, 1: No.2, Supplement 1, 40-57, 1969.

30. Davis, T. R. A., N. Adler, and J. C. Opsahl, with the technical assistance of J. P. Schepis, J. M. Essigman, and R. A. Cruz-Alvarez, Excretion of Cyclohexamine in Subjects Ingesting Sodium Cyclamate, Toxicology and Applied Pharmacology, 15: 106-116, 1969.

31. Duff, R., No Sort of Iron, Caxton Press, Christchurch, New Zealand, 1969.

32. Ellis, W., Polynesian Researches, J. & J. Harper, New York, 1833.

33. Fairbairn, T. I. J., Island Economies, Institute of Pacific studies, University of the South Pacific, Suva, 1985.

34. Finney, B. R., Hokule'a, The Way to Tahiti., Dodd, Mead & Company, New York, 1979.

35. Friedman, Milton and Rose, Free to Choose, Avon Books, Hearst Corporation, New York, New York 10019, 1979.   36. Galbraith, J. K., Economics and the Public Purpose, Penguin Books Ltd, Harmondsworth, Middlesex, England, 1977.

37. George, N., Organising the Exiles, in Cook Islands Politics, Polynesian Press, Auckland, New Zealand, 167-186, 1979.

38. Green, R., Polynesian Ancestors, in Taratai. James Siers, Millwood Press Ltd., Wellington, New Zealand, 1977.

39. Haddon, A. C., and J. Hornell, Canoes of Oceania, Vol. 1, Special Publication 27, Bernice P. Bishop Museum, Hawaii, 1936.

40. Heilbroner, R. L., The Worldly Philosophers, Simon and Schuster, New York, New York, 1972.

41. Holmes, T., The Hawaiian Canoe, Editions Limited, Hanalei, Kauai, Hawaii, 1981.

42. Jourdain, P.,Pirogues Anciennes de Tahiti, Societe des Oceanistes Dossier, Paris, 1970.

43. Joy, R. J. T., R. H. Poe, R. F. Berman, and T. R. A. Davis, Some Physiological Responses to Arctic Living, Arch. Env, Health, 3. 4: 22-26, 1962.

44. Kane, H. K., Voyage, Island Heritage Ltd, Honolulu, Hawaii, 1976.

45. Kyselka, W., An Ocean in Mind, University of Hawaii Press, Honolulu, 1987.

46. Langdon, R., The Lost Caravel, Pacific Pty Ltd., Sydney, Australia, 1975.

47. Lopdell, J., Chief medical Officer, Western Samoa, Personal Communications, 1949.

48. Malo, D., Hawaiian Antiquities, Bernice P. Bishop Museum, Special Publication 2, Translated from the Hawaiian by N. B. Emerson, 1898.

49. Murray-Oliver, A, Captain Cook's Hawaii, Millwood Press, Wellington, New Zealand, 1975.

50. Parsonson, G. S., The settlement of Oceania: An Examination of the Accidental Voyage Theory, in Polynesian Navigation, Edited by Jack Golson, Published for The Polynesian Society by A. H. & A. W. Reed, Wellington and Auckland, New Zealand, 1963.

51. The Polynesian Journal of Captain Henry Byam Martin, R.N., Peabody Museum of Salem, Salem, Mass. U.S.A. 1981.

52. Savage, S, Manuscript, circa 1905, and, Tuatua Taito, Bishop Museum Library, 1908.

53. Savage, S., A Dictionary of the Maori Language of Rarotonga, Government Printing Office, Rarotonga, Cook Islands, 1962.

54. Sharp, A., Polynesian Navigation: Some Comments, J. of the Polynesian Society, 72: 384-396, 1963.

55. Short, I., The 1978 Election Petitions, in Cook Islands Politics, Polynesian Press, Auckland, New Zealand, 227-241, 1979.

56. Simmons, D. R., The Great New Zealand Myth, A. H. & A. W. Reed, Wellington Sydney London, 1976.

57. Smith, A., The Wealth of Nations, vol. 1, p16.

58. Williams, J., A Narrative of Mission Enterprises in the South Seas, J. Snow, London, 1837.

59. Williams, Joseph., A Cabinet Minister Resigns, in Cook Islands' Politics, Polynesian Press, Auckland, New Zealand, pp 68-75, 1979.

Abbreviations:

AAL	Arctic Aeromedical Laboratories
ADL	Arthur D. Little Inc.
ADLer	A staff member of ADL
AMP	Assistant Medical practitioner
ANZUS	Australia, New Zealand and United States Treaty
CCOP-SOPAC	Committee for the Co-ordination of Off-shore Prospecting in the South Pacific
CIA	Control Intelligence Agency
CIP	Cook Islands Party
CIPA	Cook Islands Progressive Association
C&W	Cable and Wireless
FDA	Food and Drug Administration
GDP	Gross Domestic Product
GHP	General Health Purposes
GNP	Gross National Product
GST	Goods and Services Tax
KBE	Knight Commander of the British Empire
MBChB	Bachelor of Medicine and Bachelor of Surgery
MD	Doctor of Medicine
MIT	Massachusetts Institute of Technology
NASA	National Aeronautics and Space Administration
PhD	Doctor of Philosophy
PIC	Pacific Islands Conference
PIDP	Pacific Islands Development Programme
PIPA	Pacific Islands Producers Association
QC	Queen's Counsel
RNZAF	Royal New Zealand Air Force
SCCA	Sports Car Club Of America
SPARTECA	South Pacific Regional Trade and Economic Co-operation Agreement
SPC	South Pacific Commission
SPEC	South Pacific Bureau for Economic Cooperation (now Forum Secretariat)
SPREP	South Pacific Regional Environment Programme
SPTC	
SRO	Single Regional Organisation
THC	Tourist Hotel Corporation
TOT	Turnover Tax
UK	United Kingdom
USAMRL	United States Army Medical Research Laboratories
US	United States (adjective)
USA	United States of America
USP	University of the South Pacific

| USSCO | Union Steamship Company |
| USSR | Union of Soviet Socialist Republic |

Index